Liver Pathology

Edited by Vijay Gayam and Omer Engin

Published in London, United Kingdom

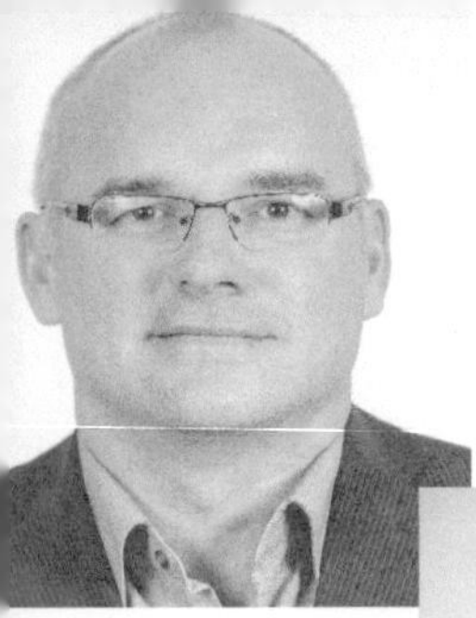
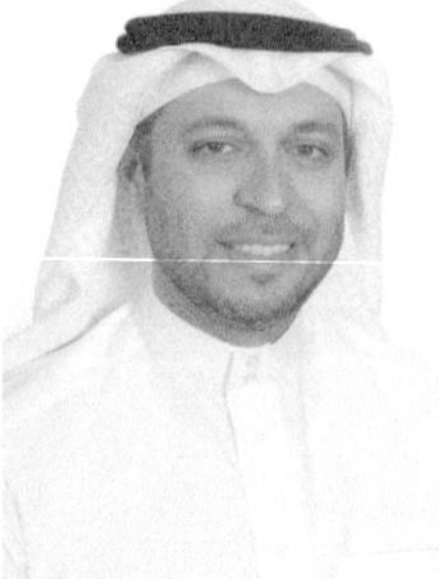
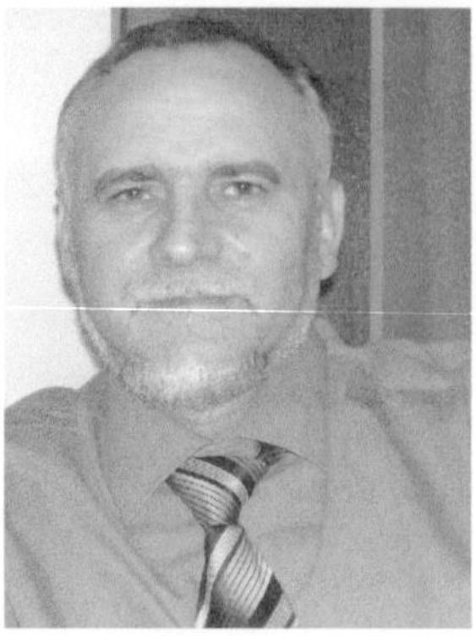
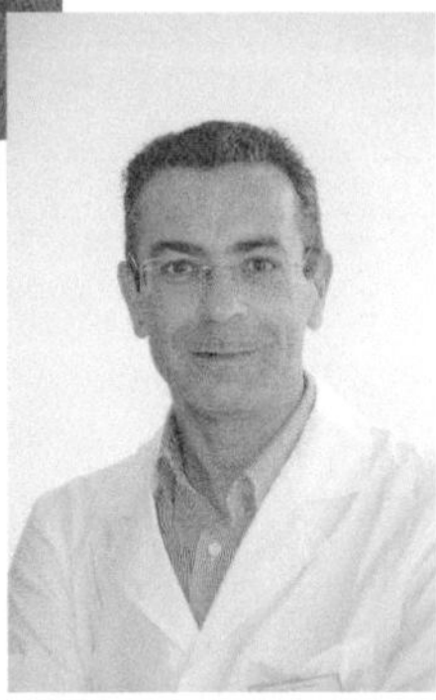
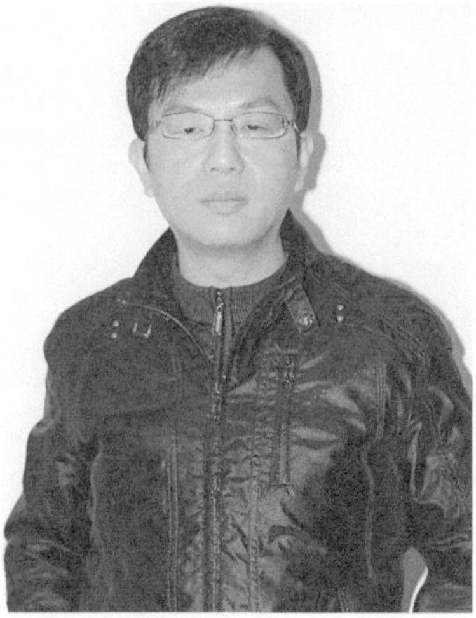
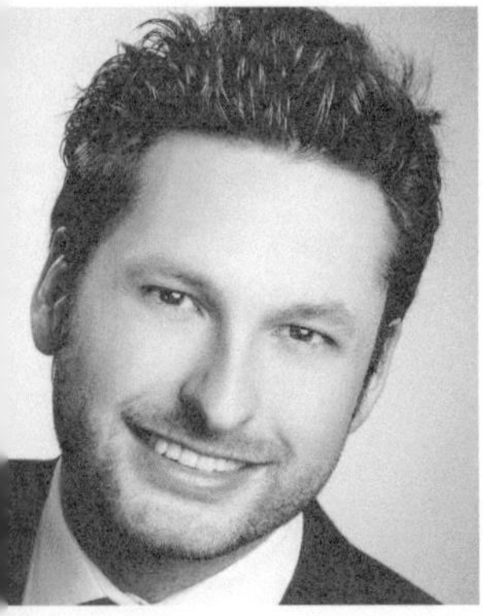
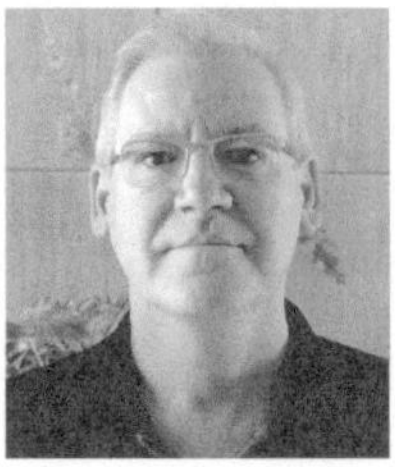

IntechOpen

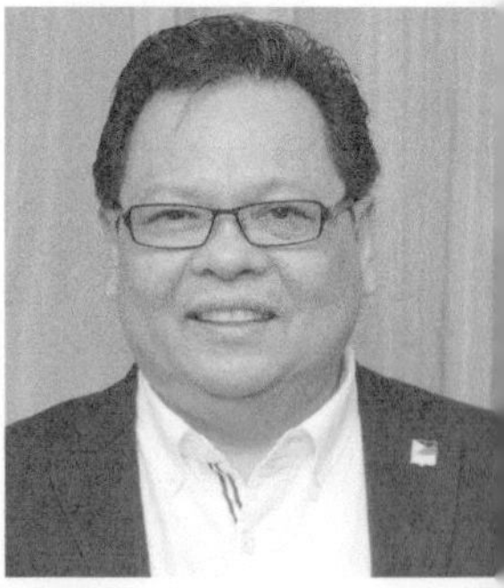
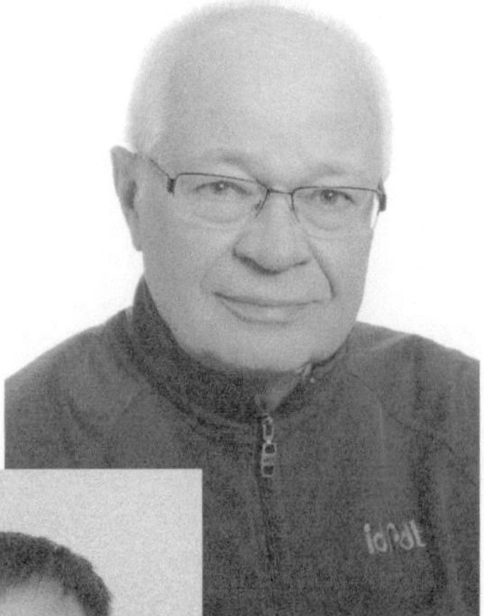
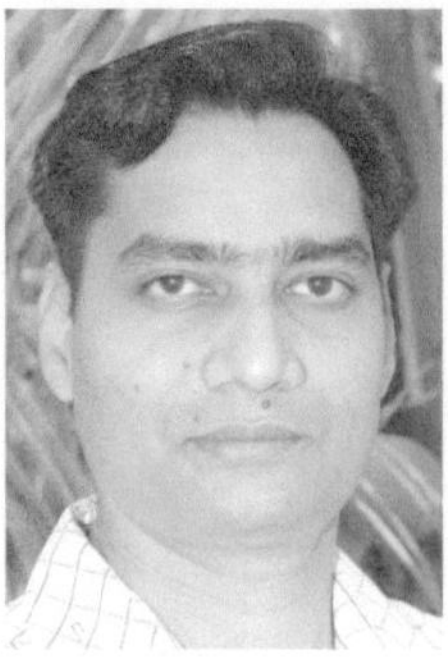
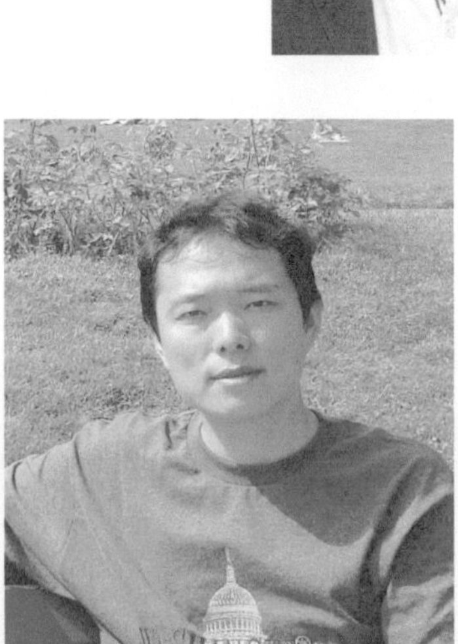
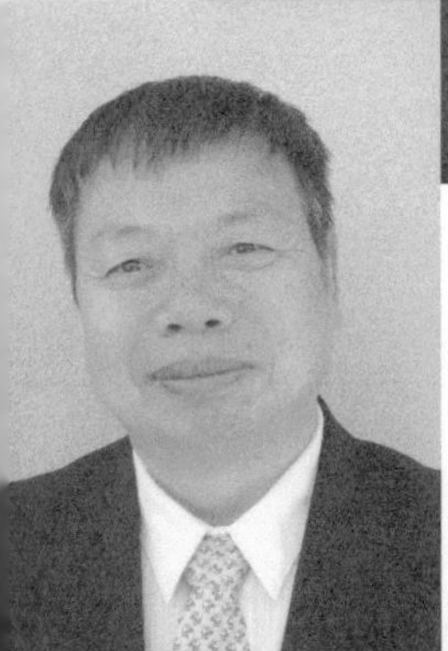
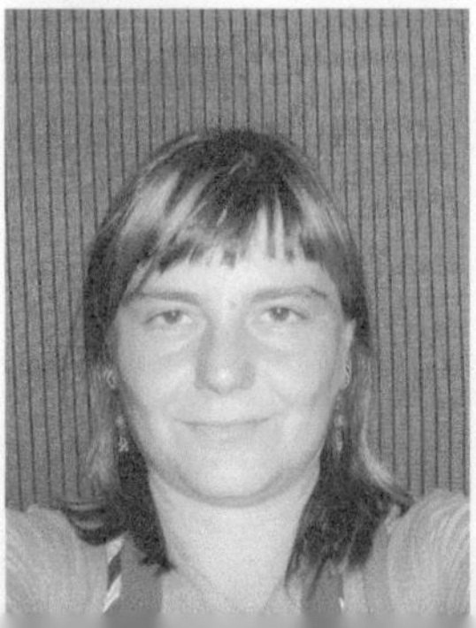

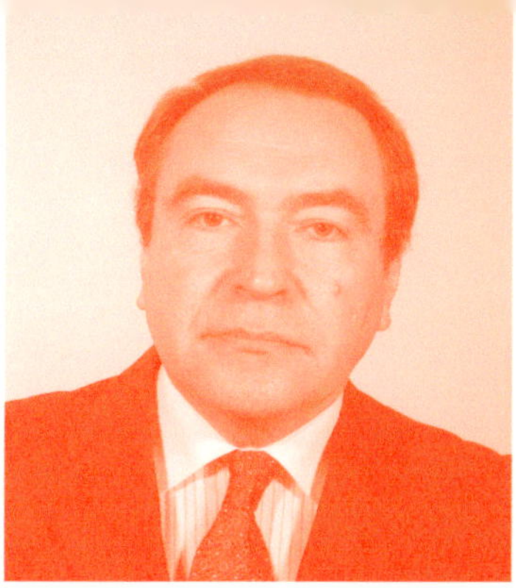
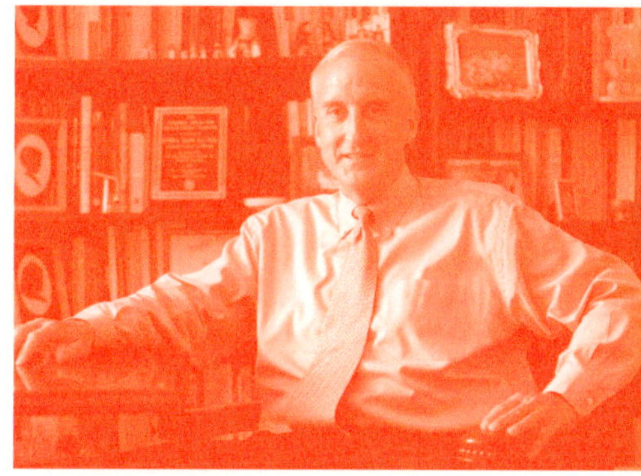
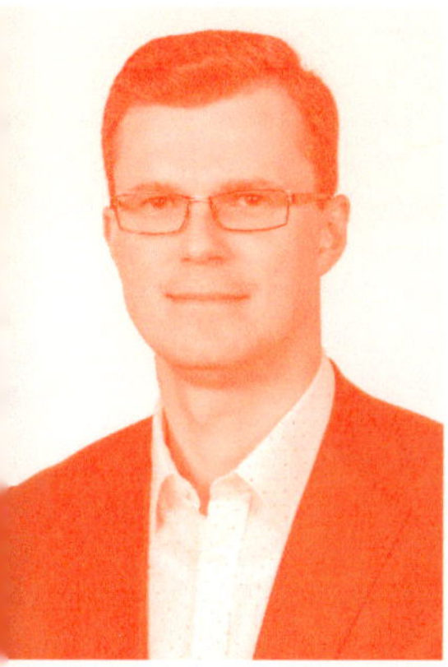
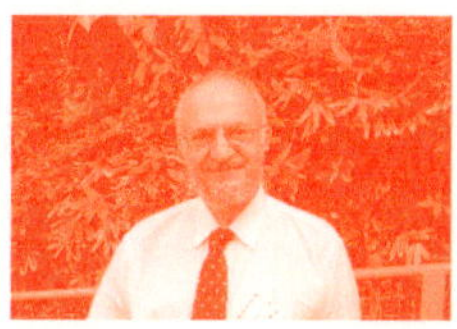
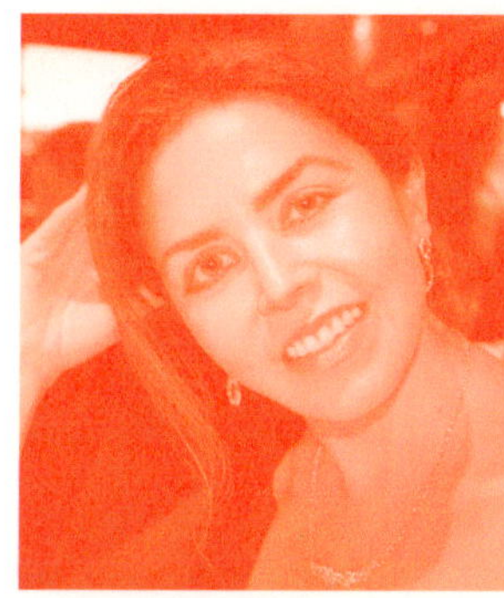

Supporting open minds since 2005

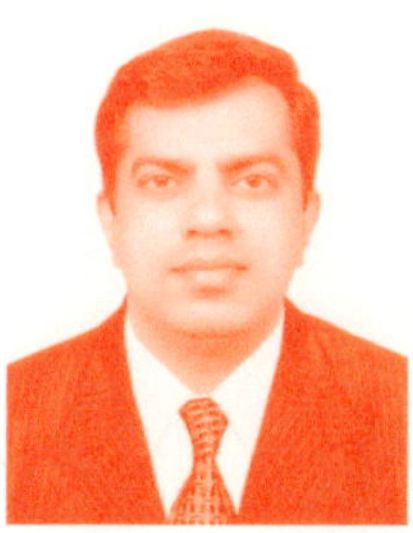
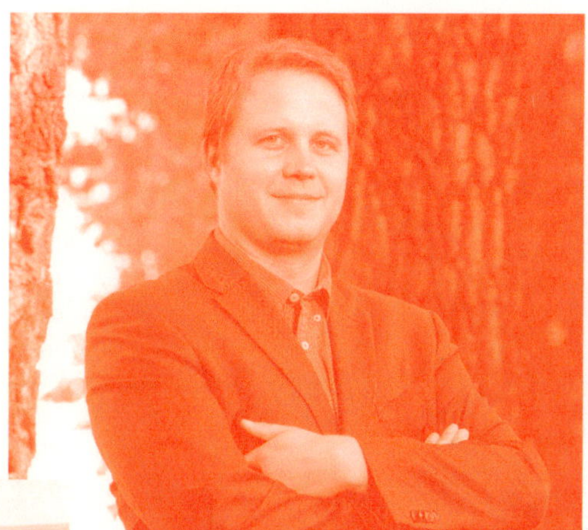
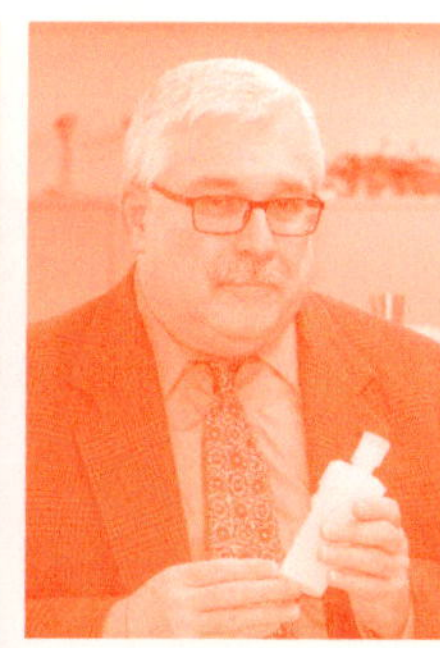
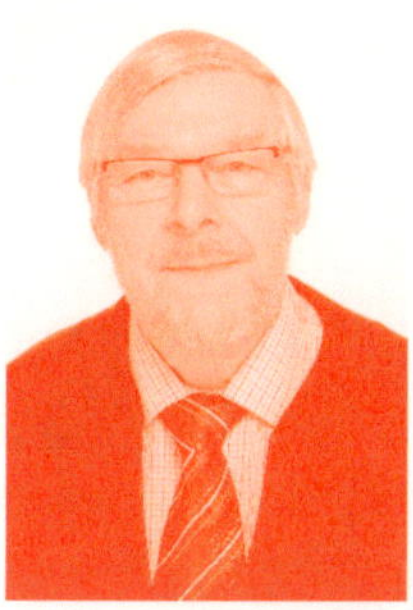
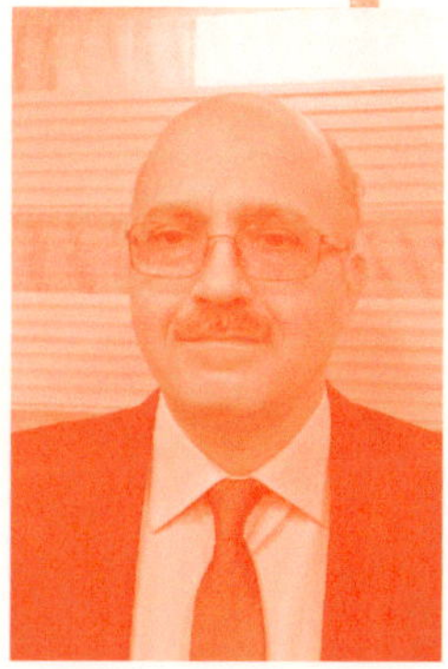
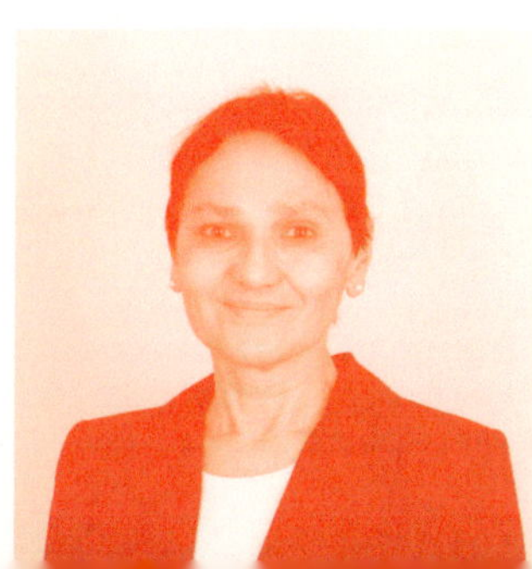
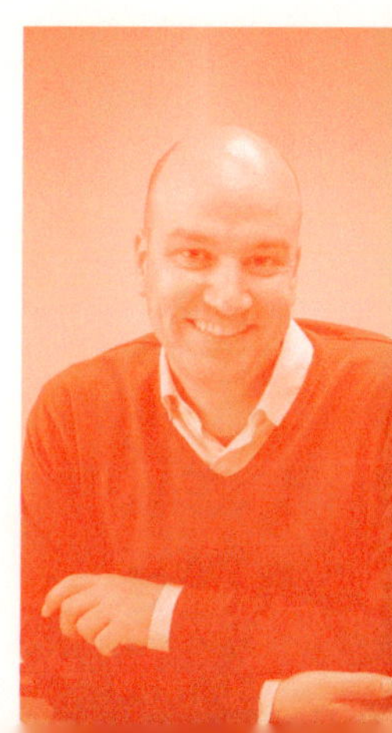

Liver Pathology
http://dx.doi.org/10.5772/intechopen.73790
Edited by Vijay Gayam and Omer Engin

Contributors
Demetrio Víctor Pérez Civantos, Alicia Muñoz-Cantero, M Ángeles Santiago Triviño, M Dolores Pérez Frutos, Emilio Fabrega, Jose Ignacio Fortea, Angela Puente, Antonio Cuadrado, Patricia Huelin, Javier Crespo, Marta Mayorga Fernandez, Raul Pellon Daben, Mauro Borzio, Elena Dionigi, Iwan Paolucci, Raluca Sandu, Pascale Tinguely, Corina Kim-Fuchs, Martin Maurer, Daniel Candinas, Stefan Weber, Anja Lachenmayer, Balasubramaniyan Vairappan, Amit Kumar Ram, Gavin Wright, Maria Jose Lizardo, Nalú Navarro, Eduardo Cervantes Alvarez, Vijay Gayam, Pavani Garlapati, Amrendra Kumar Mandal, Benjamin Tiongson, Chengzhan Zhu, Bingzi Dong, Qian Dong, Xin Chen, Xingshun Qi, Mani Sharma, Neeraj Kumar Chouhan, Sandeep Vaidya, Filippo Banchini, Patrizio Capelli, Adriana Turculeanu, Adianto Nugroho, Neşe Karadağ Soylu, Manuel Robles Marcos, Francisco Fuentes Morillas, María O. Cerezo Arias, Alberto Córdoba López, Kexin Zheng, Xiaozhong Guo, Xinhong Wang, Inés García

First published in London, United Kingdom, 2021 by IntechOpen
IntechOpen is the global imprint of INTECHOPEN LIMITED, registered in England and Wales, registration number: 11086078, 5 Princes Gate Court, London, SW7 2QJ, United Kingdom
Printed in Croatia

British Library Cataloguing-in-Publication Data
A catalogue record for this book is available from the British Library

Additional hard and PDF copies can be obtained from orders@intechopen.com

Liver Pathology
Edited by Vijay Gayam and Omer Engin
p. cm.
Print ISBN 978-1-83880-243-1
Online ISBN 978-1-83880-244-8
eBook (PDF) ISBN 978-1-83969-553-7

For EU product safety concerns:
IN TECH d.o.o., Prolaz Marije Krucifikse Kozulić 3, 51000 Rijeka, Croatia, info@intechopen.com or visit our website at intechopen.com.

Meet the editors

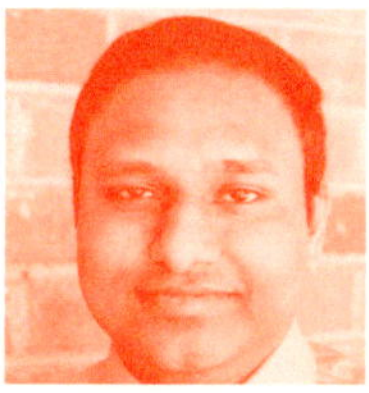

Dr. Vijay Bhaskar Reddy Gayam is currently practicing as an internist at Interfaith Medical Center in Brooklyn, New York, USA. He is also a Clinical Assistant Professor at the SUNY Downstate University Hospital and Adjunct Professor of Medicine at the American University of Antigua. He is a holder of an M.B.B.S. degree bestowed to him by Osmania Medical College and received his M.D. at Interfaith Medical Center. His career goals thus far have heavily focused on direct patient care, medical education, and clinical research. He currently serves in two leadership capacities; Assistant Program Director of Medicine at Interfaith Medical Center and as a Councilor for the American Federation for Medical Research. As a true academician and researcher, he has more than 50 papers indexed in international peer-reviewed journals. He has also presented numerous papers in multiple national and international scientific conferences. His areas of research interest include general internal medicine, gastroenterology and hepatology. He serves as an editor, editorial board member and reviewer for multiple international journals. His research on Hepatitis C has been very successful and has led to multiple research awards, including the 'Equity in Prevention and Treatment Award" from the New York Department of Health Viral Hepatitis Symposium (2018) and the 'Presidential Poster Award" awarded to him by the American College of Gastroenterology (2018). He was also awarded 'Outstanding Clinician in General Medicine" by Venus International Foundation for his extensive research expertise and services, perform over and above the standard expected in the advancement of healthcare, patient safety and quality of care.

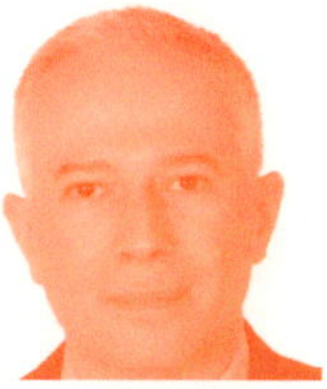

Dr. Omer Engin is an Associate Professor of General Surgery at Health Sciences University, Tepecik Training and Research Hospital, Surgery Department, Turkey. He has authored many international articles, chapters, and congress papers and has served as a book editor for internationally published books and as an organizing committee member in a number of international conferences. He is an Organisation Scientific Committee Member in the International Medical Society Scientific Committee and Athens Institute for Education and Research. He serves as an editorial board member and as a reviewer in several international medical and surgical scientific journals. His specializations are: endocrine surgery, hepatobiliary surgery, bariatric surgery, gastrointestinal surgery, and oncologic surgery.

Contents

Preface

The liver is the major organ in which our body's metabolic activities are carried out. Food is digested in the gastrointestinal tract and absorbed by the small intestines. These absorbed foods come to the liver through the venous circulation of the small intestines. The liver takes these foods through the portal vein and transforms them into a shape that the body can use, and delivers them to the vena cava and from there to the systemic circulation via hepatic veins. This circulation between the intestines and the liver is called Hepatic Portal Circulation.

The vena porta is the main venous structure that brings blood flow from the intestines to the liver. The vena porta is formed by the union of three venous structures. These structures are splenic vein, vena mesenterica superior, and vena mesenterica inferior.

This portal circulation is an important way to carry the absorbed foods to the liver, as well as for infections and cancer to metastasize by the venous spread. In appendicitis, the infection reaches the liver, causing pylephlebitis. In bowel cancer, cancer cells entering the mesenterica inferior vein or mesenterica superior vein go towards the liver due to portal venous flow, therefore the place where colon cancer most metastasizes is the liver. When these metastatic masses reach a certain size, they enter the venous circulation of the liver, from here to the vena cava and from there to the right ventricle. The blood entering the right ventricle goes from here to the lungs via the pulmonary artery. Cancer cells are retained in the lung microcirculation and metastatic masses form in the lung.

Metabolic events in the liver increase the temperature of the liver. The liver is a warmer organ than normal body temperature. The heat that occurs as a result of metabolic events is distributed throughout the body due to blood circulation.

Some organs in our body are double and some organs are single. For example, there are two kidneys in the body. The liver is a single. An amazing feature of the liver is that each tissue part of the liver performs the same function. In other words, if a part of the liver is removed, the other parts of the liver do the same job, so there will be no significant change in function. In order for the remaining liver to function properly after liver resection, the remaining liver (FLR) must be of sufficient volume.

There are many diseases of the liver. Metabolic diseases, neoplastic diseases, hepatopathy due to cardiac pathologies, infective diseases such as Hepatitis E, cirrhosis, etc. are present. These diseases can lead to impaired liver function and cause metabolic complications in the human body.

Neoplastic diseases can be benign or malignant. Malignant diseases can be primary or secondary. The most common secondary malignant neoplastic disease is metastatic cancer caused by colorectal cancer. Diagnosis can be made by radiological imaging. These methods include computerised tomography and MRI. A percutaneous liver biopsy may be required for diagnosis. Surgical metastasectomy or regular resection can be performed in the treatment. Interventional radiological procedures are another option used in the treatment of liver tumors. Chemotherapy has an important place in the treatment of liver tumors.

Various diseases of the liver that require surgical and medical treatment are examined in our book. Our authors wrote their subjects by combining their knowledge with their experiences.

Have a pleasant reading experience.

Omer Engin
Izmir Tepecik Eğitim ve Araştırma Hastanesi,
Turkey

Vijay Gayam
Interfaith Medical Center,
United States of America

Chapter 1

Diagnosis and Treatment of Hepatoblastoma: An Update

Chengzhan Zhu, Bingzi Dong, Xin Chen and Qian Dong

Abstract

Hepatoblastoma is a rare but the most common solid tumor in children. The incidence is gradually increasing. The international collaboration among four centers in the world has greatly improved the prognosis of hepatoblastoma. They formed the Children's Hepatic Tumor International Collaboration (CHIC) to standardize the staging system (2017 PRETEXT system) and the risk factors for tumor stratification. Multimodal therapy has become the standard for the management of hepatoblastoma, including surgical resection, liver transplantation, chemotherapy, and so on. Surgery is the primary treatment of early stage hepatoblastoma. Three-dimensional reconstruction is helpful for preoperative evaluation of large tumors, assisting extended hepatectomy for patients in PRETEXT III or IV. Neoadjuvant therapy is useful for reducing the tumor volume and increasing the resectability. Primary liver transplantation is recommended for advanced hepatoblastoma. The lungs are the most common metastatic organ, the treatment of which is critical for the patient's long-term survival. We reviewed the recent progress in the diagnosis and treatment of hepatoblastoma.

Keywords: hepatoblastoma, PRETEXT, stratification, neoadjuvant, surgical resection, liver transplantation

1. Introduction

Hepatoblastoma is the third most commonly diagnosed intra-abdominal solid tumor [1]. It is also the most common primary hepatic malignancy in children [2]. More than 90% of hepatoblastoma occur in children under the age of 5 years [3, 4]. Although its absolute incidence is very low, its growth rate is gradually increasing, which increased from 1.89 per 1,000,000 in 2000 to 2.16 per 1,000,000 in 2015, with an annual percentage change of 2.2%. This increase mainly occurs in male children between 2 and 4 years of age, which was found to be an independent predictor for short overall survival [5]. With the development of multimodal treatment and cooperation between international organizations, the prognoses have been greatly improved in recent years [6].

2. Diagnosis

Clinical manifestations are not typical at the early stage of hepatoblastoma. There would be epigastric or total abdominal distention, nausea, vomit, loss of appetite, abdominal pain, diarrhea, jaundice, even varicosity of abdominal wall, and dyspnea. Another clinical feature is often accompanied by fever, and the temperature can reach 39–40°C. About 3% of patients have sex hormone and sexual organ development abnormalities. And a few children have obvious osteoporosis and pathological fracture.

Physical examination could find diffuse or nodular enlargement of the liver, of which the volume varies, sometimes with splenomegaly and varicosity of the abdominal wall. Abdominal pain and abdominal muscle tension may be due to tumor rupture. In the late stage, the hepatoblastoma progresses rapidly and cachexia appeared soon.

Alpha fetoprotein (AFP) increases in more than 90% of patients, which is a specific indicator for hepatoblastoma and important for disease follow-up. Age should be considered when analyzing the clinical significance of AFP. The average AFP of the newborn is about 62.7ng/ml, and it reaches the peak in the first month after birth, the average AFP is about 1200 ng/ml. After three months, it decreases to 3.15ng/ml (the level of normal adult). In addition, the LDH, cholesterol, and alkaline phosphatase are also increased. The liver function is normal at early stage, middle, and late stage.

Imaging is necessary for diagnosis and preoperative evaluation, including tumor location, number, and the relationship with peripheral blood vessels and organs. The commonly used examination includes ultrasound, CT, MRI, angiography, etc.

Enhanced CT and MRI are important imaging studies, which are recommended. However, due to the difficulty of MRI examination for children, we usually choose enhance CT and reconstruct the images into three-dimensional images to understand the spatial structure of the tumor and the anatomical relationship with the blood vessels.

Additionally, the deep exploration of CT/MRI images is also important for the overall evaluation of hepatoblastoma. Identifying the CT/MRI image features of hepatoblastoma will help distinguish the more malignant tumor, which is potentially useful for guiding the clinical treatment. A study of 34 patients, aimed at studying contrast-enhanced CT characteristics of hepatoblastoma associated with metastatic disease and patient outcomes, found that irregular tumor margins, vascular invasion, capsule retraction, and PRETEXT staging are associated with poor patient prognosis. Among them, irregular tumor margins are the only imaging features that are significantly associated with more aggressive tumor subtypes [7]. For investigating the image characteristics, artificial intelligence has demonstrated remarkable progress in image recognition tasks. Radiomics is used to investigate the quantitative features that are invisible to the naked eye from conventional image with methods of artificial intelligence. The image features could be used to predict the pathology characteristics, therapeutic response, and survival. Previous studies have evaluated the value of radiomics in adult liver cancer. The results were achieved, particularly in the preoperative prediction of pathological features and postoperative recurrence [8, 9].

3. International collaboration

3.1 The children's hepatic tumor international collaboration (CHIC)

The four centers in the world that have performed prospective controlled studies of hepatoblastoma joined forces to form the CHIC. It includes the International Childhood Liver Tumor Strategy Group (SIOPEL), the Children's Oncology Group (COG), the German Society for Pediatric Oncology and Hematology (GPOH), and the Japanese Study Group for Pediatric Liver Tumors (JPLT). Such international cooperation provides a large-scale database for clinical trials. The CHIC has developed a centralized online platform that combines data from eight completed clinical trials to form a database of 1605 hepatoblastoma cases treated between 1988 and 2008. The resulting data set has been used for investigating the relationship between the patient prognosis and the tumor characteristics and patient stratification for treatment selection and follow-up. And the collaboration has led to a uniform implementation of staging system (PRE-Treatment EXTent of tumor, PRETEXT), which is helpful for systemically evaluating the hepatoblastoma at diagnosis and useful for establishing consensus classification. Moreover, pathologists in the collaboration have established a new histopathological consensus classification for pediatric liver tumors. There have also been advances in chemotherapy treatments and liver transplantation for unresectable tumors. These advances will be further evaluated in the upcoming Pediatric Hepatic International Tumor Trial (PHITT) [10].

3.2 2017 PRETEXT and risk stratification

Imaging is an important basis for disease assessment and treatment selection. The PRETEXT system has been firstly proposed for staging and risk stratification for hepatoblastoma in 1992 [11]. The PRETEXT system is used to classify the tumor extent before treatment, which has a good prognostic value in patients with hepatoblastoma. The PRETEXT system has been widely used to evaluate the hepatoblastoma in recent years, which could stratify patients into groups with different prognosis.

The 2017 PRETEXT has updated the 2005 PRETEXT definitions [12]. The liver was divided into four sections. For PRETEXT I, II, and IV groups, there were no obvious differences between 2017 PRETEXT and 2005 PRETEXT. For PRETEXT I group, the tumor involves only one of the two lateral sections (right posterior and left lateral section). For PRETEXT II group, the tumor involves the left lobe, right lobe, left medial section only, and right anterior section only; two separate tumors involves the two lateral sections or the caudate lobe only. For PRETEXT III group, the tumor involves three sections of the liver, leaving only one normal section. For PRETEXT IV group, the tumor involves all four sections. The 2017 PRETEXT has mainly standardized the PRETEXT annotation factors, preparing the future clinical trials. It includes hepatic venous/inferior vena cava involvement (V), portal venous involvement (P), extrahepatic disease contiguous with the main liver tumor (E), multifocality (F), and tumor rupture (R) [12].

Many single centers have put effort to investigate the prognostic factor of hepatoblastoma [13–16]. But the results were limited due to the small patients' number and the use of multiple disparate staging systems. CHIC has created a new staging system to staging and risk stratification in children with hepatoblastoma, named the Children's Hepatic tumors International Collaboration-Hepatoblastoma Stratification (CHIC-HS). Based on a 5-year event-free survival and clinical applicability, the system was established with risk factors including PRETEXT groups, metastatic disease, age, AFP concentration, PRETEXT annotation factors (VPEFR), and surgically resectable at diagnosis [17]. PRETEXT group is the primary and most important for risk stratification. If the tumor is resectable at diagnosis for patients of PRETEXT I/II group, they are in very low or low risk. After PRETEXT group, metastatic disease is the first risk factor for stratification. All patients with metastatic disease were defined as high risk. Then, age $\geq$ 8 years in PRETEXT I, II, and III group and age $\geq$ 3 years in PRETEXT IV group were high-risk factor. For younger patients, AFP $\leq$100 ng/mL was defined as high-risk group. And VPEFR+ patients were in intermediate-risk group. In PRETEXT I/II group, older patients showed a relatively poor prognosis. But many of these tumors can be surgically resected; they defined the patients at 3–7 year age in the lower-risk group; patients who had low

PRETEXT and positive VPEFR were placed in the intermediate-risk group; patients with PRETEXT I and low AFP (≤100 ng/mL) should not be stratified into high-risk group due to surgically resectable small tumors; patients with PRETEXT III group (younger than 8 years, no metastasis (M−) and AFP 100–1000 ng/mL) were defined as intermediate risk due to the poor 5-year event-free survival. CHIC-HS is by far the most complete system for risk stratification of pediatric hepatoblastoma and has important guiding significance for guiding individualized treatment [17]. Further study should also pay attention to the prognostic effect of treatment selection, such as anatomical or nonanatomical partial hepatectomy [18] and the dosage of chemotherapy [19, 20].

4. Treatment

Multimodal therapy is recommended for the management of hepatoblastoma, including surgical resection, liver transplantation, chemotherapy, or radiofrequency ablation [21]. Multimodal therapy can improve tumor remission rate of children with advanced hepatoblastoma and prolong the survival. Surgical resection is the preferred treatment of resectable hepatoblastoma at the time of diagnosis. Neoadjuvant chemotherapy could improve the rate and safety of complete surgical resection for unresectable hepatoblastoma. Liver transplantation is one of the main treatments for unresectable hepatoblastoma [22, 23]. Prognosis has been greatly improved due to advances in chemotherapeutic agents and dosing regimens as well as innovations in surgical procedures, including the preoperative three-dimensional reconstruction, the usage of energy device, and liver transplantation. The management of high-risk patients and patients with recurrent or metastatic disease remains challenging [21].

4.1 Surgical resection for hepatoblastoma

Hepatectomy is the first choice for hepatoblastoma. It is suitable for PRETEXT I, II, and part of III patients. For most PRETEXT III and IV patients, chemotherapy is preferred first. Then, reevaluate the tumor and decide the treatment, hepatectomy or liver transplantation. However, there is still controversy about whether surgery should be performed first or chemotherapy first and the selection of extended hepatectomy or liver transplantation.

4.1.1 Preoperative or postoperative chemotherapy

Over the past 40 years, the management of hepatoblastoma has changed significantly. For patients with unresectable tumors, neoadjuvant chemotherapy has become the standard treatment which can lead to a significant reduction in preoperative tumors and sometimes even complete ablation [24]. Neoadjuvant chemotherapy may facilitate partial hepatectomy by withdrawal of the tumor boundary from the confluence of portal vein bifurcation, hepatic veins, and inferior vena cava. And the tumor volume of hepatoblastoma could be significantly resolved with increasing neoadjuvant chemotherapy cycles [25]. For patients who underwent cisplatinum-based neoadjuvant and postoperative chemotherapy, microscopically positive resection margin did not affect the overall survival rate. And the "wait-and-see policy" is recommended [26].

For patients with hepatoblastoma that could be resected at diagnosis, postoperative chemotherapy with cisplatin, fluorouracil, and vincristine is useful to control the disease progression [27]. And for the subtype of pure fetal histology hepatoblastoma, complete surgical resection can achieve good survival without additional chemotherapy. Further study should be performed to identify the patients for whom chemotherapy is not necessary [28].

4.1.2 Extended hepatectomy or liver transplantation

The management of patients in PRETEXT III or IV was difficult, including the selection between an aggressive liver resection and liver transplantation. There has been several study comparing the prognosis of partial hepatectomy and liver transplantation, the 5-year overall survival rate was 92% in patients who were performed partial hepatectomy, and about 83% in patients who underwent liver transplantation [29–32].

Although primary liver transplantation is recommended for POSTTEXT III and IV hepatoblastoma, some of the patients may be possible to perform extended hepatectomy after careful preoperative evaluation. In a prospective study that involved 18 patients with PRETEXT III and IV, extended major hepatic resection is safe and feasible with a comparable prognosis. The prognosis was similar with liver transplantation, while patients could avoid long-term immunosuppressive treatment. But there should always be a potential donor for salvage liver transplantation [33, 34]. A study including 24 patients performed liver transplantation or extensive liver resection. Two patients in five who underwent liver transplantation experienced tumor recurrence and death within a mean period of 6 months, while 6 patients were recurrent in the extended hepatectomy group, with 63.2% event-free survival and 94.7% overall survival rate. The results support extensive surgical resection in patients of advanced tumor [35]. Although the surgical resection is complicated and sometimes remains positive or close negative margins, the patients could have good outcomes. Combined with neoadjuvant therapy, extensive surgical resection may spare the morbidity of orthotopic liver transplantation. And it will offer an alternative treatment for patients who are ineligible for liver transplantation [36].

In our center, we have performed extended hepatectomy for 27 cases of PRETEXT or POSTEXT III and IV, the 3-year disease-free survival was 75.0%, and the overall survival was 87.5%.

4.1.3 Does postoperative complication affect prognosis

Neoadjuvant therapy has become the standard treatment for unresected hepatoblastoma. After neoadjuvant therapy, tumor volume may reduce, and surgical resection could be safely performed [37]. Although the patients may have good survival, neoadjuvant therapy may be related with postoperative complications. A study assessing the surgical outcomes focusing on resection margins, postoperative complications, 30-day mortality, and overall survival found that patients who underwent partial hepatectomy after chemotherapy experienced high rate of surgical complications (58%). But the complications were not detrimental to survival [29]. In another report, the incidence of complications after surgical resection following adjuvant chemotherapy is high and is associated with overall survival in high-risk hepatoblastoma. One of the possible reasons is that postoperative complication will delay the chemotherapy [38]. In our experience, precise preoperative evaluation of the anatomy of tumor and intrahepatic vascular with three-dimensional (3D) reconstruction and compare with the intraoperative situation will ensure the safety of surgery.

4.2 3D reconstruction facilitates surgical resection

Three-dimensional reconstruction has been widely used in preoperative evaluation and assisting hepatectomy [39] or living donor liver transplantation [40].

3D simulation software could reconstruct the whole liver, tumor, and intrahepatic vascular, clearly displaying the anatomical variation and the correlation of tumor with the surrounding vascular. It is helpful for making the precise surgical plan and enables individualized anatomic hepatectomy for each pediatric patient with hepatoblastoma. For surgical resection, precisely understanding the location of tumor and the relation of tumor with the surrounding vascular and accurately evaluating the remnant liver volume are important for safe hepatectomy of giant hepatoblastoma. In our center, we have used a novel virtual hepatectomy simulation software named Hisense CAS for preoperative evaluation. The Hisense CAS software could simulate a 3D liver image quickly and accurately with DICOM files of contrast-enhanced CT. With the Hisense CAS, we could confirm the anatomical relationship of tumor with the surrounding vascular from any direction, preoperatively mimic hepatectomy by extracting Glisson territory for anatomical liver resection or nonanatomical hepatectomy, automatically calculate the remnant liver volume, and navigate the liver resection during operation [41, 42]. As shown in **Figure 1**, with the help of 3D reconstruction, we performed extended hepatectomy for the patients. In total, we have performed extended hepatectomy for 27 patients in PRETEXT or POSTTEXT III and IV. All the hepatoblastoma were successfully removed with no complications. There were shorter operation time and less intraoperative bleeding in the reconstructing group. And the postoperative hospital stays tended to be shorter [41, 42].

4.3 Liver transplantation in unresectable hepatoblastoma

Although extended hepatectomy for advanced hepatoblastoma has achieved favorable results, liver transplantation is still the only treatment for unresectable hepatoblastoma.

Liver transplantation can achieve a good prognosis for patients with hepatoblastoma, with a 5-year survival rate of 86% and a 10-year survival rate of about 80% [32, 43]. Compared with deceased donor transplantation, the prognosis of living liver transplantation was a little better (5-year survival rates were 83.3 and 77.6%). And compared with salvage liver transplantation, primary liver transplantation has a better prognosis (5-year survival rates were 82 and 30%) [31]. Compared with liver transplantation performed before 2010, patients who received liver transplantation after 2010 have a better prognosis (5-year survival rates were 82.6 and 75.1%) [43]. Preoperative liver metastasis, tumor lysis after chemotherapy, and perioperative anticoagulation can significantly improve the prognosis of patients with liver transplantation. And the outcome was not affected by tumor pathology [44]. For unresectable hepatoblastoma, vascular infiltration and poor resection are often present, and liver transplantation has become the first choice [45]. Adjuvant chemotherapy after transplantation can significantly improve the long-term prognosis of patients [22]. For unresectable hepatoblastoma, the pretransplantation trend of alpha-fetoprotein levels after live donor liver transplantation can be used as an indicator of predictive recurrence. Since the AFP response cannot be accurately predicted before each chemotherapy cycle, liver transplantation may be appropriate if the AFP level does not decrease after the last cycle and before AFP levels are found to rise again [46].

4.4 Treatment after metastasis

The lung is the most common metastatic organ of hepatoblastoma. In addition to lung, brain and bone metastases have also been reported [12, 47]. At the first diagnosis of hepatoblastoma, 17% of patients had pulmonary metastases [48]. Patients with lung

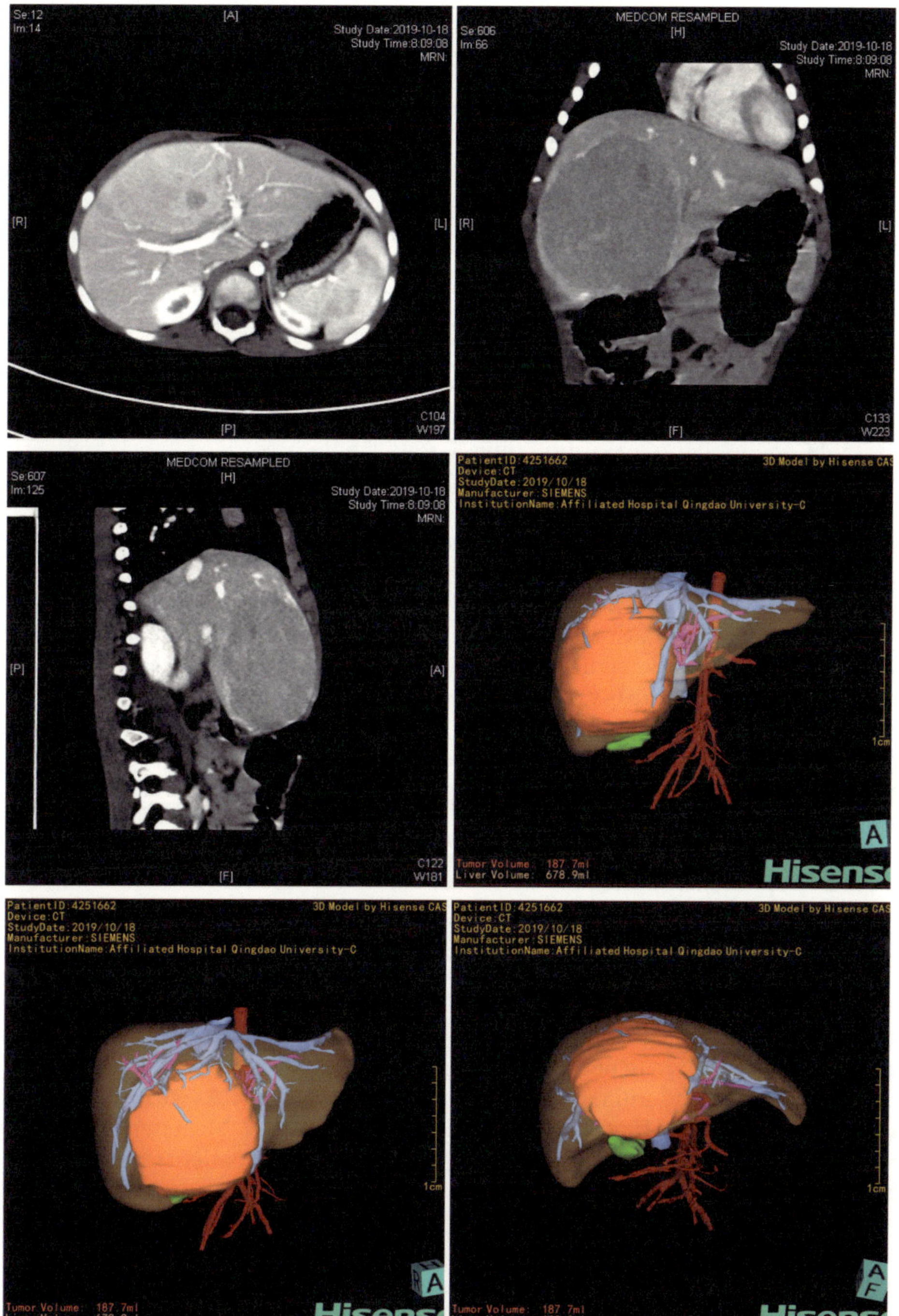

Figure 1.
Precise evaluation of hepatoblastoma with 3D reconstruction software.

metastasis will have a poor overall prognosis. Therefore, a CT scan of the lung should be performed before treatment to determine whether there is lung metastasis. Treatment after lung metastasis is also critical to extend the prognosis of patients. Comprehensive treatment of primary and metastatic lesions can improve the prognosis of patients.

The treatment of patients with synchronous lung metastasis and hepatoblastoma has been systemically reviewed [49]. To summarize, if the primary lesions and metastases are resectable, combine resection; if unresectable, eradicate or reduce the metastasis by neoadjuvant chemotherapy and then flowing combined resection. For single lung metastatic nodule, surgical resection is safe and feasible for the treatment [50]. Neoadjuvant chemotherapy combined with surgical resection of primary and metastatic lesions can achieve a better prognosis for patients with lung metastases. Most lung metastatic lesions are sensitive to chemotherapy. About half (26/60) of patients can achieve complete remission by chemotherapy. Then flowing surgical removal of primary lesion, the patient's survival could be significantly improved (3-year survival rate 67.2%) [51]. For the patients whose lung metastasis cannot be completely eradicated by chemotherapy, the prognosis is relatively poor [52]. For patients who cannot achieve complete remission, increasing the intensity of chemotherapy or expanding the scope of surgical resection may prolong the patient's prognosis. In addition, the patients will experience poor prognosis if it occurs as lung metastases while on treatment [52]. If the primary liver lesion is resectable, chemotherapy-resistant lung lesions should be surgically removed before, after, or at the same time as liver tumor surgery. In patients with unresectable primary liver tumor, liver transplantation combined with metastasectomy can be performed after chemotherapy, the 5-year survival rate of which can reach 86%. For patients with an unremovable hepatoblastoma and residual lung metastasis, overall tumor burden may be an important prognostic factor for these patients [53]. Local treatment (e.g., transcatheter arterial chemoembolization or radiofrequency ablation) may be considered to reduce tumor size [49, 54]. Sometimes it is difficult to diagnose whether there is viability of residual lung lesions after chemotherapy; it will affect the operation for the primary tumor. It is difficult to determine the pathology of tiny lesions in imaging and find the lesions during intraoperative exploration; indocyanine green fluoroscopy may be helpful. But further study is necessary to verify the usefulness [55].

4.5 Adult hepatoblastoma

Compared with pediatric hepatoblastoma, adult hepatoblastoma has a lower incidence and a higher degree of malignancy [56]. There is no significant gender difference in the incidence of adult hepatoblastoma, and the average age of onset is 42 years [57]. About 25% of adult hepatoblastomas are associated with hepatitis and cirrhosis, while it is rare in pediatric patients. Abdominal pain is the main clinical manifestation, and abdominal mass is the most common sign. As with children, surgical resection is the first choice for adult hepatoblastoma. Most hepatoblastomas are unresectable at diagnosis; chemotherapy can be used for patients who cannot be resected to gain opportunities for surgery [58]. Chemotherapy protocols are not standardized, and there was no statistically significance in survival rate between patients treated with drugs or TACE and patients not treated [57]. Due to low incidence, liver transplantation has yet to be fully evaluated. The prognosis of adult hepatoblastoma is extremely poor. The median survival time was 8 months and a 1-year survival rate of 39.2% after treatment [59]. And patients had a longer survival if operation was performed [59]. Compared with nonsurgical treatment, surgery has a better prognosis. Hepatic multilobed involvement, embryonic histology, multifocal nodules, and AFP <100 or AFP > 1000 are the poor prognostic factors [60].

5. Conclusions

In summary, surgical resection is the primary treatment for hepatoblastoma. Preoperative three-dimensional reconstruction can improve the resection rate of the tumor and the safety of the resection. For patients who cannot be directly resected, the tumor volume can be reduced by neoadjuvant therapy and then surgically treated. Liver transplantation is the best treatment for unresectable hepatoblastoma and has a good prognosis. For patients with distant metastasis, chemotherapy or metastasis resection combined with primary resection can effectively control disease progression.

Acknowledgements

This research was funded by the National Natural Science Foundation of China (81600490 and 81600691), the Research and Development Project of Shandong Province (2016GSF201221), China Postdoctoral Science Foundation (2016M602098 and 2018M640615), and Qingdao Postdoctoral Science Foundation (2016046).

Conflict of interest

The authors declare no conflict of interest.

Author details

Chengzhan Zhu[1,2], Bingzi Dong[2], Xin Chen[3] and Qian Dong[2,3*]

1 Department of Hepatobiliary and Pancreatic Surgery, The Affiliated Hospital of Qingdao University, Qingdao, China

2 Shandong Key Laboratory of Digital Medicine and Computer Assisted Surgery, The Affiliated Hospital of Qingdao University, Qingdao, China

3 Pediatric Surgery Department, The Affiliated Hospital of Qingdao University, Qingdao, China

*Address all correspondence to: 18661801885@163.com

References

[1] Hung GY, Lin LY, Yu TY, et al. Hepatoblastoma incidence in Taiwan: A population-based study. Journal of the Chinese Medical Association. 2018;**81**(6):541-547. DOI: 10.1016/j.jcma.2017.11.012

[2] Hadzic N, Finegold MJ. Liver neoplasia in children. Clinics in Liver Disease. 2011;**15**(2):443-462, vii-x. DOI: 10.1016/j.cld.2011.03.011

[3] Allan BJ, Parikh PP, Diaz S, et al. Predictors of survival and incidence of hepatoblastoma in the paediatric population. HPB: The Official Journal of the International Hepato Pancreato Biliary Association. 2013;**15**(10):741-746. DOI: 10.1111/hpb.12112

[4] Hung GY, Horng JL, Lee YS, et al. Cancer incidence patterns among children and adolescents in Taiwan from 1995 to 2009: A population-based study. Cancer. 2014;**120**(22):3545-3553. DOI: 10.1002/cncr.28903

[5] Feng J, Polychronidis G, Heger U, et al. Incidence trends and survival prediction of hepatoblastoma in children: A population-based study. Cancer Communications (London). 2019;**39**(1):62. DOI: 10.1186/s40880-019-0411-7

[6] Ismail H, Broniszczak D, Kalicinski P, et al. Changing treatment and outcome of children with hepatoblastoma: Analysis of a single center experience over the last 20 years. Journal of Pediatric Surgery. 2012;**47**(7):1331-1339. DOI: 10.1016/j.jpedsurg.2011.11.073

[7] Baheti AD, Luana Stanescu A, Li N, et al. Contrast-enhanced CT features of hepatoblastoma: Can we predict histopathology? Clinical Imaging. 2017;**44**:33-37. DOI: 10.1016/j.clinimag.2017.03.023

[8] Miranda Magalhaes Santos JM, Clemente BO, Araujo-Filho JAB, et al. State-of-the-art in radiomics of hepatocellular carcinoma: A review of basic principles, applications, and limitations. Abdominal Radiology(NY). 2019. DOI: 10.1007/s00261-019-02299-3

[9] Hosny A, Parmar C, Quackenbush J, et al. Artificial intelligence in radiology. Nature Reviews. Cancer. 2018;**18**(8):500-510. DOI: 10.1038/s41568-018-0016-5

[10] Aronson DC, Meyers RL. Malignant tumors of the liver in children. Seminars in Pediatric Surgery. 2016;**25**(5):265-275. DOI: 10.1053/j.sempedsurg.2016.09.002

[11] MacKinlay GA, Pritchard J. A common language for childhood liver tumours. Pediatric Surgery International. 1992;**7**(4):325-326

[12] Towbin AJ, Meyers RL, Woodley H, et al. 2017 PRETEXT: Radiologic staging system for primary hepatic malignancies of childhood revised for the paediatric hepatic international tumour trial (PHITT). Pediatric Radiology. 2018;**48**(4):536-554. DOI: 10.1007/s00247-018-4078-z

[13] Liu APY, Ip JJK, Leung AWK, et al. Treatment outcome and pattern of failure in hepatoblastoma treated with a consensus protocol in Hong Kong. Pediatric Blood and Cancer. 2019;**66**(1):e27482. DOI: 10.1002/pbc.27482

[14] Qiao GL, Chen Z, Wang C, et al. Pure fetal histology subtype was associated with better prognosis of children with hepatoblastoma: A Chinese population-based study. Journal of Gastroenterology and Hepatology. 2016;**31**(3):621-627. DOI: 10.1111/jgh.13165

[15] Yuan XJ, Wang HM, Jiang H, et al. Multidisciplinary effort in treating

children with hepatoblastoma in China. Cancer Letters. 2016;**375**(1):39-46. DOI: 10.1016/j.canlet.2016.02.051

[16] Shi Y, Commander SJ, Masand PM, et al. Vascular invasion is a prognostic indicator in hepatoblastoma. Journal of Pediatric Surgery. 2017;**52**(6):956-961. DOI: 10.1016/j.jpedsurg.2017.03.017

[17] Meyers RL, Maibach R, Hiyama E, et al. Risk-stratified staging in paediatric hepatoblastoma: A unified analysis from the children's hepatic tumors international collaboration. The Lancet Oncology. 2017;**18**(1):122-131. DOI: 10.1016/S1470-2045(16)30598-8

[18] Hiyama E, Hishiki T, Watanabe K, et al. Resectability and tumor response after preoperative chemotherapy in hepatoblastoma treated by the Japanese study group for pediatric liver tumor (JPLT)-2 protocol. Journal of Pediatric Surgery. 2016;**51**(12):2053-2057. DOI: 10.1016/j.jpedsurg.2016.09.038

[19] Wang TY, Pan C, Tang JY, et al. A follow-up report of childhood hepatoblastoma from 74 cases in a single center. Zhonghua Er Ke Za Zhi. 2017;**55**(5):364-368. DOI: 10.3760/cma.j.issn.0578-1310.2017.05.011

[20] Zsiros J, Brugieres L, Brock P, et al. Dose-dense cisplatin-based chemotherapy and surgery for children with high-risk hepatoblastoma (SIOPEL-4): A prospective, single-arm, feasibility study. The Lancet Oncology. 2013;**14**(9):834-842. DOI: 10.1016/S1470-2045(13)70272-9

[21] Kremer N, Walther AE, Tiao GM. Management of hepatoblastoma: An update. Current Opinion in Pediatrics. 2014;**26**(3):362-369. DOI: 10.1097/MOP.0000000000000081

[22] Pham TA, Gallo AM, Concepcion W, et al. Effect of liver transplant on long-term disease-free survival in children with Hepatoblastoma and hepatocellular cancer. JAMA Surgery. 2015;**150**(12):1150-1158. DOI: 10.1001/jamasurg.2015.1847

[23] Perilongo G, Malogolowkin M, Feusner J. Hepatoblastoma clinical research: Lessons learned and future challenges. Pediatric Blood and Cancer. 2012;**59**(5):818-821. DOI: 10.1002/pbc.24217

[24] Sharma D, Subbarao G, Saxena R. Hepatoblastoma. Seminars in Diagnostic Pathology. 2017;**34**(2):192-200. DOI: 10.1053/j.semdp.2016.12.015

[25] Murphy AJ, Ayers GD, Hilmes MA, et al. Imaging analysis of hepatoblastoma resectability across neoadjuvant chemotherapy. Journal of Pediatric Surgery. 2013;**48**(6):1239-1248. DOI: 10.1016/j.jpedsurg.2013.03.019

[26] Aronson DC, Weeda VB, Maibach R, et al. Microscopically positive resection margin after hepatoblastoma resection: What is the impact on prognosis? A childhood liver tumours strategy group (SIOPEL) report. European Journal of Cancer. 2019;**106**:126-132. DOI: 10.1016/j.ejca.2018.10.013

[27] Katzenstein HM, Langham MR, Malogolowkin MH, et al. Minimal adjuvant chemotherapy for children with hepatoblastoma resected at diagnosis (AHEP0731): A children's oncology group, multicentre, phase 3 trial. The Lancet Oncology. 2019;**20**(5):719-727. DOI: 10.1016/S1470-2045(18)30895-7

[28] Malogolowkin MH, Katzenstein HM, Meyers RL, et al. Complete surgical resection is curative for children with hepatoblastoma with pure fetal histology: A report from the children's oncology group. Journal of Clinical Oncology. 2011;**29**(24):3301-3306. DOI: 10.1200/JCO.2010.29.3837

[29] Busweiler LA, Wijnen MH, Wilde JC, et al. Surgical treatment

of childhood hepatoblastoma in the Netherlands (1990-2013). Pediatric Surgery International. 2017;**33**(1):23-31. DOI: 10.1007/s00383-016-3989-8

[30] Finegold MJ, Egler RA, Goss JA, et al. Liver tumors: Pediatric population. LiverTransplantation.2008;**14**(11):1545-1556. DOI: 10.1002/lt.21654

[31] Otte JB, Pritchard J, Aronson DC, et al. Liver transplantation for hepatoblastoma: Results from the International Society of Pediatric Oncology (SIOP) study SIOPEL-1 and review of the world experience. Pediatric Blood and Cancer. 2004;**42**(1):74-83. DOI: 10.1002/pbc.10376

[32] Triana Junco P, Cano EM, Dore M, et al. Prognostic factors for liver transplantation in unresectable hepatoblastoma. European Journal of Pediatric Surgery. 2019;**29**(1):28-32. DOI: 10.1055/s-0038-1668148

[33] El-Gendi A, Fadel S, El-Shafei M, et al. Avoiding liver transplantation in post-treatment extent of disease III and IV hepatoblastoma. Pediatrics International. 2018;**60**(9):862-868. DOI: 10.1111/ped.13634

[34] Fuchs J, Cavdar S, Blumenstock G, et al. POST-TEXT III and IV hepatoblastoma: Extended hepatic resection avoids liver transplantation in selected cases. Annals of Surgery. 2017;**266**(2):318-323. DOI: 10.1097/SLA.0000000000001936

[35] de Freitas Paganoti G, Tannuri ACA, Dantas Marques AC, et al. Extensive hepatectomy as an alternative to liver transplant in advanced hepatoblastoma: A new protocol used in a pediatric liver transplantation center. Transplantation Proceedings. 2019;**51**(5):1605-1610. DOI: 10.1016/j.transproceed.2019.03.004

[36] Fonseca A, Gupta A, Shaikh F, et al. Extreme hepatic resections for the treatment of advanced hepatoblastoma: Are planned close margins an acceptable approach? Pediatric Blood and Cancer. 2018;**65**(2). DOI: 10.1002/pbc.26820

[37] Sunil BJ, Palaniappan R, Venkitaraman B, et al. Surgical resection for hepatoblastoma-updated survival outcomes. Journal of Gastrointestinal Cancer. 2018;**49**(4):493-496. DOI: 10.1007/s12029-017-0005-z

[38] Becker K, Furch C, Schmid I, et al. Impact of postoperative complications on overall survival of patients with hepatoblastoma. Pediatric Blood and Cancer. 2015;**62**(1):24-28. DOI: 10.1002/pbc.25240

[39] Aoki T, Murakami M, Fujimori A, et al. Routes for virtually guided endoscopic liver resection of subdiaphragmatic liver tumors. Langenbeck's Archives of Surgery. 2016;**401**(2):263-273. DOI: 10.1007/s00423-016-1385-4

[40] Mochizuki K, Takatsuki M, Soyama A, et al. The usefulness of a high-speed 3D-image analysis system in pediatric living donor liver transplantation. Annals of Transplantation. 2012;**17**(1):31-34

[41] Zhang G, Zhou XJ, Zhu CZ, et al. Usefulness of three-dimensional(3D) simulation software in hepatectomy for pediatric hepatoblastoma. Surgical Oncology. 2016;**25**(3):236-243. DOI: 10.1016/j.suronc.2016.05.023

[42] Zhao J, Zhou XJ, Zhu CZ, et al. 3D simulation assisted resection of giant hepatic mesenchymal hamartoma in children. Computer Assisted Surgery (Abingdon, England). 2017;**22**(1):54-59. DOI: 10.1080/24699322.2017.1358401

[43] Ezekian B, Mulvihill MS, Schroder PM, et al. Improved contemporary outcomes of liver transplantation for pediatric hepatoblastoma and hepatocellular

carcinoma. Pediatric Transplantation. 2018;**22**(8):e13305. DOI: 10.1111/petr.13305

[44] Cruz RJ Jr, Ranganathan S, Mazariegos G, et al. Analysis of national and single-center incidence and survival after liver transplantation for hepatoblastoma: New trends and future opportunities. Surgery. 2013;**153**(2):150-159. DOI: 10.1016/j.surg.2012.11.006

[45] Uchida H, Sakamoto S, Sasaki K, et al. Surgical treatment strategy for advanced hepatoblastoma: Resection versus transplantation. Pediatric Blood and Cancer. 2018;**65**(12):e27383. DOI: 10.1002/pbc.27383

[46] Isono K, Ohya Y, Lee KJ, et al. Pretransplant trends in alpha-fetoprotein levels as a predictor of recurrence after living donor liver transplantation for unresectable hepatoblastoma: A single-institution experience. Pediatric Transplantation. 2018;**22**(5):e13221. DOI: 10.1111/petr.13221

[47] Yadav SS, Lawande MA, Patkar DA, et al. Rare case of hemorrhagic brain metastasis from hepatoblastoma. Journal of Pediatric Neurosciences. 2012;**7**(1):73-74. DOI: 10.4103/1817-1745.97634

[48] Czauderna P, Haeberle B, Hiyama E, et al. The children's hepatic tumors international collaboration (CHIC): Novel global rare tumor database yields new prognostic factors in hepatoblastoma and becomes a research model. European Journal of Cancer. 2016;**52**:92-101. DOI: 10.1016/j.ejca.2015.09.023

[49] Angelico R, Grimaldi C, Gazia C, et al. How do synchronous lung metastases influence the surgical management of children with hepatoblastoma? An update and systematic review of the literature. Cancers (Basel). 2019;**11**(11):1693. DOI: 10.3390/cancers11111693

[50] Shi Y, Geller JI, Ma IT, et al. Relapsed hepatoblastoma confined to the lung is effectively treated with pulmonary metastasectomy. Journal of Pediatric Surgery. 2016;**51**(4):525-529. DOI: 10.1016/j.jpedsurg.2015.10.053

[51] Hishiki T, Watanabe K, Ida K, et al. The role of pulmonary metastasectomy for hepatoblastoma in children with metastasis at diagnosis: Results from the JPLT-2 study. Journal of Pediatric Surgery. 2017;**52**(12):2051-2055. DOI: 10.1016/j.jpedsurg.2017.08.031

[52] Wanaguru D, Shun A, Price N, et al. Outcomes of pulmonary metastases in hepatoblastoma—Is the prognosis always poor? Journal of Pediatric Surgery. 2013;**48**(12):2474-2478. DOI: 10.1016/j.jpedsurg.2013.08.023

[53] O'Neill AF, Towbin AJ, Krailo MD, et al. Characterization of pulmonary metastases in children with hepatoblastoma treated on children's oncology group protocol AHEP0731 (the treatment of children with all stages of hepatoblastoma): A report from the children's oncology group. Journal of Clinical Oncology. 2017;**35**(30):3465-3473. DOI: 10.1200/JCO.2017.73.5654

[54] Yevich S, Calandri M, Gravel G, et al. Reiterative radiofrequency ablation in the management of pediatric patients with hepatoblastoma metastases to the lung, liver, or bone. Cardiovascular and Interventional Radiology. 2019;**42**(1):41-47. DOI: 10.1007/s00270-018-2097-7

[55] Kitagawa N, Shinkai M, Mochizuki K, et al. Navigation using indocyanine green fluorescence imaging for hepatoblastoma pulmonary metastases surgery. Pediatric Surgery International. 2015;**31**(4):407-411. DOI: 10.1007/s00383-015-3679-y

[56] Rougemont AL, McLin VA, Toso C, et al. Adult hepatoblastoma: Learning

from children. Journal of Hepatology. 2012;**56**(6):1392-1403. DOI: 10.1016/j.jhep.2011.10.028

[57] Celotti A, D'Amico G, Ceresoli M, et al. Hepatoblastoma of the adult: A systematic review of the literature. Surgical Oncology. 2016;**25**(3):339-347. DOI: 10.1016/j.suronc.2016.07.003

[58] Nakamura S, Sho M, Kanehiro H, et al. Adult hepatoblastoma successfully treated with multimodal treatment. Langenbeck's Archives of Surgery. 2010;**395**(8):1165-1168. DOI: 10.1007/s00423-010-0630-5

[59] Duan XF, Zhao Q. Adult hepatoblastoma: A review of 47 cases. ANZ Journal of Surgery. 2018;**88**(1-2):E50-E54. DOI: 10.1111/ans.13839

[60] Brotto M, Finegold MJ. Distinct patterns of p27/KIP 1 gene expression in hepatoblastoma and prognostic implications with correlation before and after chemotherapy. Human Pathology. 2002;**33**(2):198-205. DOI: 10.1053/hupa.2002.31294

Chapter 2

Early Postoperative Monitoring of the Liver Graft

Demetrio V. Pérez Civantos, Alicia Muñoz Cantero, Manuel Robles Marcos, Francisco Fuentes Morillas, María A. Santiago Triviño, María O. Cerezo Arias, María D. Pérez Frutos and Alberto Córdoba López

Abstract

Liver transplantation (LT) is a common current technique for end-stage liver disease. Complications after the surgical procedure, though uncommon, can be of very different origin and can also be severe enough to lead to liver and multiorgan failure and finally graft loss and/or recipient's death. Intensivists and the surgical team must be familiarized with these early complications to detect them as soon as possible in order to use the best diagnostic tools and take the best therapeutic measures to restore anatomical integrity and organ function to optimize the liver graft. In this chapter, we present an updated state of the art for efficiently tackling with all different, most usual complications that an LT patient can present during early postoperative period.

Keywords: liver transplantation, liver graft dysfunction, liver posttransplant complications, liver function monitoring, posttransplant critical care

1. Introduction

Liver transplantation (LT) is the only therapy for end-stage liver disease. It has become a common surgical procedure. The postoperative severe complications may compromise both patient's graft and life survival, so an early suspicion, detection, and therapeutic solution are the only way to change the threatening of post-LT complications.

The need of allografts has largely extended the set of criteria (ECD) for organ acceptability, increasing the risk of complications and adverse outcomes [1, 2].

Little is known about the parameters that can alert of early complications of liver graft function, need of retransplantation, vascular complications, reinterventions, and long intensive care stay.

Hereby we present the state of the art on the early detection and management of the most frequently complications found during the postoperative period of liver transplantation in the intensive care unit (ICU). We discuss the management of clinical, laboratory, and ancillary tests' findings that can help medical and surgical staff to tackle and take decisions when suspecting early hepatic graft malfunctioning. Early diagnosis could allow medical and surgical teams to take most difficult decisions to salvage the graft and to restore severe deteriorated patient's health condition.

Laboratory tests as well as scores (model for end-stage liver disease, MELD; acute physiology and chronic health evaluation, APACHE II; sequential organ failure assessment, SOFA; and model of early allograft function, MEAF) have good performance but can only do a late evaluation of patient status and graft function. The indocyanine green plasma disappearance rate is an interesting liver function test but produces some ambiguous results during the first days after transplantation. The liver maximal function capacity test is a novel and promising method for evaluating metabolic liver activity, but its use is limited for economic reasons and extrahepatic factors.

Recently somatic near-infrared spectroscopy of liver graft (LSrO2) has shown to be helpful to early monitor vascular graft supply after LT [3].

2. Vascular complications of the liver graft

Vascular complications after LT though seldom found are dreaded ones, as they carry high incidence of both loss of the graft and patient morbimortality [1].

Complications that affect the hepatic artery (HA) after LT can lead to ischemia of the liver graft which can result in graft morbidity, loss, or even patient death. The clinical feature of these complications varies and depends on the type (thrombosis or stenosis) and timing (early or late presentation) and the promptness of diagnosis [4–10]. Despite continuous improvements of the surgical technique, these complications represent one of the main causes of the failure of LT, with an incidence ranging from 2.6 to 20% in adult recipients [4–10].

2.1 Early monitoring of vascular graft supply and vascular complications

As it is hard to establish an effective screening of the risk of each patient undergoing LT, it is of paramount importance to bear in mind the possibility of early appearance as most studies and clinical experience have failed to demonstrate clear risk factors [4–12].

At the ICU it is difficult to monitor early graft vascular supply. Duplex ultrasound (DUS) is the usual tool used for this purpose, but it only provides information at a given point of time of the study but no continuous information.

Adequate perfusion and oxygenation to liver graft after transplantation are essential for its viability. LSrO2 through near-infrared spectroscopy (NIRS) can help by showing real-time oxygen content of the graft. Recently, our group carried out a study on post-LT patients for evaluating the efficacy of NIRS on detecting early vascular graft complications [12, 13]. Impairment of the liver graft microcirculation and tissue hypoxia are both a common pathology in all these complications with eventual loss of the graft without early intervention [14]. Early detection of this impairment could reduce the overall morbidity and mortality of LT by allowing earlier treatment. Measurement of hepatic LSrO2 has been shown to correlate significantly with the microcirculatory impairment and liver dysfunction induced by ischemia and reperfusion injury [12, 15].

The mean initial value of LSrO2 that our group observed was 74 (SD 5.7) with a tendency of a slight progressively increment along the following hours, showing a mean value of 76 (SD 4.1) at hour 24. When studying correlation of LSrO2, relevant and significant findings at hour 3 were found between this parameter and hemoglobin (Hb) ($p = .004$), as well as with cardiac index (CI) ($p = .044$). It was also found with the Apache II scale ($p = .041$) but not with SOFA ($p = .069$).

At hour 24, we also found significant correlation between LSrO2 and Hb ($p = .002$). No correlation was met with lactate at any moment (hour 1, hour 8, and hour 24) of the study ($p = .113$, $p = .293$, and $p = .141$, respectively).

Importantly, neither at the beginning nor at the end of the study was there a correlation observed between LSrO2 and liver biochemistry.

Finally, among hemodynamic parameters, a correlation was encountered between LSrO2 and CI at hour 3 ($p = .044$). DUS data expressed as resistive index and pulsatility index (RI and PI) did not correlate with LSrO2 at hour 24 ($p = .738$ and $p = .799$, respectively). We could not also find any statistical connection between LSrO2 and cold-warm ischemia time and at arrival after 24 hours ($p = .780$ and $p = .951$).

LSrO2 could early detect all severe vascular complications and all events that led to a decrease in blood or oxygenation supply to the liver graft, permitting to advance in taking diagnostic and therapeutic measures.

LSrO2 is a new monitoring tool that brings valuable information about hepatic flow and oxygenation early after liver transplant that deserves to be weighed.

2.1.1 Arterial complications

2.1.1.1 HAT

Hepatic artery thrombosis (HAT) [16] differs depending on time of presentation, usually ranging from 1 to 28 days (mean 7.4 days) [4].

HAT represents the most common vascular complication, accounting for more than 50% of all vascular complications [13]. Late reports show a lower HAT incidence, ranging from 1 to 25% [13, 17, 18]. It is the first cause of non-function of the graft [13].

The clinical presentation of HAT ranges from a mild elevation of liver function tests (LFT) and bilirubin levels in 75% of patients to fulminant hepatic necrosis. Other symptoms vary from biliary complications in 15%, fever and sepsis in 6%, and graft dysfunction or failure in 4% [13]. The clinical expression depends on the timing and the existence of collaterals. Early HAT is mostly expressed as a non-functioning graft, and late HAT is associated with biliary tract complications (bile duct strictures and/or biliary leaks).

Early HAT usually is manifested with fever, increased leukocytosis, and important elevation in liver enzyme levels. The natural history of early HAT can be summarized as biliary tract necrosis followed by uncontrolled septic shock in the immunosuppressed population and even the patient's death [6, 13, 19–22]. The cause of early HAT is still under debate and remains unknown [6, 19, 21–23]. Up to 20% of HAT cases are due to surgical causes [6, 19, 21–23].

Early diagnosis is mandatory to allow immediate treatment. Elevation of transaminase levels, LSrO2 monitoring [3] showing a > 10% reduction from basal data, duplex ultrasound (DUS will show absence of HA signal sensibility of 92%) and increased resistive index (RI). Visceral angiography will confirm the diagnosis [19, 22, 24].

Approximately 20% of them can be treated successfully with surgical revascularization with a Fogarty balloon-tip catheter and refashioning of the arterial anastomosis the very same day of diagnosis [4]. Percutaneous endovascular interventions including intra-arterial thrombolysis (IAT), percutaneous transluminal angioplasty (PTA), and stent placement have shown hopeful outcomes in the literature [13]. Anticoagulant or antiplatelet therapy is also advisable [13, 16]. Survival rates are 40% in symptomatic vs. 82% in asymptomatic patients [13]. Sylva et al. reported an overall mortality of 23% [20].

Different factors that cannot be involved in the appearance of HAT are etiology of recipient end-stage liver disease, previous LT, donor sex and age, cause of donor death, recipient sex and age, type of preservation solution, cold ischemia time, experience of the surgeon, type of arterial anastomosis, intraoperative transfusion requirement of red blood cells and fresh frozen plasma, acute rejection, and CMV infection. Donor age of greater than 60 years and back-table artery reconstruction have been found significantly associated with this complication [4].

2.1.1.2 HAS

Hepatic artery stenosis (HAS) is not rarely found and its incidence ranges 2–13% [13, 16]. It is defined as a narrowing of the transverse diameter of the HA, resulting in ischemia mainly revealed by elevated liver function tests [13, 25–31]. Significant HAS is defined as a reduction of >50% on angiogram associated with a resistive index (RI) <0.5 and a peak systolic velocity >400 cm/s by Duplex ultrasound (DUS) [8, 13, 26, 32]. LSrO2 reduction of >10% from basal levels and maintained during first hours can alert of HAC [3]. HAS also carries a high rate in morbidity and mortality. It has been postulated that HAT and HAS are two contiguous components of the broader allotransplant ischemic complications [13, 25–28, 30–35].

2.1.1.3 HAP

Hepatic artery pseudoaneurysm (HAP) is defined as a dilated hepatic artery, which occurs after iatrogenic injury in most cases, causing blood leaking and pool outside the artery wall into surrounding tissue with a persistent communication between the HA and the adjacent cavity [13].

Volpin et al. [36] informed of an incidence of 2.5% and Boleslawski et al. of 0.64% [37].

The clinical presentation varies from an asymptomatic state to an incidental finding upon abdominal pain associated with fever and gastrointestinal bleeding (25%), massive bleeding through abdominal drain (31%), and hemorrhagic shock (81%).

Several predisposing factors have been suggested, including peritoneal infections, technical difficulties during anastomosis, and biliary leak [24, 27, 35–62]. The rate of microorganisms cultured from HAP is 50% and from abdominal fluid 31% [36]. Diagnosis of HAP is based on DUS, contrast-enhanced CT scan, or angiography [36]. Treatment is based on reoperation or interventional radiology [36, 37, 42, 45, 63]. Urgent ligation of HA has a mortality that ranges from 28 to 85% [36, 40, 41, 45]. Boleslawski et al. [37] reported good results with HA ligation without revascularization.

2.1.1.4 HAR

HAR is defined as a severe hemorrhage from the trunk or from the main branch of the HA. It is a very serious complication that results in the disruption of blood supply to the graft. This is an exceptional but dramatic complication that carries a very high rate incidence of graft loss and mortality.

In most cases, this condition complicates a pseudoaneurysm of the HA, leading to major bleeding that requires emergency operation. Many authors report the role of infectious pathogens as causative agents of pseudoaneurysms [13]. Diagnosis of HAP is available with different radiological techniques, but in half of cases, HAP is not recognized before rupture, requiring immediate surgery [37].

In case of rupture and acute bleeding, there are many therapeutic possibilities: endovascular intervention with embolization with or without stenting, surgical intervention for anastomotic revision, aorto-hepatic grafting, HA ligation, or emergency retransplantation. Mortality remains very high, and no consensus exists about indication for the type of procedure [13, 37, 40, 45, 47, 64].

Boleslawski et al. [37] reported the largest series of ruptured posttransplant HAP and highlighted the efficacy of primary HA ligation with good (70–80%) early and late survival.

2.1.2 Venous complications

Compared to arterial complications, venous complications (VC) are less frequent, with an estimated overall incidence of <3% [65–72]. They can be potentially devastating, leading to graft failure and representing an important source of morbidity and mortality, especially if they occur in early period of post-LT [68, 71, 72].

Incidence is higher in pediatric population [68, 69, 73, 74].

The etiology of VC mostly involves venous anastomosis; those are portal, cava, and hepatic veins.

Portal vein complications (PVCs) are relative uncommon, occurring in 1–3% of LT [65–68, 70–72, 75]. These complications are related to high morbidity and graft loss [67, 68]. These complications are more common with split liver and living donor LT and in pediatric LT [72, 76].

Regarding PVCs we can make the diagnosis by DUS, contrast-enhanced ultrasound (CEUS), contrast-enhanced computed tomography (CECT), and magnetic resonance venography (MRV) [67, 68, 77]. Therapeutic management of PVCs ranges from endovascular procedures (as the first-line treatment) with highly successful results [50, 69, 74, 78] to surgical thrombectomy and anastomosis revision.

2.1.2.1 Portal vein thrombosis (PVT)

Incidence ranges from 0.3 to 2.6% [51, 71]. The clinical presentation depends on the time of thrombosis. Early thrombosis (<72 h) is presented as acute liver insufficiency or graft failure. If PVT occurs late (>day 30), clinical symptoms depend on the portocaval collateral circulation existence. Portal hypertension manifestations including upper gastrointestinal bleeding due to esophagogastric varices and ascites are the most frequent symptoms, and liver failure is rare [35, 71, 75]. PVC usually occurs during the first week after LT [27, 35, 52, 79]. The most common causes of PVT are technical errors related to venous redundancy, kinking, or stenosis of the anastomosis [71].

Therapeutic options for PVT range from systemic anticoagulation, catheter-based thrombolytic therapy via transjugular intrahepatic portosystemic shunt (TIPS), to surgical revision until retransplantation. The best three percutaneous options in literature are transhepatic vein angioplasty (with or without stent placement), percutaneous thrombolytic treatment via TIPS, and transsplenic approach [53, 54].

In clinical practice, the treatment depends on timing of appearance, if early liver failure or multiorgan failure appear, it compels surgical revision and if PVT is late to occur and no alteration in liver function test, observation, or medical treatment and complementary percutaneous treatment is required. If PVT is late in developing and with clinical manifestation of acute gastroesophageal bleeding or ascites, that will require percutaneous or TIPS procedures [55].

2.1.2.2 PVS

The true incidence of portal vein stenosis (PVS) is not known. The only data in literature concerning the incidence of venous complications is <3% [72].

When PVS is diagnosed, it can be present with acute graft failure or portal hypertension [56]. In practice the vast majority of patients are asymptomatic, and the finding is incidental on routine scanning ultrasound. In the case of symptomatic PVS, clinical signs will be those of portal hypertension as gastrointestinal bleeding due to gastroesophageal varices, ascites, and splenomegaly. Abnormal liver function tests are not constant.

Risk factor for developing PVS is the same as for PVT. The significant size mismatch is likely a cause of developing a stenosis [72].

DUS is the first tool for PVS diagnosis; it is highly sensitive but not specific. Some authors as Wei et al. [57] consider a pre- and post-stenosis gradient of >5 as compatible with PVS. Other authors prefer to rely on portal caliper diameter, and a reduction of >75% is suggestive [58].

In case there are no important clinical signs, the patient may be solely observed. If clinical picture is progressively deteriorating, a therapeutic access as transhepatic approach or transjugular access [58] must be done. A single balloon dilatation is sufficient to maintain patency in 77.7% of patients. In selected cases, a stent can be placed to prevent recurrence [59]. The use of three anticoagulant therapies (low-molecular-weight heparin, warfarin, and aspirin) may reduce the recurrence of thrombosis [60].

2.1.2.3 CVC

Caval vein complications (CVC) are extremely infrequent. They can be due to kinking, stenosis, or thrombosis and clinically appear as lower limb edema, ascites, pleural effusion, Budd-Chiari syndrome, and liver or renal failure [61, 65, 70].

Technical errors are the leading cause of CVC. Diagnosis should be made by DUS, contrast-enhanced CT, or cavography. Percutaneous radiological interventions are the methods of choice for therapeutical approach [59, 62, 80–83].

3. Biliary complications after liver transplantation

The most frequent and important causes of morbidity and mortality in LT recipients are stenosis, biliary leaks, and stones. The estimated incidence is 10–25% [84]. Most can be managed successfully with endoscopic retrograde cholangiography (ERC).

3.1 Types of complications

Biliary complications (stenosis, leaks, and stones) after LT can be classified as early (within 4 weeks) or late. Biliary strictures can be further divided into intrahepatic anastomotic stenoses, not anastomotic and diffuse stenoses. Other complications, such as bile emptying, Oddi sphincter dysfunction, mucocele, and hemobilia, are rare (**Table 1**).

3.2 Risk factors

There are several risk factors for development of biliary complications after LT (**Table 2**):

- Type of biliary reconstruction: ductal choledochocholedochostomy versus choledochojejunostomy in Roux-en-Y; the complication rate is similar [85].

- Routine tube placement in T: it is associated with a higher incidence of biliary complications, such as stenosis, biliary leaks, and cholangitis [86].

Bile leaks and biloma
Strictures
Anastomotic
Nonanastomotic
Diffuse intrahepatic
Common bile duct filling defects
Stones
Sludge
Casts
Sphincter of Oddi dysfunction
Other complications
Hemobilia
Mucocele
Bactobilia

Table 1.
Biliary complications after liver transplantation.

Roux-en-Y anastomosis
Use of T-tubes
Improper surgical technique
Inappropriate suture material or excessive tension at the anastomosis
Excessive use of electrocauterization for control of bile duct bleeding
Mismatch in size between donor and recipient bile ducts
ABO mismatched grafts
Acute hepatic artery thrombosis
Hepatic artery stenosis
Ischemia/reperfusion injury (ischemic-type biliary lesions)
Infections
Non heart-beating donors
Primary sclerosing cholangitis

Table 2.
Risk factors for the development of biliary complications after liver transplantation.

- Other risk factors (especially stenosis): acute thrombosis of the hepatic artery, stenosis of the hepatic artery, biliary leak, technical factors during surgery (excessive dissection of the periductal tissue during acquisition, excessive use of electrocautery for the control of bile duct bleeding) both in the donor and the recipient, the tension of the anastomosis, small caliber of the bile duct and the size of the donor and recipient not matching, ischemia injury/reperfusion, pre-LT diagnosis of cytomegalovirus infection, donation after cardiac death, ABO blood mismatch in the group, increased donor age, prolonged periods of cold and warm ischemia, and primary sclerosing cholangitis (**Table 2**) [85].

3.3 Diagnostic approach

In asymptomatic LT recipients that have elevations in serum levels of aminotransferases, bilirubin, alkaline phosphatase, and/or gamma-glutamyl transferase. Occasionally, they have nonspecific symptoms (fever and anorexia), abdominal pain in the right upper quadrant (especially with biliary leaks), pruritus, jaundice, and biliary ascites. However, pain may be absent due to immunosuppression and hepatic denervation [85].

The initial evaluation should include hepatic ultrasound (US) with Doppler of the hepatic vessels (**Figure 1**). If US Doppler suspects stenosis or occlusion of the hepatic artery, a computed tomographic (CT) angiogram should be obtained or a liver angiogram should be performed.

Liver biopsy is performed to exclude rejection, although it is usually deferred in patients with bile dilation and/or the presence of stones in the common bile duct due to the risk of causing a bile leak [87].

The abdominal US may not be sensitive enough (sensitivity 38–66%) to detect biliary obstruction [88]. Therefore, an additional evaluation with more sensitive techniques is recommended in patients with clinical suspicion.

If there is a strong clinical suspicion and US that indicates an obstruction of the bile duct with or without stones or a bile leak, cholangiography should be obtained [85]. Although ERC or percutaneous transhepatic cholangiography (PTC) remains the gold standard, magnetic resonance cholangiopancreatography (MRCP) is a reliable technique (96% sensitivity and 94% specificity) [89]. Currently, MRCP is considered an optimal noninvasive diagnostic tool for the evaluation of biliary complications after TL, if the abdominal US is normal and there is a high suspicion of a biliary complication [89].

ERC is perhaps the best diagnostic/therapeutic intervention in patients with conduit-to-conduit anastomosis. We reserved PTC for patients in whom ERC was not successful and in patients with Roux-en-Y choledochojejunostomy [90].

3.4 Stenosis

The incidence ranges from 4 to 16% [85]. Stenoses that occur early after TL are due to technical problems, while late stenoses are due to vascular insufficiency and scarring and fibrosis problems. Bile leakage is an independent risk factor for the development of anastomotic stenoses. Stenoses were more common with reconstruction with Roux-en-Y choledochojejunostomy.

They are classified as anastomotic or non-anastomotic, according to the place.

3.4.1 Anastomotic stenosis (AS)

It occurs within the first 12 months after LT. It has a good response to short-term stenting (3–6 months). However, patients require long-term surveillance, since the restrictions are often repeated.

The cholangiographic appearance characteristic of an AS is that of a narrowing of the area of the biliary anastomosis. In some patients, it may manifest itself in the first or second month after TL due to postoperative edema and inflammation [85]. This type responds to endoscopic balloon dilation and placement of the plastic stent; in most patients, it will be resolved in 3 months. The majority of patients with AS require continuous ERC (every 3 months) with balloon dilation and long-term stenting (12–24 months). Due to the high success rates, we suggest that endoscopic management be considered.

There is growing experience in the temporary placement (3–12 months) of self-expanding metal stents (cSEMS) covered to reduce the need for repeated stent exchanges [91]. There is insufficient data to support the systematic use, but the cSEMS may be beneficial in patients who fail therapy with plastic stents and dilatation [91].

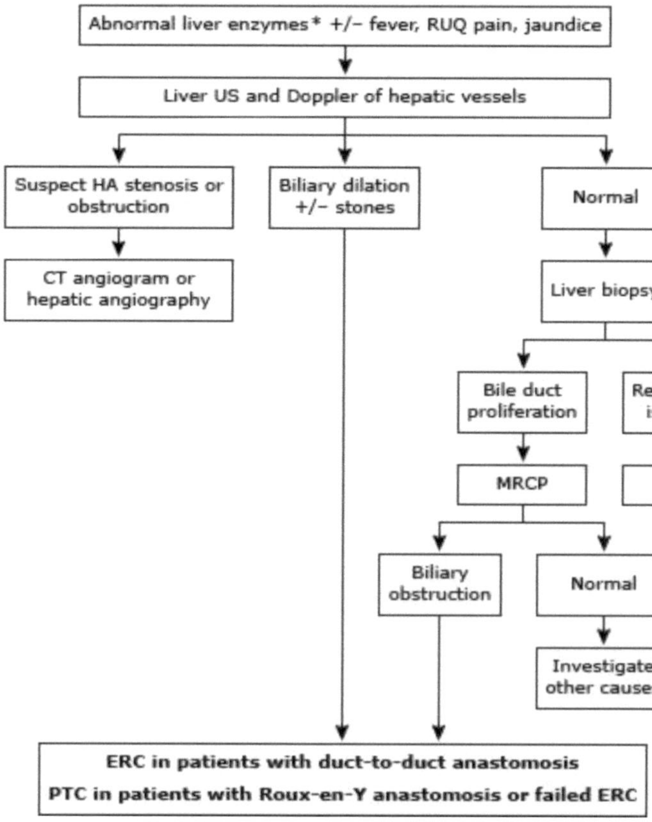

Figure 1.
Algorithm for the diagnosis and evaluation of suspected biliary obstruction after liver transplantation.

In 4–17% of cases, ERC cannot be performed successfully because the AS could not be crossed with a guidewire. Previous leaks of bile and high blood transfusion requirements during surgery are risk factors for the initial failure of ERC. The majority of these patients will require surgery. In patients with Roux-en-Y choledochojejunostomy, ERC is often unsuccessful, and we suggest treatment with PTC and dilation, followed by placement of a percutaneous transhepatic catheter [92]. Surgical revision (usually a repair or conversion to a Roux-en-Y choledochojejunostomy) may be an alternative in stable patients with a duct-to-duct stenosis that is difficult to treat.

3.4.2 Non-anastomotic stenoses (NAS)

These are mainly due to thrombosis of the hepatic artery or other forms of ischemia. Less commonly, they may be due to the recurrence of the underlying disease, such as primary sclerosing cholangitis. Its incidence is 0.5–10%.

NAS can occur proximal to the anastomosis in the extrahepatic or intrahepatic bile duct. There may be multiple stenoses that affect the hilum and intrahepatic ducts, causing a cholangiographic appearance that resembles primary sclerosing cholangitis. Bile sludge can accumulate proximal to the stenosis, leading to recurrent episodes of cholangitis.

NAS are more difficult to treat than AS. NAS endoscopic therapy consists of a balloon dilatation followed by sphincterotomy and plastic stents with replacement every 3 months. NAS results are not as favorable as AS. Only 50% have a long-term response with endoscopic therapy with dilatation and stent placement. In addition, up to 50% undergo a transplant or die [93]. As a general rule, ischemic events that lead to diffuse stenosis of the intrahepatic bile duct are associated with poor graft survival.

Surgical revision may finally be necessary in strictures that are refractory to endoscopic or percutaneous treatment. A Roux-en-Y choledochojejunostomy is performed in patients with conduit-to-conduit anastomoses. In those who already have a Roux-en-Y anastomosis, it may be necessary to reposition the bile duct of the graft in a better vascularized area.

3.5 Biliary leaks

They have an incidence between 2 and 25%. The presence of a bile leak is an independent risk factor for the development of early or late stenoses. Leakage of the anastomosis, the cystic duct, the T-tube tract, or (in living donor or an LH divided into the liver) the cut surface of the liver may occur. Biliary leaks can be divided into early and late.

3.5.1 Early bile leaks

They occur at the site of the anastomosis and are often related to technical problems. Predisposing factors include the lack of perfusion of the hepatic artery and other technical reasons. They must be suspected in case of peritonitis or fluid collections in imaging tests.

In cases where a T-tube is placed, small anastomotic leaks can be diagnosed with a T-tube cholangiogram and can be controlled by leaving the tube open. In patients without a T-tube, ERC is the standard diagnostic method. Hepatobiliary scintigraphy (HIDA) can be useful in cases where there is a low suspicion of leakage [94].

The placement of a plastic stent, with or without biliary sphincterotomy, is successful in 90 to 95%. As a result, ERC is the treatment of choice. In some cases, small leaks can be treated with biliary sphincterotomy alone. The stent remains 2 months and is not changed during this period unless there is a clinical suspicion of obstruction.

Anastomotic leaks from Roux-en-Y choledochojejunostomy are less common. It can be diagnosed with a HIDA scan if the patient does not have a drainage catheter in place. ERC is often not feasible due to anatomical difficulties. Management is usually performed with internal-external percutaneous drainage and more frequently requires surgical treatment.

3.5.2 Late leaks of bile

They are usually related to the removal of the tube in T. It should be suspected in patients who develop pain when the tube is removed in T. ERC is indicated (with or without sphincterotomy) with transpapillary stenting [95]. Surgery or a percutaneous transhepatic approach is reserved for patients in whom the endoscopic approach is unsuccessful. Some centers use nasobiliary tubes instead of stents.

3.6 Biloma

They are produced by rupture of the duct and extravasation of bile in the hepatic parenchyma or abdominal cavity, in patients with necrosis of the bile duct secondary to thrombosis of the hepatic artery. Most post-LT bilomas occur in the perihepatic area, outside the liver. If the biloma occurs in the hepatic parenchyma and communicates with the biliary tree, it may resolve spontaneously or, in some cases, be treated with endoscopy and a transpapillary stent. Large bilomas that do not communicate with the bile ducts should be treated with percutaneous drainage and antibiotics. Surgery is indicated when it cannot be effectively controlled with nonsurgical methods.

3.7 Filling defects of the common bile duct

They can be due to gallstones, sludges, blood clots, cylinders, and/or migrated stents [88]. Gallstones, cylinders, and sludge are relatively common after TL, with an incidence between 2.5 and 12%. The related mechanisms are stenosis, warm and cold ischemia, bacterial infection, and obstruction [95].

3.7.1 Stones

They appear late after the TL. In the majority of cases (59–66%), a session of ERC with biliary sphincterotomy was sufficient for cleaning the canal.

3.7.2 Molds

They are seen more frequently in the context of ischemia (e.g., thrombosis of the hepatic artery), when there is a diffuse stenosis of the hilum [96]. Mold cleaning can be difficult to achieve with endoscopic methods. Combined endoscopic and percutaneous methods can be performed successfully [96]. Often several combinations of sphincterotomy, balloon and basket extraction, stent placement, and lithotripsy are necessary, and many patients will eventually require treatment with PTC. Patients with Roux-en-Y choledochojejunostomy should be treated with a percutaneous method.

3.8 Sphincter of Oddi dysfunction

It has been described in 2–7% [79]. The pathogenesis is not clear; one hypothesis is that the denervation of the common bile duct in the ampullary region (secondary to surgery) leads to the development of a hypertonic sphincter, which causes dilatation of the ducts and cholestasis. In most studies, the diagnosis was based on clinical suspicion and response to biliary sphincterotomy [79].

3.9 Other complications

3.9.1 Mucocele

It is a rare complication after LT caused by an accumulation of mucus from the cells lining the remnant of the cystic duct, leading to extrinsic compression of the bile duct. Its formation is insidious and therefore difficult to diagnose. A CT scan or US will reveal the mucocele as an accumulation of fluid in the region of the hepatic portal. The diagnosis can be confirmed with MRCP [95]. Most patients will require surgical or radiological drainage.

3.9.2 Hemobilia

It may occur in patients undergoing percutaneous liver biopsy or percutaneous transhepatic cholangiography. This condition can cause transpapillary bleeding, along with biliary obstruction, due to the formation of clots. The treatment is conservative but may require angiography with embolization. Biliary obstruction can be treated with percutaneous drainage or ERC.

3.9.3 Bactobilia

Patients who have undergone LT are predisposed to bacterial colonization of the bile ducts. Mechanical obstruction, plastic stents, gallstones, and sphincterotomy significantly increased the risk of bactobilia. The majority are asymptomatic. It is possible that bactobilia is a predisposing factor for the development of biliary complications after LT.

3.9.4 Biliary plaster syndrome

It refers to the presence of biliary cylinders and debris that cause biliary obstruction. Associated risk factors include hepatic artery stenosis and biliary stenosis [97]. Patients who develop biliary emptying syndrome have poor graft survival and a worse post-LT result than LT recipients without biliary emptying syndrome. Several endoscopic approaches have been described with varying success.

4. Rejection in liver transplant

4.1 Introduction

The human immune system is a host defense mechanism against the invasion of pathogens. However, a side effect of the ability of the host immune system to recognize and attack "nonself" tissues is rejection of grafted tissues posttransplantation. The exogenous modulation of the host immune system to allow sustained graft function has proceeded along with—and often preceded—our understanding of the physiologic mechanism of rejection and tolerance [98, 99].

The immunologic disparity among members of the same species of mammals that leads to recognition of "self" tissue and to rejection of nonself tissue is based on the differences in cell surface molecules that are expressed. In humans, these major histocompatibility antigens are termed human leukocyte antigens (HLAs). HLAs are subdivided into two classes: class I (HLA-A, HLA-B, and HLA-C), expressed on the surface of all nucleated cells, and class II (HLA-DR, HLA-DQ, and HLA-DP), expressed on the surface of antigen-presenting cells (APCs) [98–101].

The recognition of nonself tissue occurs via two distinct immunologic pathways: direct and indirect allorecognition. Direct allorecognition consists of host T-helper cells recognizing donor HLA disparity expressed on the donor cell surface. Indirect allorecognition consists of recipient APCs (e.g., activated macrophages, dendritic cells, and B lymphocytes) phagocytosing donor cellular debris, including HLAs, which are then processed and re-presented on the APC surface to be recognized by recipient T-helper cells (CD4+ lymphocytes) (**Figure 2**) [100].

In either pathway, co-stimulation signals between CD4+ T-helper lymphocytes and CD8+ cytotoxic T lymphocytes trigger a cascade of immunologic events. Interleukin (IL)-2, an important and early signal in immune activation, is secreted by activated CD4+ T-helper lymphocytes, stimulating increased T-cell responsiveness, clonal expansion of alloreactive T lymphocytes, and acquisition of the cytolytic phenotype by host T lymphocytes. Direct allorecognition leads to a more immediate and vigorous immune response against foreign tissue, but, in both pathways, additional helper T lymphocytes are recruited and secrete a wide array of cytokines (e.g., IL-1, interferon-γ, tumor necrosis factor-α), facilitating the further

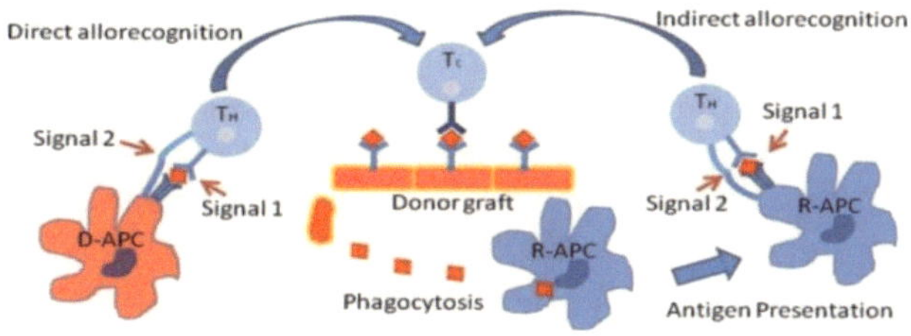

Figure 2.
Direct and indirect pathways of allorecognition (modified Ref. [100]).

recruitment of cytotoxic T lymphocytes, natural killer cells, and B lymphocytes. B lymphocytes begin to secrete antibody directed against the allogeneic tissue in ever-increasing quantities. B lymphocytes also play an antibody-independent role in graft rejection through the secretion of proinflammatory cytokines and chemokines and the participation in antigen presentation [98–102].

Rejection mechanistically occurs by infiltration of the graft by effector cells, the binding of antibody, and the activation of complement. Unchecked, the phenomenon inexorably leads in graft loss (**Table 1**) [100].

Rejection is classified according to the temporal relation between the implantation of the graft and its dysfunction supported by the histologic features seen in allograft: hyperacute (HAR), acute (AR), and chronic (CR). Each type is mediated by a different host immune mechanism.

4.2 Hyperacute rejection

HAR occurs within a few minutes to a few hours after the reperfusion of the graft. Preformed antibodies directed against antigens presented by the graft mediate activation of complement activation of endothelial cells, and formation of microvascular thrombi, leading to graft thrombosis and loss. The process is irreversible and, currently, no treatment is available.

HAR is mediated by circulating preformed antibodies, normally directed against ABO system (comprising the four main blood types, i.e., A, B, AB, and O) antigens or against major HLA antigens. The screening of potential transplant recipients and strict adherence to ABO verification prevent nearly all HAR [101].

In pretransplantation study, crossmatch testing is performed to identify preformed antibodies against class I HLAs (T-lymphocyte crossmatch testing) and class II HLAs (B-lymphocyte crossmatch testing). Crossmatch testing helps clinicians to identify the presence of antibodies against potential donor antigens and to assess the risks of posttransplant rejection and subsequent graft loss. However, these crossmatching assays are not standardized [98, 101, 102].

At most centers, heart and liver transplantations are performed without a crossmatch (except with system ABO compatibility between donor and recipient), unless the recipient is highly sensitized or has previously received a graft possessing major antigens in common with the current donor.

In *liver transplant* recipients, anti-HLA antibody-mediated HAR has been described, but HAR due to ABO-incompatible blood groups is seen in up to 33% and described as a more delayed form of antibody-mediated rejection, but even this barrier appears surmountable with the use of plasmapheresis along with aggressive immunosuppression. Unlike the renal graft, the hepatic graft can undergo HAR over a number of days, probably secondary to its ability to absorb a large amount of antibody and its functional reserve before the onset of the significant microthrombosis and vascular damage [100–102].

The *diagnosis of HR* in liver transplant recipients is normally suggested by fever and rapid deterioration in graft function: AST >1000, coagulopathy, acidosis, encephalopathy, and distributive shock. The *differential diagnosis* may be that of primary non-function/delayed function and hepatic artery thrombosis [101].

The *histological features* of hyperacute rejection are vascular congestion, fibrin-platelet thrombi within capillaries, neutrophilic vasculitis with fibrinoid necrosis, prominent interstitial edema, and neutrophil infiltrates [98, 100].

In unsuccessful cases the only treatment is *retransplantation*.

4.3 Acute rejection

AR is the most common form of graft rejection. It may develop at any time but is most frequent during the first several months posttransplant. Rarely, it occurs within the first several days posttransplant, a process termed accelerated acute rejection, most likely a combination of amnestic immune response driven by sensitized memory B lymphocytes and activation of the direct allorecognition pathway [99].

AR may be cell mediated, antibody mediated (AMR), or very occasionally mixed. Histologically, AR generates an infiltration of activated T lymphocytes into the graft, resulting in gradually progressive endothelial damage, microvascular thrombosis, and parenchymal necrosis. Pathologic grading schemes have been developed regarding the extent to which AR involves vascular damage, cellular infiltration, or a combination of both [98, 99, 101].

Without intervention, AR inevitably progresses to graft loss. The clinical presentation of AR varies markedly, depending on the specific organ, on the level of immunosuppression, and on the attendant level of inflammation in the affected tissues.

Unless the host immune system is adequately suppressed pharmacologically, transplantation inevitably leads to AR.

A combination of immunosuppressive agents is typically used chronically to prevent AR, including a lymphocyte antagonist (usually a calcineurin inhibitor such as cyclosporine or tacrolimus) and an antiproliferative agent (such as azathioprine or mycophenolate mofetil), with or without corticosteroids. Antilymphocyte antibody therapy is often added during induction of immunosuppression or for treatment of "steroid-resistant" AR. The most common *liver transplantation* regimen consists of two doses of a monoclonal anti-IL2 receptor (basiliximab) as induction therapy and dual maintenance therapy with the CNI, tacrolimus, and the antimetabolite mycophenolate mofetil, which lessens the incidence and severity of rejection without increasing infection rates [100, 101].

AR remains an important clinical problem in liver transplantation. Incidence of AR ranges from 30 to 80%. Various risk factors for its development are known, such as low concentrations of immunosuppressants, prolonged cold ischemia time, and young receptor [102].

The *diagnosis of AR* in liver transplant recipients is normally suggested by fever and elevated levels of transaminases, bilirubin, or alkaline phosphatase. Among patients with T-tube drainage (which is increasingly uncommon), the biliary drainage may be seen to thicken, darken, and decrease in amount. The suspicion of AR mandates graft biopsy and studies to eliminate other possible causes of early hepatic graft failure as Doppler ultrasonography and, in some cases, cholangiography resonance. Biopsy findings are classified, according to a standardized set of criteria, as mild, moderate, and severe, with clear implications for prognosis. Microscopic observation reveals interstitial infiltrates of lymphocytes and macrophages, arteritis, fibrinoid necrosis, and thrombosis. The involvement of the blood vessels is a poor sign because its usual meaning is that of an episode of rejection that will be refractory to treatment. Biopsy may be relatively contraindicated due to coagulopathy. In some circumstances transjugular biopsy offers a solution to this problem (**Table 3**) [100–102].

The *differential diagnosis* may be that of sepsis or problems with vascular integrity.

AR is normally *treated* with high-dose corticosteroids, but 5–10% of cases are steroid resistant; such recipients are then treated with an antilymphocyte antibody or tacrolimus at higher levels [100].

5. Primary graft liver dysfunction

Primary graft liver dysfunction is defined as the liver dysfunction that occurs from the moment of liver transplantation, which is not explained by the existence of another etiology, neither vascular nor bile.

Although there is improvement on preservation solutions and surgical techniques [103], its incidence varies from 2 to 23% in several studies. It also seems to be the cause of 20–30% of the retransplants. The mortality without it is close to 80%.

The clinical suspect is established during the first hours after the liver transplant due to the presence of hemodynamic instability, metabolic acidosis, severe coagulopathy (prothrombin time >20 seconds), hypertransaminasemia (>1000 U/l), and encephalopathy.

When primary dysfunction does not threaten patient life immediately, it is known as "poor early graft function." On those several cases whose patient dies if the transplantation is not done, it is known as "primary graft failure" [104].

The pathogenesis of primary graft liver dysfunction is nearly related to the ischemia-reperfusion injury, so there are some predisposing donor factors that impact on recipient outcome [105, 106]. Prophylaxis includes a thorough donor selection and an exhaustive ischemia time control [107–109].

These premises are very important because of the fact that retransplantation is the isolated efficacy treatment.

Diagnosis is encouraged by additional examinations which discard secondary graft dysfunction. Transhepatic cholangiography must demonstrate a permeable bile duct as Doppler ultrasound and arteriography must demonstrate the absence of vascular complications. Liver biopsy is useful to discard a hyperacute rejection [104].

Nowadays the shortage of available donor organs is the major limiting factor in liver transplantation. Optimal deceased donors are generally young, previously healthy persons who develop a fatal brain injury due to causes such as head trauma, intracerebral hemorrhage, or anoxia. The relative paucity of donor organs has led transplant centers to consider organs from marginal donors (**Table 4**) [109–113].

Aside from the marginal donors, there are other factors associated with graft failure (**Table 5**) [113].

5.1 Treatment

As we have commented, the isolated efficacy treatment is retransplant and goes on identifying donors and recipient factors that lead to this kind of injury as avoiding large ischemic times. The proper donor maintenance at the intensive care unit is at most important [103, 107, 108].

Prostaglandins type E1 come be used as preventing treatment.

	Comment	Characteristics	Liver biopsy	Differential diagnosis	Treatment options
Hyperacute rejection	Rare in OLT 1–10 days posttransplant	Rapid deterioration in graft function: AST >1000 Coagulopathy, acidosis	Hemorrhagic necrosis	Primary non-function/ delayed function Hepatic artery thrombosis	Retransplantation Rarely: OKT3, cyclophosphamide, plasmapheresis
Acute rejection	30–70% occurs at mean of 7–9 days	Often clinically silent apart from fever and RUQ pain High AST and bilirubin Coagulation and acid-base undisturbed	Portal inflammation Endotheliitis Bile duct damage	Sepsis Vascular Viral	Methylprednisolone 1 g daily for 3 days

Table 3.
AST, aspartate aminotransferase; MMF, mycophenolate mofetil; OLT, orthotopic liver transplantation; RUQ, right upper quadrant.

Marginal liver graft outcomes
• Donor age > 70 years
• Hepatitis C-positive donors
• Cold ischemia time > 12 hours
• Donations after cardiac death donors
• More than 30% steatosis
• Liver splits between two recipients

Table 4.
Marginal liver graft outcomes.

Donor factors	Recipient factors
• Hepatitis B core antibody positivity	• Hepatitis C virus infection
• A mean arterial pressure lower than 60 mmHg more than 20 minutes after life support withdrawal (after cardiac death)	• Presence of malignancy
	• Previous liver transplantation
	• BMI > 30
	• Non-Caucasian race

Table 5.
Donor and recipient factors.

6. Early infection in liver transplantation

Despite advances in liver transplantation, morbidity and mortality due to infectious complications remain the biggest problem [114, 115]. In many centers, infection is the leading cause of death after liver transplantation, particularly after the first year [116]. In series of autopsies, it has been announced that the infection was the cause of death in 64% of the 321 patients studied who died between 1982 and 1997 [117]. Recent advances include in standardized and condoned protocols molecular research of viruses, demonstrating the binding between genetic polymorphisms of the immune response and the risk for specific infections and treatment with new antibiotics, including the latest advances in C virus therapy [118].

The most common infections are bacterial (48%), followed by fungal (22%) and viral (12%). Some series observe an incidence of up to 1–2.5 episodes of infection per patient [119–121], this being the most common cause of fever in liver transplant recipients [122].

It is important to recognize a number of general principles [118, 123]:

1. Signs and symptoms of infection are attenuated by immunosuppression; therefore, the infection may be more difficult to diagnose.

2. Noninfectious causes of fever, such as rejection, medications, etc., can simulate an infection.

3. The variety of possible pathogens is extensive but is influenced by the timing of the infection in relation to transplantation.

4. Antibiotics have interactions with immunosuppressive medication.

5. The infection may be more severe and progress faster than an immunocompetent host.

6. The risks of infection are determined by the balance between factors related to immunosuppressive treatment at full dose (dose, type, and duration of immunosuppressive therapy) and the existence of catheters, nutritional status, condition function of grafting, and the presence of underlying diseases.

Identifying risk factors before transplantation optimizes strategies to prevent infections. Although our ability to predict the risk of infection after transplantation remains limited, there are risk factors that can be modified, such as cytomegalovirus (CMV) positivity and donor and receiver.

An important risk factor is the presence of a latent or unrecognized infection either from the donor or recipient. These infections can be reactivated and cause morbidity after the introduction of immunosuppressants. Therefore, both donors and recipients are routinely tested for infections such as CMV, other herpes viruses, tuberculosis, hepatitis B and C, syphilis, and human immunodeficiency virus.

Colonization of transplant recipients with organisms, such as methicillin-resistant *Staphylococcus aureus* (MRSA) or vancomycin-resistant *Enterococcus* (VRE), can lead to infection posttransplant of these organisms. A significant prevalence of multiresistant gram-negative bacilli, such as expanded betalactase enterobacteria (BLEES) and *Escherichia coli* and *carbapenem-resistant Klebsiella pneumoniae*, has been observed in both the general population and *solid organ transplant recipients, as they present risk factors for acquiring multi-resistant bacteria such as previous antibiotic therapy, catheter presence, exposure to the hospital environment, and presence of underlying diseases* [124].

Other risk factors have been described, for example, those related to surgical complications. In a series of 101 patients, the risk factors associated with these infections were prolonged surgery of more than 12 hours and reoperation.

Among those related to pretransplantation were predictive infection, a serum value of alanine aminotransferase above 60 IU/L for all types of infections, and a T-helper ratio of 2.8, for fungal and viral infections [125].

Bacterial infections are seen more in those Roux-type y-procedures than with cholecystectomy, when there were multiple abdominal surgeries or there was a concomitant CMV infection in the postoperative period [126]. Graft dysfunction and the presence of critical pre-surgery diseases also confer an increased risk to acquire posttransplant infections.

The presence of CMV infection increases the risk of other infections, partly due to the immunomodulatory effects of this virus. Likewise, those who have rejection or those who have poor graft function after implantation increase the risk because they receive a more aggressive regimen of immunosuppressants.

The risk and type of infection found differ from the elapsed time after the implant and can be grouped into three major periods: first month, 1–6 months, and after 6 months.

Focusing on the first period or early infections, these are similar to those seen by an immunocompetent patient after surgery. Bacterial infections of nosocomial origin predominate, such as catheter infection, external drainage, or are related to foreign bodies, presence of necrotic tissue, or prolonged tracheal intubation [127]. We must also consider donor transmitted infections when there is an unexplained syndrome consistent with the infection.

Abdominal and lung infection are the most common, both associated with the presence of bacteremias [115].

Abdominal abscess and peritoneal abscess are the result of postoperative complications including gallbladder or surgical hematomas, with the predominant pathogens being enteric organisms [119]. Intrahepatic abscess and bile duct ischemia manifest as a consequence of hepatic artery thrombosis, occurring in the immediate postoperative period. And cholangitis is caused by blockage of the bile tract, including blockage of the Kher tube. Abdominal wall infections are also common.

Regarding lung infections, they are common in those who require intubations with prolonged mechanical ventilation. *Pseudomonas aeruginosa* and *Enterobacter* are most commonly grown. *Other common bacteria include S. aureus*, *K. pneumoniae*, *Stenotrophomonas maltophilia*, and *Citrobacter freundii* [119].

Colitis related with *Clostridium difficile* can occur in early periods, especially herethat have prolonged hospitalization. More than half of cases occur in the first posttransplant month. In fact, liver transplantation is identified as a risk factor for acquiring a *C. difficile* infection at the hospital due to immunosuppression and antibiotic treatment among other factors [128, 129].

Candida species are common pathogens identified in the first month. Bacteremia, surgical wounds, as well as urinary tract infection are common places of primary infection and can be subsequently disseminated [130]. The presence of esophagitis, oral cavity infection, and folliculitis is usually common. Due to the high mortality in candidemias, these should be treated aggressively, having to take into account the high incidence of *Candida albicans* reported in recent years.

Except for herpes simplex virus (HSV), viral infections are uncommon in the first month after transplantation. Without adequate prophylaxis, HSV reaction reaches up to 50%, in those HIV-positive patients prior to transplantation, usually manifesting as oral or genital ulcers.

7. Extrahepatic complications after liver transplantation

Patients undergoing a liver transplant may have long-term complications in different devices and systems. The most common are infections, de novo tumors, cardiovascular disease (including high blood pressure, hyperlipidemia, obesity, and metabolic syndrome), kidney disease, and diabetes.

These complications usually have a more or less direct relationship with the need for immunosuppressive drugs after implantation to prevent rejection of the implant. The use of high doses of corticosteroids for a long period promotes the onset of diabetes and increases the risk of cardiovascular disease, while the rest of immunosuppressants are associated with more common long-term complications, the appearance of tumors, cardiovascular disease, and kidney failure.

The management of these pathologies does not differ from that received by patients not undergoing a transplant, so they can be detected and treated by different specialists, having direct communication with the hepatologists for the adjustment of medication in the different complications.

Next, we will further develop each of them.

7.1 De novo tumors

The incidence of de novo tumors is three times higher in liver transplant recipients than the rest of the population, making the first or second leading cause of long-term death in the liver implant patient (frequency varies according to the different series) [131].

The most commonly developed tumor is the skin epithelioma, directly related to sun exposure. Other de novo tumors associated with prolonged immunosuppressive treatment in liver transplants include non-Hodgkin lymphoma, Kaposi lymphoma, and oropharyngeal, bladder, cervix, and lung cancers, 10–20% at 10 years of transplantation.

However, the incidence of breast, prostate, or colon tumors has not been increased with respect to the incidence in the general population, except if the etiology of transplantation has been led to primary sclerosing cholangitis associated with ulcerative colitis, in which case the incidence of colon neoplasm increases.

The flattering factors do not differ from the rest of the population, but we must make special impact on primary and secondary prevention in this type of patients, given the situation of immunosuppression. That is why we must make special focus on the prevention of smoking habit, safe sex, and, of course, alcohol withdrawal.

7.2 Cardiovascular disease

Liver transplant recipients have a frequency three times higher than the general population suffering from a major cardiovascular event, considering in this group coronary heart disease, heart failure, sudden death, vascular brain accident, or severe occlusive peripheral artery disease. So the likelihood of suffering a cardiovascular event increases over the years, being 5% in the first 2 years posttransplant, 15% at 10 years after transplantation, and greater than 20% more than 10 years posttransplant. It is considered to be the second or first cause of death in liver transplants according to the different series. This increase in incidence, in addition to immunosuppressive treatment, has been associated with increased cardiovascular risk factors over time, especially metabolic syndrome (HTA, obesity, and dyslipidemia) and diabetes.

Other habits that contribute to the development of cardiovascular disease are smoking and alcohol intake [130].

7.3 Metabolic syndrome

It is defined by the onset of diabetes, dyslipidemias, obesity, and HTA. Up to 50–60% of patients undergoing HT will develop metabolic syndrome [132].

7.3.1 HTA

The incidence of HTA in liver transplant patients is related, in particular, to the vasoconstrictor effect of calcineurin inhibitors and to the mineralocorticoid effect of corticosteroids. It usually occurs in 40–60% of patients in the late period of liver transplantation.

We consider optimal voltage figures between 130 and 80 mmHg of systolic and diastolic blood pressure, respectively, being a little more restrictive than with the limits set for the general population (140 and 90 mmHg), adopting the same established limits as for diabetic patients with renal impairment. We must be restrictive in terms of these figures, always maintaining lower levels in liver transplant patients.

We should avoid drugs such as NSAIDs as soon as possible, as in patients treated with calcineurin inhibitors tend to increase blood pressure levels.

Patients treated with calcineurin inhibitors should receive their antihypertensive treatment late in the afternoon or evening, as these drugs have a nightly blood pressure rhythm, and therefore most of them we found at night. If, however, we cannot decrease tension levels, one might consider reducing the dose of these immunosuppressants [133, 134].

7.3.2 Obesity

Approximately 30% of TH receptors will develop obesity (BMI greater than 30). This is due to the increase in sedentariness due to the situation of pretransplant disease, the corticoid treatment, the release of restrictive diets once transplanted, and the decrease of physical exercise. The treatment is the same as in any non-immunocompromised patient: physical exercise and low-calorie diets. If necessary, lipase inhibitors could be administered as adjuvant drugs in weight loss; in which case, it would be necessary to monitor immunosuppressant levels more thoroughly to prevent possible interactions that decrease their absorption [132].

7.3.3 Dyslipidemias

The administration of immunosuppressants such as calcineurin inhibitors, mTOR inhibitors, and corticosteroids, independently or in addition to each patient's genetic predisposition, may contribute to rising levels of plasma cholesterol and triglycerides, with increased LDL and decreased HDL, resulting in hypercholesterolemia and hypertriglyceridemia in up to 40% liver transplant recipients. The treatment is using hypolipidizing drugs (statins and fibrates) and diet, as in the rest of the population. Keep in mind that patients who take cyclosporine and need treatment with statin are at higher risk of developing severe myopathy [132].

7.3.4 Diabetes

It has an incidence between 20 and 35% development in transplant patients. Factors that contribute to its emergence are advanced age, obesity, existing pretransplant diabetes, immunosuppressants with diabetic effects, especially tacrolimus, the development of insulin resistance of corticosteroids, and the insulin secretion deficit of calcineurin inhibitors.

Treatment is based on insulin and oral antidiabetics, although most patients with HT will need insulin because of the lower efficacy of ADOs, with the highest insulin needs being in the morning and noon in those patients with corticosteroids, since the pattern is usually in the morning [132].

7.4 Chronic renal failure

The incidence of renal impairment in liver transplant patients is 50–70% higher [135]. The most directly related cause is treatment with calcineurin inhibitors, due to its nephrotoxic effect, although factors such as HTA, diabetes, or other infections that secondarily affect the correct kidney filtration, such as HCV infection, may also contribute. Of these patients treated with calcineurin inhibitors, 10% will develop a chronic end-stage renal disease (glomerular filter age less than 30 ml/min/1.73 m^2), in need of hemodialysis therapy or even renal transplantation in 1–2% of cases. This percentage, fortunately, has been declining in recent years coinciding with the lower use of this family of immunosuppressants. Clearly, for patients who develop renal impairment, we must readjust immunosuppressive treatment, reducing the dose of calcineurin inhibitors or substitutes or other non-nephrotoxic immunosuppressants such as inhibitors mTOR or mycophenolate. Similarly, the use of nonsteroidal anti-inflammatory drugs and all drugs that may contribute to worsening kidney function will be avoided [135].

7.5 Other complications

Apart from the most important complications in both frequency and clinical impact, liver transplant recipients may develop other types of related complications in whole or in total or with the intake of immunosuppressive drugs. In this way, patients taking calcineurin inhibitors may develop neurological problems, especially headache, migraine, insomnia tremor, and paresthesia.

Corticoids: Ostearticular pathology, especially osteoporosis (50%), Cushingoid facies, alteration in body fat distribution, hirsutism.

Mycophenolate: diarrhea and vomiting, especially with mofetil mycophenolate, less common with sodium mycophenolate, bone marrow depression also favored by concomitant administration of interferon for any other reason.

mTOR inhibitors: bone marrow depression, respiratory problems such as pulmonary fibrosis and organizational pneumonia, difficulty healing wounds.

And all of them can lead to more or less sexual dysfunction.

So it is necessary to do a complete scan and anamnesis to be able to detect these side effects and assess modification of pattern or replacement of it [133, 134].

7.6 Survival

Annual mortality after the first year after liver transplantation is 2–3% per year, higher than in the general population of the same age and gender. The principal causes of death are cardiovascular diseases, appearance of novo tumors, and relapse of hepatitis C [136–139].

The quality of life posttransplantation is not fully satisfactory although it is better than the quality of pretransplant life. Only a percentage of lower patients presents a quality of life lower than the general population, about everything in aspects related with the function staff on paper partner-work family.

8. Conclusions

LT is nowadays a common surgical technique in many hospitals and is undoubtedly the most definitive treatment for end-stage liver disease. Early monitoring and a correct treatment of this kind of patients at the ICU are of utmost importance. The success lies in early detection and treating of complications by using the proper diagnostic and medical or surgical techniques that all intensivists need to know and manage. All the surgical and medical team need to deploy their best competencies to save the graft and the patient's life.

Author details

Demetrio V. Pérez Civantos[1,2*], Alicia Muñoz Cantero[1], Manuel Robles Marcos[1,2], Francisco Fuentes Morillas[1], María A. Santiago Triviño[1], María O. Cerezo Arias[1], María D. Pérez Frutos[1] and Alberto Córdoba López[1]

1 Intensive and Critical Care Department, Badajoz University Hospital, University of Extremadura, Badajoz, Spain

2 Intensive and Critical Care Medicine, Faculty of Medicine, University of Extremadura, Badajoz, Spain

*Address all correspondence to: demetrio.perez@salud-juntaex.es; dpcivantos@gmail.com

References

[1] Maluf DG, Edwards EB, Kauffman HM. Utilization of extended donor criteria liver allograft: Is the elevated risk of failure independent of the model for end-stage liver disease score of the recipient? Transplantation. 2006;**82**:1653-1657. DOI: 10.1097/01.tp.0000250571.41361.21

[2] Bonney GK, Aldersley MA, Asthana S, Toogood GJ, Pollard SG, Lodge JP, et al. Donor risk index and MELD interactions in predicting long-term graft survival: A single-centre experience. Transplantation. 2009;**87**:1858-1863. DOI: 10.1097/TP.0b013e3181a75b37

[3] Pérez Civantos D, Muñoz Cantero A, Robles Marcos M, Fuentes Morillas F, Cerezo Arias M, Fariñas Seijas H. Utility of basal regional oximetry as an early predictor of graft failure after liver transplant. Transplantation Proceedings. 2019;**51**(2):353-358. DOI: 10.1016/j.transproceed.2018.10.023

[4] Vivarelli M et al. Ischemic arterial complications after liver transplantation in the adult: Multivariate analysus of the risk factros. Archives of Surgery. 2004;**139**:1069-1074

[5] Langs AN, Marujo W, Stratta RJ, Wood RP, Shaw BW Jr. Vascular complications after orthotopic liver transplantation. American Journal of Surgery. 1991;**161**:76-82; discussion 82-83

[6] Drazan K, Shaked A, Olthoff KM, et al. Etiology and management of symptomatic adult hepatic artery thrombosis after orthotopic liver transplantation (OLT). The American Surgeon. 1996;**62**:237-240

[7] Settmancher U, Stange B, Haase R, et al. Arterial complications after liver transplantation. Transplant International. 2000;**13**:372-378

[8] Abbasoglu O, Levy MF, Vodapally MS, et al. Hepatic artery stenosis after liver transplantation—Incidence, presentation, treatment, and long term outcome. Transplantation. 1997;**63**:250-255

[9] Bhattacharjya S, Gunson BK, Mirza DF, et al. Delayed hepatic artery thrombosis in adult orthotopic liver transplantation—A 12-year experience. Transplantation. 2001;**71**:1592-1596

[10] Oh CK, Pelletier SJ, Sawyer RG, et al. Uni-andmulti-variate análisis of risk factors for early and late hepatic artery thrombosis afte rliver transplantation. Transplantation. 2001;**71**:767-772

[11] Gunsar F, Rolando N, Pastacaldi S, et al. Late hepatic artery thrombosis after orthotopic liver transplantation. Liver Transplantation. 2003;**9**:605-611

[12] Stange BJ, Glanemann M, NuesslerNC, SettmacherU, SteinmullerT, Nehaus P. Hepatic artery thrombosis after adult liver transplantation. Liver Transplantation. 2003;**9**:612-620

[13] Piardi T, Lhuaire M, Bruno O, Memeo R, Pessaux P, Kianmanesh R, et al. Vascular complications following liver transplantation: A literature review of advances in 2015. World Journal of Hepatology. 2016;**8**(1):36-57

[14] Boyvat F, Aytekin C, Firat A, Harman A, Karakayali H, Haberal M. Diagnostic and therapeutic management of hepatic artery thrombosis and stenosis after orthotopic and heterotopic liver transplantation. Transplantation Proceedings. 2003;**35**:2791-2795

[15] Zhou J, Fan J, Wang JH, Wu ZQ, Qiu SJ, Shen YH, et al. Continuous transcatheter arterial thrombolysis for early hepatic artery thrombosis after

liver transplantation. Transplantation Proceedings. 2005;**37**:4426-4429

[16] Gad EH, Abdelsamee MA, Kamel Y. Hepatic arterial and portal venous complications after adult and pediatric living donor liver transplantation, risk factors, management and outcome (a retrospective cohort study). Annals of Medicine and Surgery. 2016;**8**:28-39

[17] Pinna AD, Smith CV, Furukawa H, Starzl TE, Fung JJ. Urgent revascularization of liver allografts after early hepatic artery thrombosis. Transplantation. 1996;**62**:1584-1587

[18] Panaro F, Ramos J, Gallix B, Mercier G, Herrero A, Niampa H, et al. Hepatic artery complications following liver transplantation. Does preoperative chemoembolization impact the postoperative course? Clinical Transplantation. 2014;**28**:598-605. DOI: 10.1111/ctr.12358

[19] Singhal A, Stokes K, Sebastian A, Wright HI, Kohli V. Endovascular treatment of hepatic artery thrombosis following liver transplantation. Transplant International. 2010;**23**:245-256. DOI: 10.1111/j.1432-2277.2009.01037.x

[20] Silva MA, Jambulingam PS, Gunson BK, Mayer D, Buckels JA, Mirza DF, et al. Hepatic artery thrombosis following orthotopic liver transplantation: A 10-year experience from a single centre in the United Kingdom. Liver Transplantation. 2006;**12**:146-151

[21] Bekker J, Ploem S, de Jong KP. Early hepatic artery thrombosis after liver transplantation: A systematic review of the incidence, outcome and risk factors. American Journal of Transplantation. 2009;**9**:746-757

[22] Pareja E, Cortes M, Navarro R, Sanjuan F, López R, Mir J. Vascular complications after orthotopic liver transplantation: Hepatic artery thrombosis. Transplantation Proceedings. 2010;**42**:2970-2972

[23] Tzakis AG, Gordon RD, Shaw BW, Iwatsuki S, Starzl TE. Clinical presentation of hepatic artery thrombosis after liver transplantation in the cyclosporine era. Transplantation. 1985;**40**:667-671

[24] Pastacaldi S, Teixeira R, Montalto P, Rolles K, Burroughs AK. Hepatic artery thrombosis after orthotopic liver transplantation: A review of nonsurgical causes. Liver Transplantation. 2001;7:75-81

[25] Wozney P, Zajko AB, Bron KM, Point S, Starzl TE. Vascular complications after liver transplantation: A 5-year experience. AJR. American Journal of Roentgenology. 1986;**147**:657-663

[26] Saad WE, Davies MG, Saad NE, Westesson KE, Patel NC, Sahler LG, et al. Catheter thrombolysis of thrombosed hepatic arteries in liver transplant recipients: Predictors of success and role of thrombolysis. Vascular and Endovascular Surgery. 2007;**41**:19-26

[27] Saad WE, Davies MG, Sahler L, Lee DE, Patel NC, Kitanosono T, et al. Hepatic artery stenosis in liver transplant recipients: Primary treatment with percutaneous transluminal angioplasty. Journal of Vascular and Interventional Radiology. 2005;**16**:795-805

[28] da Silva RF, Raphe R, Felício HC, Rocha MF, Duca WJ, Arroyo PC, et al. Prevalence, treatment, and outcomes of the hepatic artery stenosis after liver transplantation. Transplantation Proceedings. 2008;**40**:805-807. DOI: 10.1016/j.transproceed.2008.02.041

[29] Hamby BA, Ramirez DE, Loss GE, Bazan HA, Smith TA,

Bluth E, et al. Endovascular treatment of hepatic artery stenosis after liver transplantation. Journal of Vascular Surgery. 2013;**57**:1067-1072. DOI: 10.1016/j.jvs.2012.10.086

[30] Rostambeigi N, Hunter D, Duval S, Chinnakotla S, Golzarian J. Stent placement versus angioplasty for hepatic artery stenosis after liver transplant: A meta-analysis of case series. European Radiology. 2013;**23**:1323-1334. DOI: 10.1007/s00330-012-2730-9

[31] Sommacale D, Aoyagi T, Dondero F, Sibert A, Bruno O, Fteriche S, et al. Repeat endovascular treatment of recurring hepatic artery stenoses in orthotopic liver transplantation. Transplant International. 2013;**26**:608-615. DOI: 10.1111/tri.12089

[32] Sabri SS, Saad WE, Schmitt TM, Turba UC, Kumer SC, Park AW, et al. Endovascular therapy for hepatic artery stenosis and thrombosis following liver transplantation. Vascular and Endovascular Surgery. 2011;**45**:447-452. DOI: 10.1177/1538574411407088

[33] Blumhardt G, Ringe B, Lauchart W, Burdelski M, Bechstein WO, Pichlmayr R. Vascular problems in liver transplantation. Transplantation Proceedings. 1987;**19**:2412

[34] Denys AL, Qanadli SD, Durand F, Vilgrain V, Farges O, Belghiti J, et al. Feasibility and effectiveness of using coronary stents in the treatment of hepatic artery stenoses after orthotopic liver transplantation: Preliminary report. AJR. American Journal of Roentgenology. 2002;**178**:1175-1179

[35] Langnas AN, Marujo W, Stratta RJ, Wood RP, Shaw BW. Vascular complications after orthotopic liver transplantation. American Journal of Surgery. 1991;**161**:76-82 discussion 82-83

[36] Volpin E, Pessaux P, Sauvanet A, Sibert A, Kianmanesh R, Durand F, et al. Preservation of the arterial vascularisation after hepatic artery pseudoaneurysm following orthotopic liver transplantation: Long-term results. Annals of Transplantation. 2014;**19**:346-352. DOI: 10.12659/AOT.890473

[37] Boleslawski E, Bouras AF, Truant S, Liddo G, Herrero A, Badic B, et al. Hepatic artery ligation for arterial rupture following liver transplantation: A reasonable option. American Journal of Transplantation. 2013;**13**:1055-1062. DOI: 10.1111/ajt.12135

[38] Houssin D, Ortega D, Richardson A, Ozier Y, Stephan H, Soffer M, et al. Mycotic aneurysm of the hepatic artery complicating human liver transplantation. Transplantation. 1988;**46**:469-472

[39] Lerut J, Gordon RD, Iwatsuki S, Starzl TE. Surgical complications in human orthotopic liver transplantation. Acta Chirurgica Belgica. 1987;**87**:193-204

[40] Madariaga J, Tzakis A, Zajko AB, Tzoracoleftherakis E, Tepetes K, Gordon R, et al. Hepatic artery pseudoaneurysm ligation after orthotopic liver transplantation—A report of 7 cases. Transplantation. 1992;**54**:824-828

[41] Bonham CA, Kapur S, Geller D, Fung JJ, Pinna A. Excision and immediate revascularization for hepatic artery pseudoaneurysm following liver transplantation. Transplantation Proceedings. 1999;**31**:443

[42] Lowell JA, Coopersmith CM, Shenoy S, Howard TK. Unusual presentations of nonmycotic hepatic artery pseudoaneurysms after liver transplantation. Liver Transplantation and Surgery. 1999;**5**:200-203

[43] Stange B, Settmacher U, Glanemann M, Nuessler NC, Bechstein WO, Neuhaus P. Aneurysms of the hepatic artery after liver transplantation. Transplantation Proceedings. 2000;**32**:533-534

[44] Leonardi LS, Soares C, Boin IF, Oliveira VC. Hemobilia after mycotic hepatic artery pseudoaneurysm after liver transplantation. Transplantation Proceedings. 2001;**33**:2580-2582

[45] Marshall MM, Muiesan P, Srinivasan P, Kane PA, Rela M, Heaton ND, et al. Hepatic artery pseudoaneurysms following liver transplantation: Incidence, presenting features and management. Clinical Radiology. 2001;**56**:579-587

[46] Turrión VS, Alvira LG, Jimenez M, Lucena JL, Ardaiz J. Incidence and results of arterial complications in liver transplantation: Experience in a series of 400 transplants. Transplantation Proceedings. 2002;**34**:292-293

[47] Leelaudomlipi S, Bramhall SR, Gunson BK, Candinas D, Buckels JA, McMaster P, et al. Hepatic-artery aneurysm in adult liver transplantation. Transplant International. 2003;**16**:257-261

[48] Jarzembowski TM, Sankary HN, Bogetti D, Manzelli A, Ong E, Oberholzer J, et al. Living donor liver graft salvage after rupture of hepatic artery pseudoaneurysm. International Surgery. 2008;**93**:300-303

[49] Panaro F, Miggino M, Bouyabrine H, Carabalona JP, Berthet JP, Canaud L, et al. Reversed saphenous bypass for hepatic artery pseudoaneurysm after liver transplantation. Annals of Vascular Surgery. 2013;**27**:1088-1097. DOI: 10.1016/j.avsg.2013.01.007

[50] CharcoR,FusterJ,FondevilaC,FerrerJ, Mans E, GarcíaValdecasas JC. Portal vein thrombosis in liver transplantation. Transplantation Proceedings. 2005;**37**:3904-3905

[51] Khalaf H. Vascular complications after deceased and living donor liver transplantation: A single-center experience. Transplantation Proceedings. 2010;**42**:865-870. DOI: 10.1016/j.transproceed.2010.02.037

[52] Kyoden Y, Tamura S, Sugawara Y, Matsui Y, Togashi J, Kaneko J, et al. Portal vein complications after adultto-adult living donor liver transplantation. Transplant International. 2008;**21**:1136-1144. DOI: 10.1111/j.1432-2277.2008.00752.x

[53] Olcott EW, Ring EJ, Roberts JP, Ascher NL, Lake JR, Gordon RL. Percutaneous transhepatic portal vein angioplasty and stent placement after liver transplantation: Early experience. Journal of Vascular and Interventional Radiology. 1990;**1**:17-22

[54] Kensinger CD, Sexton KW, Baron CM, Lipnik AJ, Meranze SG, Gorden DL. Management of portal vein thrombosis after liver transplantation with a combined open and endovascular approach. Liver Transplantation. 2015;**21**:132-134. DOI: 10.1002/lt.24011

[55] Lodhia N, Salem R, Levitsky J. Transjugular intrahepatic portosystemic shunt with thrombectomy for the treatment of portal vein thrombosis after liver transplantation. Digestive Diseases and Sciences. 2010;**55**:529-534. DOI: 10.1007/s10620-009-0735-2

[56] Schneider N, Scanga A, Stokes L, Perri R. Portal vein stenosis: A rare yet clinically important cause of delayed-onset ascites after adult deceased donor liver transplantation: Two case reports. Transplantation Proceedings. 2011;**43**:3829-3834. DOI: 10.1016/j.transproceed.2011.09.068

[57] Wei BJ, Zhai RY, Wang JF, Dai DK, Yu P. Percutaneous portal venoplasty and stenting for anastomotic stenosis after liver transplantation. World Journal of Gastroenterology. 2009;**15**:1880-1885

[58] Shibata T, Itoh K, Kubo T, Maetani Y, Shibata T, Togashi K, et al. Percutaneous transhepatic balloon dilation of portal venous stenosis in patients with living donor liver transplantation. Radiology. 2005;**235**:1078-1083

[59] Zajko AB, Sheng R, Bron K, Reyes J, Nour B, Tzakis A. Percutaneous transluminal angioplasty of venous anastomotic stenoses complicating liver transplantation: Intermediate-term results. Journal of Vascular and Interventional Radiology. 1994;**5**:121-126

[60] Sanada Y, Kawano Y, Mizuta K, Egami S, Hayashida M, Wakiya T, et al. Strategy to prevent recurrent portal vein stenosis following interventional radiology in pediatric liver transplantation. Liver Transplantation. 2010;**16**:332-339. DOI: 10.1002/lt.21995

[61] Navarro F, Le Moine MC, Fabre JM, Belghiti J, Cherqui D, Adam R, et al. Specific vascular complications of orthotopic liver transplantation with preservation of the retrohepatic vena cava: Review of 1361 cases. Transplantation. 1999;**68**:646-650

[62] Cavallari A, Vivarelli M, Bellusci R, Jovine E, Mazziotti A, Rossi C. Treatment of vascular complications following liver transplantation: Multidisciplinary approach. Hepato-Gastroenterology. 2001;**48**:179-183

[63] Patel JV, Weston MJ, Kessel DO, Prasad R, Toogood GJ, Robertson I. Hepatic artery pseudoaneurysm after liver transplantation: Treatment with percutaneous thrombin injection. Transplantation. 2003;**75**:1755-1757

[64] Golse N, Spina A, Abdelaal A, Mennesson N, Feugier P, Dumortier J, et al. Extra-anatomical hepatic artery reconstruction following post-embolization iatrogenic dissection and arterial anastomotic rupture in two liver transplant recipients. Gastroentérologie Clinique et Biologique. 2010;**34**:111-114. DOI: 10.1016/j.gcb.2009.11.003

[65] Pawlak J, Grodzicki M, Leowska E, Małkowski P, Michałowicz B, Nyckowski P, et al. Vascular complications after liver transplantation. Transplantation Proceedings. 2003;**35**:2313-2315

[66] Duffy JP, Hong JC, Farmer DG, Ghobrial RM, Yersiz H, Hiatt JR, et al. Vascular complications of orthotopic liver transplantation: Experience in more than 4,200 patients. Journal of the American College of Surgeons. 2009;**208**:896-903; discussion 903-905. DOI: 10.1016/j.jamcollsurg.2008.12.032

[67] Pérez-Saborido B, Pacheco-Sánchez D, Barrera-Rebollo A, Asensio-Díaz E, Pinto-Fuentes P, Sarmentero-Prieto JC, et al. Incidence, management, and results of vascular complications after liver transplantation. Transplantation Proceedings. 2011;**43**:749-750

[68] Steinbrück K, Enne M, Fernandes R, Martinho JM, Balbi E, Agoglia L, et al. Vascular complications after living donor liver transplantation: A Brazilian, single-center experience. Transplantation Proceedings. 2011;**43**:196-198. DOI: 10.1016/j.transproceed.2010.12.007

[69] Uller W, Knoppke B, Schreyer AG, Heiss P, Schlitt HJ, Melter M, et al. Interventional radiological treatment of perihepatic vascular stenosis or occlusion in pediatric patients after liver transplantation. Cardiovascular and Interventional Radiology. 2013;**36**:1562-1571. DOI: 10.1007/s00270-013-0595-1

[70] Parrilla P, Sánchez-Bueno F, Figueras J, Jaurrieta E, Mir J, Margarit C, et al. Analysis of the complications of the piggy-back technique in 1,112 liver transplants. Transplantation. 1999;**67**:1214-1217

[71] Sánchez-Bueno F, Hernández Q, Ramírez P, Robles R, Acosta F, Rodríguez JM, et al. Vascular complications in a series of 300 orthotopic liver transplants. Transplantation Proceedings. 1999;**31**:2409-2410

[72] Woo DH, Laberge JM, Gordon RL, Wilson MW, Kerlan RK. Management of portal venous complications after liver transplantation. Techniques in Vascular and Interventional Radiology. 2007;**10**:233-239

[73] Yilmaz A, Arikan C, Tumgor G, Kilic M, Aydogdu S. Vascular complications in living-related and deceased donation pediatric liver transplantation: Single center's experience from Turkey. Pediatric Transplantation. 2007;**11**:160-164

[74] Orlandini M, Feier FH, Jaeger B, Kieling C, Vieira SG, Zanotelli ML. Frequency of and factors associated with vascular complications after pediatric liver transplantation. Jornal de Pediatria. 2014;**90**:169-175. DOI: 10.1016/j.jped.2013.08.010

[75] Lerut J, Tzakis AG, Bron K, Gordon RD, Iwatsuki S, Esquivel CO, et al. Complications of venous reconstruction in human orthotopic liver transplantation. Annals of Surgery. 1987;**205**:404-414

[76] Buell JF, Funaki B, Cronin DC, Yoshida A, Perlman MK, Lorenz J, et al. Long-term venous complications after full-size and segmental pediatric liver transplantation. Annals of Surgery. 2002;**236**:658-666

[77] Strovski E, Liu D, Scudamore C, Ho S, Yoshida E, Klass D. Magnetic resonance venography and liver transplant complications. World Journal of Gastroenterology. 2013;**19**:6110-6113. DOI: 10.3748/wjg.v19.i36.6110

[78] Goss JA, Shackleton CR, McDiarmid SV, Maggard M, Swenson K, Seu P, et al. Long-term results of pediatric liver transplantation: An analysis of 569 transplants. Annals of Surgery. 1998;**228**:411-420

[79] Fernandez-Simon A et al. Sphincter of Oddi dysfunction after liver transplantation: Experience in a high volume transplant center. Hepatology. 2014;**60**:466

[80] Weeks SM, Gerber DA, Jaques PF, Sandhu J, Johnson MW, Fair JH, et al. Primary gianturco stent placement for inferior vena cava abnormalities following liver transplantation. Journal of Vascular and Interventional Radiology. 2000;**11**:177-187

[81] Darcy MD. Management of venous outflow complications after liver transplantation. Techniques in Vascular and Interventional Radiology. 2007;**10**:240-245

[82] Yamagiwa K, Yokoi H, Isaji S, Tabata M, Mizuno S, Hori T, et al. Intrahepatic hepatic vein stenosis after living-related liver transplantation treated by insertion of an expandable metallic stent. American Journal of Transplantation. 2004;**4**:1006-1009

[83] Lorenz JM, van Beek D, Funaki B, Van Ha TG, Zangan S, Navuluri R, et al. Long-term outcomes of percutaneous venoplasty and gianturco stent placement to treat obstruction of the inferior vena cava complicating liver transplantation. Cardiovascular and Interventional Radiology. 2014;**37**:114-124

[84] Roos FJM, Poley J-W, Polak WG, Metselaar HJ. Biliary complications

after liver transplantation; recent developments in etiology, diagnosis and endoscopic treatment. Best Practice & Research Clinical Gastroenterology. 2017;**31**(2):227-235

[85] Verdonk RC, Buis CI, Porte RJ, Haagsma EB. Biliary complications after liver transplantation: A review. Scandinavian Journal of Gastroenterology. 2006;**41**(sup243):89-101

[86] Sotiropoulos GC, Sgourakis G, Radtke A, Molmenti EP, Goumas K, Mylona S, et al. Orthotopic liver transplantation: T-tube or not T-tube? Systematic review and meta-analysis of results. Transplantation. 2009;**87**(11):1672-1680

[87] Lefkowitch JH. The Liver in Organ Transplantation. WB Saunders; 2000. Scheuer's Liver biopsy interpretation. Elsevier

[88] Potthoff A, Hahn A, Kubicka S, Schneider A, Wedemeyer J, Klempnauer J, et al. Diagnostic value of ultrasound in detection of biliary tract complications after liver transplantation. Hepatitis Monthly. 2013;**13**(1):6003. DOI: 10.5812/hepatmon.6003

[89] Jorgensen JE, Waljee AK, Volk ML, Sonnenday CJ, Elta GH, Al-Hawary MM, et al. Is MRCP equivalent to ERCP for diagnosing biliary obstruction in orthotopic liver transplant recipients? A meta-analysis. Gastrointestinal Endoscopy. 2011;**73**(5):955-996

[90] Chahal P, Baron TH, Poterucha JJ, Rosen CB. Endoscopic retrograde cholangiography in post-orthotopic liver transplant population with roux-en-Y biliary reconstruction. Liver Transplantation. 2007;**13**(8):1168-1173

[91] Devière J, Reddy DN, Püspök A, Ponchon T, Bruno MJ, Bourke MJ, et al. Successful management of benign biliary strictures with fully covered self-expanding metal stents. Gastroenterology. 2014;**147**(2):385-395

[92] Balderramo D, Sendino O, Burrel M, Real MI, Blasi A, Martinez-Palli G, et al. Risk factors and outcomes of failed endoscopic retrograde cholangiopancreatography in liver transplant recipients with anastomotic biliary strictures: A case-control study. Liver Transplantation. 2012;**18**(4):482-489

[93] Pascher A, Neuhaus P. Biliary complications after deceased-donor orthotopic liver transplantation. Journal of Hepato-Biliary-Pancreatic Surgery. 2006;**13**(6):487-496

[94] Kanazawa A, Kubo S, Tanaka H, Takemura S, Yamazaki K, Hirohashi K, et al. Bile leakage after living donor liver transplantation demonstrated with hepatobiliary scan using 9mTc-PMT. Annals of Nuclear Medicine. 2003 Sep;**17**(6):507-509

[95] Thuluvath PJ, Pfau PR, Kimmey MB, Ginsberg GG. Biliary complications after liver transplantation: The role of endoscopy. Endoscopy. 2005;**37**(9):857-863

[96] Shah JN, Haigh WG, Lee SP, Lucey MR, Brensinger CM, Kochman ML, et al. Biliary casts after orthotopic liver transplantation: Clinical factors, treatment, biochemical analysis. The American Journal of Gastroenterology. 2003;**98**(8):1861-1867

[97] Voigtlander T et al. Biliary cast síndrome post-liver transplantation: Risk factors and outcomes. Liver International. 2013;**33**:1287-1292

[98] Copstead L-EC, Banasik JL. Pathophysiology. 5th ed. USA: Elsevier Saunders; 2013:204-205

[99] Grossman S, Mattson C. Porth's Pathophysiology: Concepts of Altered

Health States. 9th ed. USA: Wolters Kluwer; 2013:350-353

[100] Irwin RS, Rippe JM. Irwin & Rippe's Intensive Care Medicine. 8th ed. USA: Wolters Kluwer; 2018:587-589

[101] Parrillo JE, Phillip Dellinger R. Critical Care Medicine: Principles of Diagnosis and Management in the Adult. 5th ed. Philadelphia: Elsevier; 2019:1188-1190

[102] Layon AJ, Mihae Y, Gabrielli A, Wood KE. Civetta, Taylor & Kirby's Critical Care. 5th ed. Wolters Kluwer; 2017:833-835

[103] Moore DE, Feurer ID, Speroff T, Gorden DL, Wright JK, Chari RS, et al. Impact of donor, technical, and recipient risk factors on survival and quality of life after liver transplantation. Archives of Surgery. 2005;**140**(3):273

[104] Fernández-Merino FJ, Nuño-Garza J, López-Hervás P, López-Buenadicha A, Moreno-Caparrós A, Quijano-Collazo Y, et al. Impact of donor, recipient, and graft features on the development of primary dysfunction in liver transplants. Transplantation Proceedings. 2003;**35**(5):1793

[105] Condron SL, Heneghan MA, Patel K, Dev A, McHutchison JG, Muir AJ. Effect of donor age on survival of liver transplant recipients with hepatitis C virus infection. Transplantation. 2005;**80**(1):145

[106] Cuende N, Miranda B, Cañón JF, Garrido G, Matesanz R. Donor characteristics associated with liver graft survival. Transplantation. 2005;**79**(10):1445

[107] Sánchez-Perez B, Santoyo J, Fernández-Aguilar JL, Suárez MA, Pérez JA, Jiménez M, et al. Preoperative factors and models predicting mortality in liver transplantation. Transplantation Proceedings. 2005;**37**(3):1499

[108] Totsuka E, Fung U, Hakamada K, Tanaka M, Takahashi K, Nakai M, et al. Analysis of clinical variables of donors and recipients with respect to short-term graft outcome in human liver transplantation. Transplantation Proceedings. 2004;**36**(8):2215

[109] Corradini SG, Elisei W, De Marco R, Siciliano M, Iappelli M, Pugliese F, et al. Preharvest donor hyperoxia predicts good early graft function and longer graft survival after liver transplantation. Liver Transplantation. 2005;**11**(2):140

[110] Zapletal Ch FD, Wullstein C, Woeste G, Caspary WF, Golling M, Bechstein WO. Does the liver ever age? Results of liver transplantation with donors above 80 years of age. Transplantation Proceedings. 2005;**37**(2):1182

[111] Pirenne J, Monbaliu D, Van Gelder F, Van Hees D, Aerts R, Verslype C, et al. Liver transplantation using livers from septuagenarian and octogenarian donors: An underused strategy to reduce mortality on the waiting list. Transplantation Proceedings. 2005;**37**(2):1180

[112] Santori G, Andorno E, Morelli N, Gianelli Castiglione A, Casaccia M, Saltalamacchia L, et al. Impact of ischemia/reperfusion on transplanted livers procured from elderly cadaveric donors. Transplantation Proceedings. 2004;**36**(10):2909

[113] Halazun KJ, Quillin RC, Rosenblatt R, Bongu A, Griesemer AD, Kato T, et al. Expanding the margins: High volume utilization of marginal liver grafts among >2000 liver transplants at a single institution. Annals of Surgery. 2017;**266**(3):441

[114] Hernández MP, Martin P, Simkins J. Infectious complications after

liver transplantation. Gastroenterology & Hepatology. 2015;**11**(11):741-753

[115] Timsit J-F, Sonneville R, Kalil AC. Diagnostic and therapeutic approach to infectious diseases in solid organ transplant recipients. Intensive Care Medicine. 2019;**45**:573-591

[116] Baganate F, Beal EW, Tumin D, et al. Early mortality after liver transplantation: Defining the course and the cause. Surgery. 2018;**164**:694

[117] Torbenson M, Wang J, Nichols L, et al. Causes of death in autopsied liver transplantation patients. Modern Pathology. 1998;**11**:37

[118] Fishman JA. Infection in organ transplantation. American Journal of Transplantation. 2017;**17**:856-879

[119] Colonna JO 2nd, Winston DJ, Brill JE, et al. Infectious complications in liver transplantation. Archives of Surgery. 1988;**123**:360

[120] Kim YJ, Kim SI, Wie SH, et al. Infectious complications in living-donor liver transplant recipients: 9-year single-center experience. Transplant Infectious Disease. 2008;**10**:316

[121] Singh N, Wagener MM, Gayowski T. Seasonal pattern of early mortality and infectious complications in liver transplant recipients. Liver Transplantation. 2001;**7**:884

[122] Chang FY, Singh N, Gayowski T, et al. Fever in liver transplant recipients: Changing spectrum of etiologic agents. Clinical Infectious Diseases. 1998;**26**:59

[123] Fishman JA. From the classic concepts to modern practice. Clinical Microbiology and Infection. 2014;**20**(Suppl 7):4

[124] Van Duin D, van Delden C. AST infectious diseases community of practice. Multidrug-resistant gram-negative bacteria infections in solid organ transplantation. American Journal of Transplantation. 2013;**13**(Suppl 4):31

[125] Kusne S, Dummer JS, Singh N, et al. Infections after liver transplantation. An analysis of 101 consecutive cases. Medicine (Baltimore). 1988;**67**:132

[126] Paya CV, Wiesner RH, Hermans PE, et al. Risk factors for cytomegalovirus tond severe bacterial infections following liver transplantation: A prospective multivariate time-dependent analysis. Journal of Hepatology. 1993;**18**:185

[127] Fishman JA, Rubin RH. Infection in organ-transplant recipients. The New England Journal of Medicine. 1998;**338**:1741

[128] Riddle DJ, Dubberke ER. Clostridium difficile infection in solid organ transplant recipients. Current Opinion in Organ Transplantation. 2008;**13**:592

[129] Doron S, Ruthazer R, Werner BG, et al. Hypogammaglobulinemia in liver transplant recipients: Incidence, timing, risk factors, and outcomes. Transplantation. 2006;**81**:697

[130] Husain S, Tollemar J, Dominguez EA, et al. Changes in the spectrum and risk factors for invasive candidiasis in liver transplant recipients: Prospective, multicenter, case-controlled study. Transplantation. 2003;**75**:2023

[131] Herrero JI. De novo malignancies following liver transplantation: Impact and recommendations. Liver Transplantation. 2009;**15**(suppl 2):S90-S94

[132] Charlton M. Obesity, hyperlipidemia, and metabolic syndrome. Liver Transplantation. 2009;**15**(suppl 2):S83-S89

[133] Montoro MA, García Pagán JC, Castells A, Gomollón F, Mearin F,

Panés J, et al. Gastroenterology and Hepatology. Commons Problems in the Clinic Practice. 2nd ed. Madrid: Jarpyo Editores; 2012:1005-1016. ISBN: 978-84-92982-31-9

[134] Mc Guire BM, Rosenthal P, Brown CC, Busch AM, Calcatera SM, Claria RS, et al. Long-term management of the liver transplant patient: Recommendations for the primary care doctor. American Journal of Transplantation. 2009 Sep;**9**(9):1988-2003. DOI: 10.1111/j.1600-6143.2009.02733.x

[135] Charlton MR, Wall WJ, Ojo AO, Ginès P, Textor S, Shihab FS, et al. Report of the first international liver transplantation society panel consensus conference on renal insufficiency in liver transplantation. Liver Transplantation. 2009;**15**:S1S34

[136] Guichelaar MMJ, Schmoll J, Malinchoc M, Hay JE. Fractures and avascular necrosis before and after orthotopic liver transplantation: Long-term follow-up and predictive factors. Hepatology. 2007;**46**:1198-1207

[137] European Liver Transplant Registry. Available from: http://www.eltr.org

[138] Watt KDS, Pedersen RA, Kremers WK, Heimbach JK, Charlton MR, et al. Evolution of causes and risk factors for mortality post liver transplant: Results of the NIDDK long term follow up study. American Journal of Transplantation. 2010;**10**:1420-1427

[139] Karam V, Castaing D, Danet C, Delvart V, Gasquet I, Adam R, et al. Longitudinal prospective evaluation of quality of life in adult patients before and one year after liver transplantation. Liver Transplantation. 2003;**9**:703-711

Chapter 3

Stroke and Liver Cirrhosis: A Brief Review of Current Evidence

Kexin Zheng, Xiaozhong Guo, Xinhong Wang and Xingshun Qi

Abstract

Stroke and liver cirrhosis are common in our everyday clinical practice, both of which can lead to serious complications. Their association is unclear. In this chapter, we briefly summarized the epidemiology of liver cirrhosis in stroke, reviewed the current evidence regarding the association between liver cirrhosis and stroke, and discussed the potential mechanisms for explaining such an association, such as coagulopathy, hypoperfusion, cardiac diseases, diabetes, and dyslipidemia.

Keywords: liver cirrhosis, stroke, review, mechanisms, epidemiology

1. Introduction

Stroke and liver cirrhosis are two leading causes of death worldwide [1]. Patients with liver cirrhosis often have coagulopathy, hypoperfusion, cardiac diseases, diabetes, and dyslipidemia, which are associated with the development of stroke. Recent evidence also suggests a higher risk of stroke in liver cirrhosis. In the present chapter, we reviewed the current evidence regarding epidemiology of stroke in liver cirrhosis, association of stroke with liver cirrhosis, and their potential mechanisms.

2. Stroke

Stroke is the second leading cause of death and disability worldwide, which is defined as an acute episode of focal dysfunction of the brain, retina, or spinal cord [2]. It is often divided into hemorrhagic and ischemic stroke. Hemorrhagic and ischemic stroke leads to 2978 and 3348 thousands people dying until 2015, respectively [1]. Over two thirds of stroke-related deaths occur in developing countries in the world [3], especially in low-income and middle-income countries [4]. Burden of stroke in Asia is heavier than Europe or North America [5]. Patients with stroke are more susceptible to suffer systemic complications, including cardiac, pulmonary, gastrointestinal, genitourinary, musculoskeletal, and neuropsychiatric systems, venous thromboembolism, and so on [6, 7]. Prognosis of stroke is poor. About 20–30% of patients died 6 months after stroke, 20–30% had moderate to severe disability, and 20–25% had mild to moderate disability [8]. Traditional risk factors of stroke are hypertension, decreased physical activity, increased ratio of lipoprotein (Apo)B/ApoA1 and waist-to-hip, unhealthy diet, depression status, smoking, cardiac disease, alcohol intake, and diabetes mellitus [4, 9]. Additionally, our clinical practice suggested that acute upper gastrointestinal bleeding would lead to stroke [10]. Several possible explanations are as follows. First, massive blood loss leads to reduced blood supply to the brain secondary to cerebral vessel vasoconstriction. Second, massive blood loss sometimes leads to reactive thrombocytosis [11], thereby resulting in potential hypercoagulability. Third, hemocoagulase is occasionally employed for the treatment of gastrointestinal bleeding, which could reduce fibrinogen concentration [12]. Fourth, blood transfusion is an important treatment of upper gastrointestinal bleeding [13], but the ischemia reperfusion injury of brain cannot be ignored.

3. Liver cirrhosis

Liver cirrhosis is an end stage of liver disease [14]. Histologically, it is characterized by diffuse fibrosis within hepatic tissue, false lobular formation, and regenerative nodules [14, 15]. It is the 17th cause of death globally [16], and the mortality has increased steadily over the past 30 years, especially in Central Asia, North Africa, and the Middle East [17]. The major causes of liver cirrhosis are chronic hepatitis B virus (HBV) and hepatitis C virus (HCV) infection, alcoholism, nonalcoholic steatohepatitis (NASH), drug abuse, and cholestasis [18–20]. The major complications are variceal hemorrhage [21], ascites [22], cirrhotic cardiomyopathy [23], hepatic encephalopathy [24], hepatocellular carcinoma [25, 26], portal vein thrombosis [27], and other common venous thromboembolism [28]. Up-to-date concept suggests a tendency towards both bleeding and thrombotic events in cirrhotic patients due to decreased levels of both procoagulant and anticoagulant factors [29, 30].

4. Association between stroke and liver cirrhosis

Overall, it remains unclear about whether liver cirrhosis increases or reduces the risk of ischemic stroke. A majority of studies [31–35] indicated an obviously higher risk of overall, ischemic, and/or hemorrhagic stroke after adjusting the covariates in cirrhotic patients than non-cirrhotic patients. By contrast, another two studies by Chen [36] and Solaymani-Dodaran [37] suggested the protective role of liver cirrhosis in the development of ischemic stroke. Heterogeneous results regarding this association among the studies might be attributed to the selection of patients. The characteristics of study population were different. Studies by Chen and Solaymani-Dodaran et al. focused on patients with nonalcoholic cirrhosis and primary biliary

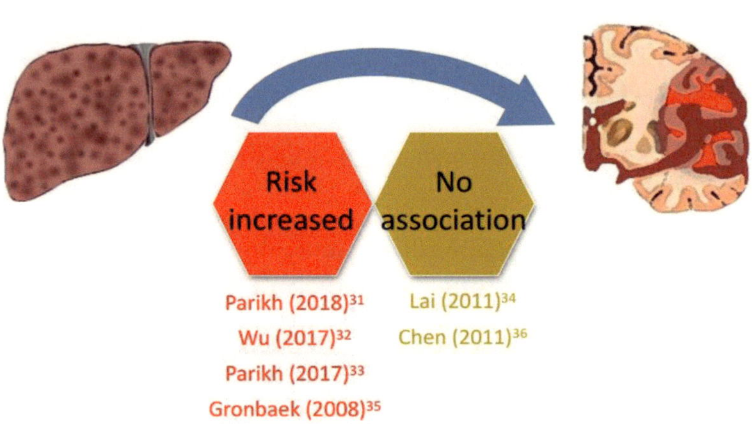

Figure 1.
The association between liver cirrhosis and hemorrhagic stroke.

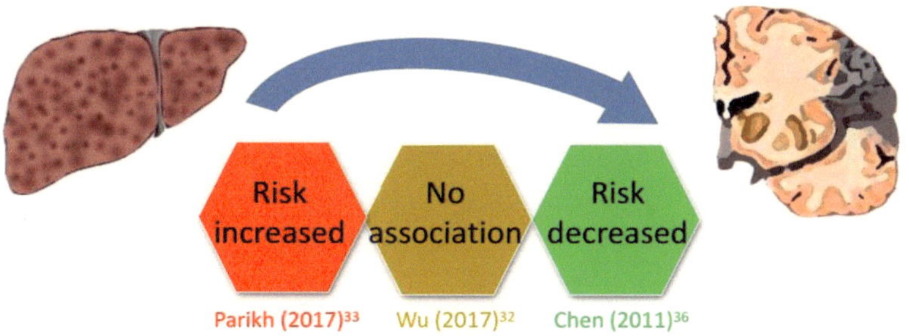

Figure 2.
The association between liver cirrhosis and ischemic stroke.

cirrhosis, respectively. By comparison, the study population had unspecified liver cirrhosis in other studies. The association between liver cirrhosis and stroke was outlined according to the evidence from abovementioned studies (**Figures 1** and **2**).

5. Incidence/prevalence of stroke in liver cirrhosis

Regardless of the type of stroke, the prevalence of stroke was from 2.06 to 53.81% [36–49] (**Figure 3**). Several subgroup populations should be further reported.

First, the prevalence of hemorrhagic stroke in liver cirrhosis seemed to be higher than that of ischemic stroke. The prevalence of hemorrhagic stroke was from 0.80 to 34.33% [34–36, 50–56] (**Figure 4**).

The prevalence of ischemic stroke was from 0.85 to 6.55% [34, 36, 57, 58] (**Figure 5**).

Second, the annual incidence of ischemic stroke in cirrhotic patients with atrial fibrillation was 1.2% [59]. The prevalence of stroke in cirrhotic patients with atrial fibrillation was 53.81 and 34.58% in the studies by Kuo [38] and Lee [44], respectively. This figure is significantly higher than that reported by studies including unclassified cirrhotic patients without atrial fibrillation.

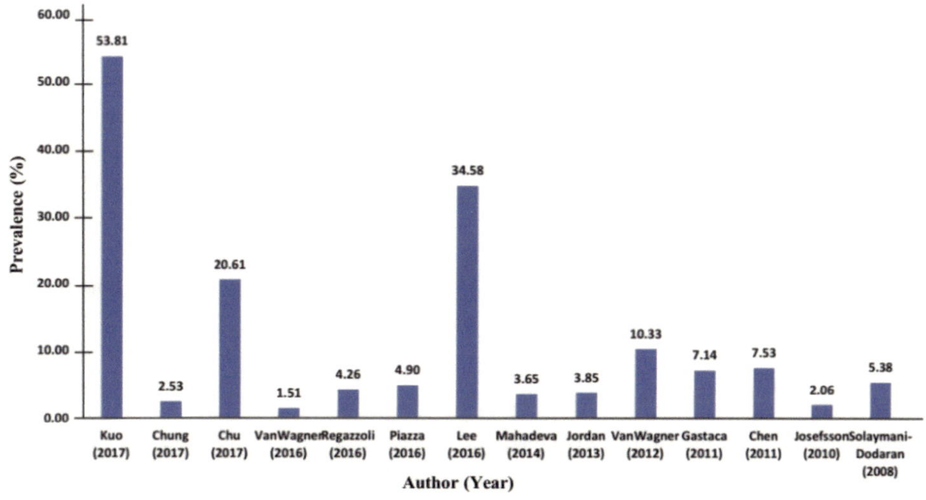

Figure 3.
The prevalence of stroke in liver cirrhosis.

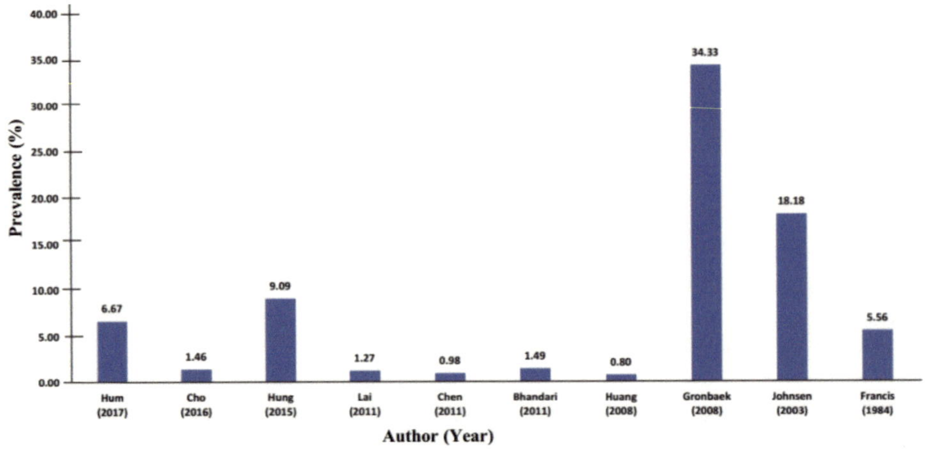

Figure 4.
The prevalence of hemorrhagic stroke in liver cirrhosis.

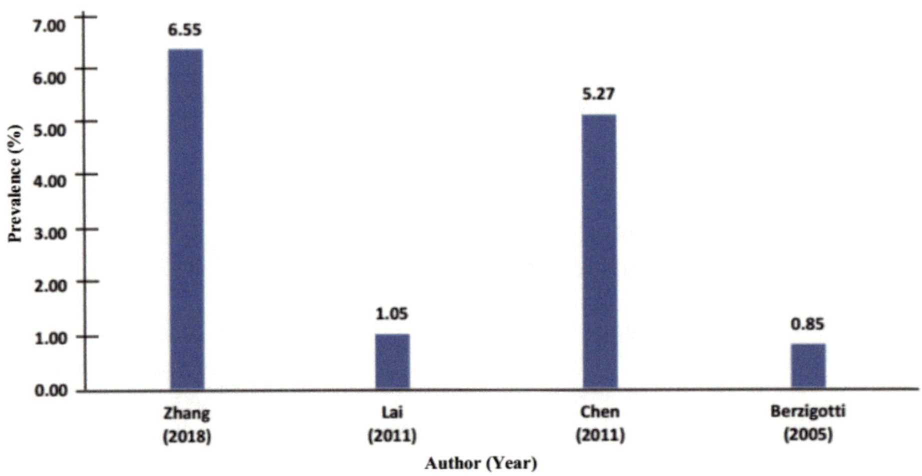

Figure 5.
The prevalence of ischemic stroke in liver cirrhosis.

Third, the annual incidence of aneurysmal subarachnoid hemorrhage (SAH) in cirrhotic patients was 0.11% [31].

6. Potential mechanisms for the association between stroke and liver cirrhosis

There are several potential mechanisms for explaining the association between stroke and liver cirrhosis.

6.1 Coagulopathy

Coagulation and anticoagulation factors maintain a dynamic balance to prevent from the development of thrombosis and hemorrhage in healthy population [60]. By comparison, coagulopathy is frequently observed in cirrhotic patients [61] due to an imbalance between coagulation and anticoagulation factors [62]. First, clotting factors are often decreased in cirrhotic patients [63] and in parallel to the progression of liver disease [64]. Second, the mean lifetime of platelet is shortened and thrombopoietin production is decreased [65]. Thrombocytopenia is also caused by hypersplenism, antiplatelet autoantibodies, toxic effects of excessive alcohol intake, and treatment with interferon [65, 66]. Third, a hypercoagulable status has been recognized in advanced cirrhosis due to increased levels of factor VIII and decreased levels of protein C [64]. Therefore, both hemorrhage and thrombosis can develop in cirrhotic patients.

6.2 Hypoperfusion

Hypoperfusion is often observed in liver cirrhosis. First, ascites is a common clinical sign in cirrhotic patients due to liver dysfunction and portal hypertension [67], in which lots of capillary fluids leak into abdominal cavity. Second, serum albumin level is often decreased in liver cirrhosis, which can decrease intravascular osmotic pressure [68]. Third, massive gastrointestinal bleeding secondary to gastroesophageal variceal rupture is a common complication of liver cirrhosis, leading to the hypoperfusion of various organs [21]. Fourth, there is a hyperdynamic circulation status in cirrhotic patients, which is characterized by arterial hypotension, high cardiac output, and low peripheral vascular resistance [69, 70].

6.3 Cardiac diseases

Cirrhotic patients often present with cirrhotic cardiomyopathy defined as cardiac systolic and/or diastolic dysfunction in the absence of previous history of heart disease [23]. Additionally, cardiac arrhythmias, especially atrial fibrillation, have been increasingly recognized in patients with chronic liver diseases [71, 72]. A nationwide population-based study suggests an increased risk of atrial fibrillation development in cirrhosis [73].

6.4 Diabetes

Up to 70% of cirrhotic patients develop diabetes or impaired glucose tolerance [74]. Evidence also suggests an association of hepatogeneous diabetes with higher portal pressure and increased risk of hepatocellular carcinoma, hepatic encephalopathy, and mortality in cirrhosis [75]. Several potential mechanisms of hepatogeneous diabetes include [1] reduced insulin clearance and hyperinsulinemia [76], [2] beta cell failure and reduced insulin secretion [77], and [3] increased secretion from alpha cells and hyperglucagonemia [75].

6.5 Dyslipidemia

Liver plays a key role in the synthesis, decomposition, and digestion of lipids, and dyslipidemia is found in patients with impaired liver function. Triglycerides, the ratio of triglycerides to high-density lipoprotein, and the ratio of apolipoprotein B to apolipoprotein A1 increase in cirrhotic patients [78, 79].

7. Conclusions

Patients with liver cirrhosis might have an increased risk of stroke probably due to their concomitant high-risk factors, such as coagulopathy, hypoperfusion, cardiac diseases, diabetes, and dyslipidemia. Once a patient was diagnosed with liver cirrhosis, the management of stroke should be initiated.

Abbreviations

Apo	apolipoprotein
HBV	hepatitis B virus
HCV	hepatitis C virus
NASH	nonalcoholic steatohepatitis
SAH	subarachnoid hemorrhage

Author contributions

Kexin Zheng: reviewed the literature and drafted the manuscript. Xiaozhong Guo, Xinhong Wang: gave critical comments. Xingshun Qi: conceived the work and drafted and revised the manuscript. All authors have made an intellectual contribution to the manuscript and approved the submission.

Author details

Kexin Zheng[1,2], Xiaozhong Guo[1*], Xinhong Wang[3] and Xingshun Qi[1*]

1 Department of Gastroenterology, General Hospital of Northern Theater Command (formerly General Hospital of Shenyang Military Area), Shenyang, Liaoning Province, China

2 Postgraduate College, Jinzhou Medical University, Jinzhou, Liaoning Province, China

3 Department of Neurology, General Hospital of Northern Theater Command (formerly General Hospital of Shenyang Military Area), Shenyang, Liaoning Province, China

*Address all correspondence to: xingshunqi@126.com
and guo_xiao_zhong@126.com

References

[1] GBD. 2015 mortality and causes of death collaborators. Global, regional, and national life expectancy, all-cause mortality, and cause-specific mortality for 249 causes of death, 1980-2015: A systematic analysis for the global burden of disease study 2015. Lancet. 2016;**388**:1459-1544

[2] Sacco RL, Kasner SE, Broderick JP, Caplan LR, Connors JJ, Culebras A, et al. An updated definition of stroke for the 21st century: A statement for healthcare professionals from the American Heart Association/ American Stroke Association. Stroke. 2013;**44**:2064-2089

[3] Freedman B, Potpara TS, Lip GY. Stroke prevention in atrial fibrillation. Lancet. 2016;**388**:806-817

[4] O'Donnell MJ, Chin SL, Rangarajan S, Xavier D, Liu L, Zhang H, et al. Global and regional effects of potentially modifiable risk factors associated with acute stroke in 32 countries (INTERSTROKE): A case-control study. Lancet. 2016;**388**:761-775

[5] Kim JS. Stroke in Asia: A global disaster. International Journal of Stroke. 2014;**9**:856-857

[6] Kumar S, Selim MH, Caplan LR. Medical complications after stroke. Lancet Neurology. 2010;**9**:105-118

[7] Hackett ML, Kohler S, O'Brien JT, Mead GE. Neuropsychiatric outcomes of stroke. Lancet Neurology. 2014;**13**:525-534

[8] Gresham GE, Fitzpatrick TE, Wolf PA, McNamara PM, Kannel WB, Dawber TR. Residual disability in survivors of stroke—the Framingham study. The New England Journal of Medicine. 1975;**293**:954-956

[9] O'Donnell MJ, Xavier D, Liu L, Zhang H, Chin SL, Rao-Melacini P, et al. Risk factors for ischaemic and intracerebral haemorrhagic stroke in 22 countries (the INTERSTROKE study): A case-control study. Lancet. 2010;**376**:112-123

[10] Qi X, Qiu J, De Stefano V, Shao X, Sun R, Guo X. Development of acute ischemic stroke in two patients with acute upper gastrointestinal bleeding. AME Medical Journal. 2017;**2**:24

[11] Qi X, De Stefano V, Shao X, Guo X. Thrombocytosis in a patient with upper gastrointestinal bleeding. Intractable & Rare Diseases Research. 2017;**6**:69-71

[12] Qi X, Wang J, Yu X, De Stefano V, Li H, Wu C, et al. Hemocoagulase might not control but worsen gastrointestinal bleeding in an elderly patient with type II respiratory failure. Translational Gastroenterology and Hepatology. 2017;**2**:71

[13] Nelamangala-Ramakrishnaiah VP, Chellappa V, Goneppanavar M. Blood transfusion strategy in cirrhotic patients with active upper GI bleeding. AME Medical Journal. 2019;**4**:1. Available from: http://amj.amegroups.com/article/view/4768/html

[14] Tsochatzis EA, Bosch J, Burroughs AK. Liver cirrhosis. Lancet. 2014;**383**:1749-1761

[15] Schuppan D, Afdhal NH. Liver cirrhosis. Lancet. 2008;**371**:838-851

[16] Lozano R, Naghavi M, Foreman K, Lim S, Shibuya K, Aboyans V, et al. Global and regional mortality from 235 causes of death for 20 age groups in 1990 and 2010: A systematic analysis for the global burden of disease study 2010. Lancet. 2012;**380**:2095-2128

[17] Mokdad AA, Lopez AD, Shahraz S, Lozano R, Mokdad AH, Stanaway J,

et al. Liver cirrhosis mortality in 187 countries between 1980 and 2010: A systematic analysis. BMC Medicine. 2014;**12**:145

[18] Ge PS, Runyon BA. Treatment of patients with cirrhosis. The New England Journal of Medicine. 2016;**375**:767-777

[19] Selmi C, Bowlus CL, Gershwin ME, Coppel RL. Primary biliary cirrhosis. Lancet. 2011;**377**:1600-1609

[20] Henriksen JH, Fuglsang S, Bendtsen F, Moller S. Arterial hypertension in cirrhosis: Arterial compliance, volume distribution, and central haemodynamics. Gut. 2006;**55**:380-387

[21] Garcia-Tsao G, Bosch J. Management of varices and variceal hemorrhage in cirrhosis. The New England Journal of Medicine. 2010;**362**:823-832

[22] Gines P, Cardenas A, Arroyo V, Rodes J. Management of cirrhosis and ascites. The New England Journal of Medicine. 2004;**350**:1646-1654

[23] Moller S, Henriksen JH. Cardiovascular complications of cirrhosis. Gut. 2008;**57**:268-278

[24] Shawcross D, Jalan R. Dispelling myths in the treatment of hepatic encephalopathy. Lancet. 2005;**365**:431-433

[25] Forner A, Reig M, Bruix J. Hepatocellular carcinoma. Lancet. 2018;**391**:1301-1314

[26] Maluccio M, Covey A. Recent progress in understanding, diagnosing, and treating hepatocellular carcinoma. CA: A Cancer Journal for Clinicians. 2012;**62**:394-399

[27] Qi X, Han G, Fan D. Management of portal vein thrombosis in liver cirrhosis. Nature Reviews. Gastroenterology & Hepatology. 2014;**11**:435-446

[28] Qi X, Ren W, Guo X, Fan D. Epidemiology of venous thromboembolism in patients with liver diseases: A systematic review and meta-analysis. Internal and Emergency Medicine. 2015;**10**:205-217

[29] Garcia-Tsao G, Bosch J. Varices and variceal hemorrhage in cirrhosis: A new view of an old problem. Clinical Gastroenterology and Hepatology. 2015;**13**:2109-2117

[30] Sogaard KK, Horvath-Puho E, Gronbaek H, Jepsen P, Vilstrup H, Sorensen HT. Risk of venous thromboembolism in patients with liver disease: A nationwide population-based case-control study. The American Journal of Gastroenterology. 2009;**104**:96-101

[31] Parikh NS, Merkler AE, Jesudian A, Kamel H. Liver cirrhosis is associated with an increased risk of aneurysmal subarachnoid hemorrhage. Stroke. 2018;**49**:ATP171

[32] Wu HY, Lin CS, Yeh CC, Hu CJ, Shih CC, Cherng YG, et al. Cirrhosis patients' stroke risks and adverse outcomes: Two nationwide studies. Atherosclerosis. 2017;**263**:29-35

[33] Parikh NS, Navi BB, Schneider Y, Jesudian A, Kamel H. Association between cirrhosis and stroke in a nationally representative cohort. JAMA Neurology. 2017;**74**:927-932

[34] Lai CH, Cheng PY, Chen YY. Liver cirrhosis and risk of intracerebral hemorrhage: A 9-year follow-up study. Stroke. 2011;**42**:2615-2617

[35] Gronbaek H, Johnsen SP, Jepsen P, Gislum M, Vilstrup H, Tage-Jensen U, et al. Liver cirrhosis, other liver diseases, and risk of hospitalisation for intracerebral haemorrhage: A Danish population-based case-control study. BMC Gastroenterology. 2008;**8**:16

[36] Chen YH, Chen KY, Lin HC. Non-alcoholic cirrhosis and the risk of stroke: A 5-year follow-up study. Liver International. 2011;**31**:354-360

[37] Solaymani-Dodaran M, Aithal GP, Card T, West J. Risk of cardiovascular and cerebrovascular events in primary biliary cirrhosis: A population-based cohort study. The American Journal of Gastroenterology. 2008;**103**:2784-2788

[38] Kuo L, Chao TF, Liu CJ, Lin YJ, Chang SL, Lo LW, et al. Liver cirrhosis in patients with atrial fibrillation: Would oral anticoagulation have a net clinical benefit for stroke prevention? Journal of the American Heart Association. 2017;**6**:e005307

[39] Chung MS, Kim HS, Lim YS, Jeon SB, Kim SO, Kim HJ, et al. Clinical impact of preoperative brain MR angiography and MR imaging in candidates for liver transplantation: A propensity score-matching study in a single institution. European Radiology. 2017;**27**:3532-3541

[40] Chu LM, Liu CC, Yeh CC, Chang YC, Hu CJ, Shih CC, et al. Increased diabetes risk and interaction with social and medical events in patients upon stroke: Two nationwide studies. Atherosclerosis. 2017;**265**:87-92

[41] VanWagner LB, Serper M, Kang R, Levitsky J, Hohmann S, Abecassis M, et al. Factors associated with major adverse cardiovascular events after liver transplantation among a national sample. American Journal of Transplantation. 2016;**16**:2684-2694

[42] Regazzoli D, Latib A, Montorfano M, Tanaka A, Jabbour R, Chieffo A, et al. Acute and medium-term outcomes of transcatheter aortic valve implantation in patients with cirrhosis. Giornale Italiano di Cardiologia. 2016;**17**:e14

[43] Piazza NA, Singal AK. Frequency of cardiovascular events and effect on survival in liver transplant recipients for cirrhosis due to alcoholic or nonalcoholic steatohepatitis. Experimental and Clinical Transplantation. 2016;**14**:79-85

[44] Lee SJ, Uhm JS, Kim JY, Pak HN, Lee MH, Joung B. The safety and efficacy of vitamin K antagonist in patients with atrial fibrillation and liver cirrhosis. International Journal of Cardiology. 2015;**180**:185-191

[45] Mahadeva S, Kadhim O. Morbidity and mortality differences between cryptogenic and non-cryptogenic cirrhosis: A retrospective cohort study. Journal of Gastroenterology and Hepatology. 2014;**29**:189-190

[46] Jordan C, Pilch N, Taber D, Meadows H, Fleming J, Mardis A, et al. Liver transplant for NASH: We need to spare the nephron. American Journal of Transplantation. 2013;**13**:72

[47] Vanwagner LB, Bhave M, Te HS, Feinglass J, Alvarez L, Rinella ME. Patients transplanted for nonalcoholic steatohepatitis are at increased risk for postoperative cardiovascular events. Hepatology. 2012;**56**:1741-1750

[48] Gastaca M, Agüero F, Montejo M, Rimola A, Miralles P, Lozano R, et al. Retransplantation in HIV-infected patients after liver transplantation: A prospective cohort study. American Journal of Transplantation. 2011;**11**:277

[49] Josefsson A, Fu M, Bjornsson E, Olausson M, Kalaitzakis E. The use of beta-blockers in patients with liver cirrhosis undergoing liver transplantation. Gastroenterology. 2010;**138**:S821

[50] Hum J, Shatzel JJ, Jou JH, Deloughery TG. The efficacy and safety of direct oral anticoagulants vs traditional anticoagulants in cirrhosis.

European Journal of Haematology. 2017;**98**:393-397

[51] Cho J, Choi SM, Yu SJ, Park YS, Lee CH, Lee SM, et al. Bleeding complications in critically ill patients with liver cirrhosis. The Korean Journal of Internal Medicine. 2016;**31**:288-295

[52] Hung TH, Hsieh YH, Tseng KC, Tseng CW, Lee HF, Tsai CC, et al. High mortality in cirrhotic patients following hemorrhagic stroke. Journal of Clinical Neuroscience. 2015;**22**:995-997

[53] Bhandari BM, Kumar S, Latimer DC, Sass DA, Rothstein K. A head CT is unnecessary in the initial evaluation of hepatic encephalopathy in patients with cirrhosis. Gastroenterology. 2011;**140**:S903

[54] Huang HH, Lin HH, Shih YL, Chen PJ, Chang WK, Chu HC, et al. Spontaneous intracranial hemorrhage in cirrhotic patients. Clinical Neurology and Neurosurgery. 2008;**110**:253-258

[55] Johnsen SP, Pedersen L, Friis S, Blot WJ, McLaughlin JK, Olsen Jø H, et al. Nonaspirin nonsteroidal anti-inflammatory drugs and risk of hospitalization for intracerebral hemorrhage: A population-based case-control study. Stroke. 2003;**34**:387-391

[56] Francis RB Jr, Feinstein DI. Clinical significance of accelerated fibrinolysis in liver disease. Haemostasis. 1984;**14**:460-465

[57] Zhang X, Qi X, Yoshida E, Méndez-Sánchez N, Hou F, Deng H, et al. Ischemic stroke in liver cirrhosis: Epidemiology, risk factors, and in-hospital outcomes. European Journal of Gastroenterology & Hepatology. 2018;**30**:233-240

[58] Berzigotti A, Bonfiglioli A, Muscari A, Bianchi G, Libassi S, Bernardi M, et al. Reduced prevalence of ischemic events and abnormal supraortic flow patterns in patients with liver cirrhosis. Liver International. 2005;**25**(2):331-336

[59] Choi J, Kim J, Shim JH, Kim M, Nam GB. Risks versus benefits of anticoagulation for atrial fibrillation in cirrhotic patients. Journal of Cardiovascular Pharmacology. 2017;**70**:255-262

[60] Jairath V, Burroughs A. Anticoagulation in patients with liver cirrhosis: Complication or therapeutic opportunity? Gut. 2013;**62**:479-482

[61] Lisman T, Leebeek FW, de Groot PG. Haemostatic abnormalities in patients with liver disease. Journal of Hepatology. 2002;**37**:280-287

[62] Drolz A, Horvatits T, Roedl K, Rutter K, Staufer K, Kneidinger N, et al. Coagulation parameters and major bleeding in critically ill patients with cirrhosis. Hepatology. 2016;**64**:556-568

[63] Everett LA, Cleuren AC, Khoriaty RN, Ginsburg D. Murine coagulation factor VIII is synthesized in endothelial cells. Blood. 2014;**123**:3697-3705

[64] Tripodi A, Primignani M, Chantarangkul V, Dell'Era A, Clerici M, de Franchis R, et al. An imbalance of pro- vs anti-coagulation factors in plasma from patients with cirrhosis. Gastroenterology. 2009;**137**:2105-2111

[65] Peck-Radosavljevic M. Thrombocytopenia in liver disease. Canadian Journal of Gastroenterology. 2000;**14**(Suppl D):60d-66d

[66] Yongxiang W, Zongfang L, Guowei L, Zongzheng J, Xi C, Tao W. Effects of splenomegaly and splenic macrophage activity in hypersplenism due to cirrhosis. The American Journal of Medicine. 2002;**113**:428-431

[67] Moore KP, Aithal GP. Guidelines on the management of ascites in cirrhosis. Gut. 2006;**55**(Suppl 6):vi1-v12

[68] Hsu SJ, Huang HC. Management of ascites in patients with liver cirrhosis: Recent evidence and controversies. Journal of the Chinese Medical Association. 2013;**76**:123-130

[69] Iwakiri Y, Groszmann RJ. The hyperdynamic circulation of chronic liver diseases: From the patient to the molecule. Hepatology. 2006;**43**:S121-S131

[70] Arroyo V, Gines P. Mechanism of sodium retention and ascites formation in cirrhosis. Journal of Hepatology. 1993;**17**(Suppl 2):S24-S28

[71] Zhao J, Qi X, Hou F, Ning Z, Zhang X, Deng H, et al. Prevalence, risk factors and in-hospital outcomes of QTc interval prolongation in liver cirrhosis. The American Journal of the Medical Sciences. 2016;**352**:285-295

[72] Zhao J, Li S, Ren L, Guo X, Qi X. Pro-brain natriuretic peptide and troponin T-hypersensitivity levels correlate with the severity of liver dysfunction in liver cirrhosis. The American Journal of the Medical Sciences. 2017;**354**:131-139

[73] Anstee QM, Mantovani A, Tilg H, Targher G. Risk of cardiomyopathy and cardiac arrhythmias in patients with nonalcoholic fatty liver disease. Nature Reviews. Gastroenterology & Hepatology. 2018;**15**:425-439

[74] Hickman IJ, Macdonald GA. Impact of diabetes on the severity of liver disease. The American Journal of Medicine. 2007;**120**:829-834

[75] Junker AE, Gluud LL, Holst JJ, Knop FK, Vilsboll T. Influence of gastrointestinal factors on glucose metabolism in patients with cirrhosis. Journal of Gastroenterology and Hepatology. 2015;**30**:1522-1528

[76] Deschenes M, Somberg KA. Effect of transjugular intrahepatic portosystemic shunt (TIPS) on glycemic control in cirrhotic patients with diabetes mellitus. The American Journal of Gastroenterology. 1998;**93**:483

[77] Petrides AS. Hepatogenic diabetes: Pathophysiology, therapeutic options and prognosis. Zeitschrift für Gastroenterologie. 1999;(Suppl 1):15-21

[78] Nderitu P, Bosco C, Garmo H, Holmberg L, Malmstrom H, Hammar N, et al. The association between individual metabolic syndrome components, primary liver cancer and cirrhosis: A study in the Swedish AMORIS cohort. International Journal of Cancer. 2017;**141**:1148-1160

[79] Sierra-Johnson J, Somers VK, Kuniyoshi FH, Garza CA, Isley WL, Gami AS, et al. Comparison of apolipoprotein-B/apolipoprotein-AI in subjects with versus without the metabolic syndrome. The American Journal of Cardiology. 2006;**98**:1369-1373

Chapter 4

Cardiac Hepatopathy

Jose Ignacio Fortea, Ángela Puente, Antonio Cuadrado, Patricia Huelin, Inés García, Marta Mayorga, Raul Pellon, Javier Crespo and Emilio Fábrega

Abstract

Liver disease resulting from heart disease has generally been referred as "cardiac hepatopathy." The two main forms of cardiac hepatopathy are acute cardiogenic liver injury (ACLI) and congestive hepatopathy (CH). ACLI most commonly occurs in the setting of acute cardiocirculatory failure, whereas CH results from passive venous congestion in the setting of chronic right-sided heart failure (HF). Both conditions often coexist and potentiate the deleterious effects of each other on the liver. In CH, the chronic passive congestion leads to sinusoidal hypertension, centrilobular fibrosis, and ultimately, cirrhosis ("cardiac cirrhosis") and hepatocellular carcinoma. The differentiation between congestion and fibrosis currently represents an unmet need and a growing research area. Although cardiac cirrhosis may only arise after several decades of ongoing injury, the long-term survival of cardiac patients due to advances in medical and surgical treatments is responsible for the increased number of liver complications in this setting. Eventually, the liver disease could become as clinically relevant as the cardiac disease and further complicate its management.

Keywords: cirrhosis, portal hypertension, heart failure, heart transplantation, hepatitis

1. Introduction

Heart failure (HF) is a systemic clinical syndrome with typical symptoms and signs (e.g., dyspnea, paroxysmal nocturnal dyspnea, orthopnea, elevated jugular venous pressure, and peripheral edema) caused by a structural and/or functional cardiac abnormality, resulting in reduced cardiac output and/or elevated intracardiac pressures. It is a major public health problem with an estimated prevalence of 1–2% of the adult population in the developed countries, rising to ≥10% among people >70 years of age [1]. Although much of the research on its systemic interactions has focused on the so-called cardio-renal syndrome, cardio-hepatic interactions are arousing great interest in recent years [2]. These cardio-hepatic interactions have been classified into three groups according to the role of each organ as culprit or victim of the other [3, 4]: (1) liver disease resulting from heart disease; (2) heart disease resulting from liver disease (e.g., cirrhotic cardiomyopathy); and (3) systemic diseases that affect both the heart and the liver (e.g., systemic amyloidosis).

This chapter seeks to make a comprehensive review of the first group: liver disease resulting from heart disease. This type of liver disease has generally been referred as "cardiac hepatopathy," although there is still no consensus on terminology [5, 6]. The two main forms of cardiac hepatopathy are acute cardiogenic liver injury (ACLI) and congestive hepatopathy (CH). ACLI most commonly occurs in the setting of acute cardiocirculatory failure, whereas CH results from passive venous congestion in the setting of chronic right-sided HF. Both conditions often coexist and potentiate the deleterious effects of each other on the liver [5–7]. In the following pages, we aim to describe their pathophysiology, clinical features, diagnosis, and treatment.

2. Hepatic circulation

The liver receives a dual blood supply from the hepatic artery and portal vein. The former delivers well-oxygenated blood and comprises approximately 25% of total hepatic blood flow, whereas the remaining 75% is deoxygenated blood supplied by the portal vein. The total hepatic blood flow ranges from 800 to 1200 ml/min, representing up to 25% of the total cardiac output [7]. As a highly vascular organ, it is sensitive to hemodynamic changes but resilient to ischemic damage through its robust vascular mechanisms of defense [3]. The hepatic artery buffer response is one of such mechanisms whereby decreased portal flow instigates compensatory up-regulation of hepatic arterial flow. It is estimated that it may be capable of compensating for up to a 60% decrease in portal flow [3, 7, 8]. The signaling pathway for this response is local, with the reduction of portal flow resulting in an increase in concentration of the vasodilator adenosine [9]. Unlike the hepatic artery, the portal vein does not have the ability to autoregulate its flow and is dependent on cardiac output and the gradient between portal and hepatic venous pressures [7, 8]. The high permeability of sinusoids represents a second mechanism of defense against hypoxia. It favors oxygen diffusion to the hepatocytes, increasing oxygen extraction to levels near 90%. It prevents any change in liver oxygen consumption despite decreases in liver blood flow up to half of its normal. It must be highlighted that this remarkable ability is exclusive to the liver [7, 10, 11].

By contrast, the protective mechanisms against congestion are less developed and mainly rely on the highly connected sinusoidal network to relieve the increase in pressure. This elevated pressure hits the sinusoidal bed without attenuation since the hepatic veins lack valves [6]. As will be explained in greater detail below, the pre-existing hepatic congestion predisposes the liver to hypoxic injury under any acute event resulting in reduced hepatic blood flow [7, 12].

3. Acute cardiogenic liver injury (ACLI)

ACLI has also been referred to as ischemic hepatitis, shock liver, or hypoxic hepatitis in medical literature. These terms reflect the long-standing debate regarding its pathogenesis [7]. In 1901, F.B. Mallory (of Mallory-Denk body fame) first described the typical pattern of centrilobular liver necrosis (CLN) characteristic of this entity based on a series of autopsies in Boston. He proposed a toxic theory whereby liver damage was secondary to toxins released by bacteria into the circulation [13]. This theory was soon challenged by Lambert and Allison who found no proof of bacterial infection in a series of 112 patients deceased from congestive HF, 30% of whom had CLN [14]. They then proposed passive congestion as its prime etiological factor, and this "congestion theory" prevailed for more than 50 years. The emergence of transaminases measurement in the early 1950s revealed the massive increase of these enzymes that come in parallel with CLN. The association between shock, CLN, and significant rise in transaminases found by different studies led some investigators to propose liver ischemia as the sole factor responsible for liver cell necrosis [15–18]. It was then that the terms "shock liver" and "ischemic hepatitis" were introduced by Birgens et al. [19] and Bynum et al. [20], respectively. Hence, by the late 1970s, the "ischemic" theory had replaced the "congestion" theory and remained unquestioned until 1990. In this year, Henrion et al. reported the first prospective series with hemodynamic data of 45 episodes of ischemic hepatitis. They observed that a shock state was only present in 47% of the episodes and proposed renaming this liver injury "hypoxic hepatitis" as hypoxia from a variety of etiologies (e.g., sepsis and respiratory failure) was present in all cases [21]. These findings were later confirmed by the final report from the same authors including 142 episodes [22] and by the series of 322 cases of ischemic hepatitis published later by Birrer et al. [23]. Thus, the term hypoxic hepatitis together with ACLI is currently used to name this entity. Some authors believe that ACLI provides more details about the underlying pathophysiological process as an acute cardiac event in a patient with an underlying congestive liver represents the most common clinical scenario [2, 5, 24, 25].

3.1 Epidemiology

The prevalence of ACLI among patients admitted to hospital varies greatly depending on the severity of illness. Indeed, in a recent meta-analysis of 1782 cases, ACLI was present in two every 1000 patients for all levels of hospital care but increased to 2.5 out of every 100 patients in intensive care units (ICUs) [26]. Studies including very critically ill patients have described maximum figures ranging from 11.9 to 21.9% [27–29]. Although previously debated [7], recent series indicate that the presence of a primary liver disease also increases the risk of ACLI. In a nationwide study including patients with hemodynamic instability, Waseem et al. observed a prevalence of acute liver injury of 22% in patients with underlying liver disease compared to only 3% in those without baseline hepatopathy [30].

These variations in frequency of ACLI not only respond to the severity of illness or the presence of a primary liver disease, as sometimes the diagnosis is overlooked clinically and variable cutoffs of transaminases are an important determinant of prevalence. Thus, in the previous meta-analysis, different liver enzyme cutoffs were used among studies as inclusion criteria, and the highest frequency of ACLI was among patients with increased serum aminotransferases above 1000 IU/L, where the prevalence reached 57% [26]. Therefore, current prevalence rates of ACLI might be underestimated [7, 12].

3.2 Pathophysiology

Liver damage in ACLI is the result of several mechanisms: passive congestion reduced hepatic blood flow, total body hypoxemia, inability to utilize oxygen, and ischemia/reperfusion injury. Necrosis, rather than apoptosis, is the main mode of death due to these mechanisms [31]. Although frequently multifactorial, the predominating mechanism of damage can be different depending on the underlying condition [7, 12]. In this regard, the most frequent diseases leading to ACLI are HF, respiratory failure, and septic shock, accounting for more than 90% of cases [7]. These diseases often coexist and lead to ACLI. Hence, Fuhrmann et al. identified more than one disease contributing to ACLI in 74% of their study population [27].

As mentioned previously, HF represents the main underlying condition in ACLI. The proportion of ACLI cases due to HF published in the literature ranges from 39 to 78% [7, 12, 22, 23, 26–28]. In this condition, the main mechanisms involved in the development of ACLI are passive congestion and ischemia of the liver. Indeed, in this scenario, ACLI is believed to reflect the extreme of a spectrum of liver injury that begins with passive hepatic congestion since the vast majority of patients have markedly elevated cardiac filling pressures [17, 22, 26, 32, 33]. Thus, several studies have shown how, despite similar hemodynamic derangements, only those with a pre-existing congestive liver developed ACLI [23, 29, 33]. This crucial role of passive congestion of the liver justifies the rare occurrence of ACLI in hemorrhagic or hypovolemic shock [7]. Most importantly, Seeto et al. showed that 15–20 minutes of hypotension is sufficient to provoke ACLI [33]. This explains why hemodynamic instability is not systematically observed, since such a brief period can easily be unrecognized.

Respiratory failure accounts for approximately 15% of ACLI cases [7]. Severe hypoxemia resulting from an exacerbation of chronic respiratory disease is the main mechanism leading to ACLI. Very low levels of arterial pressure in oxygen (i.e., under 40 mmHg) are commonly observed, as well as the coexistence of hepatic venous congestion. In this setting, cardiac output and hepatic blood flow are normal or even increased [22, 23].

Septic shock is the cause of ACLI in 15–30% of cases. The prime factor leading to hypoxia is both the increased demands of oxygen and the decreased ability of hepatocytes to utilize oxygen [7]. It has been postulated that inflammatory mediators and endotoxins may be behind this abnormal oxygen utilization [7, 34, 35]. Although at the initial phases of septic shock hepatic blood flow is increased, the progression from high to low cardiac output may occur rapidly and aggravate the hypoxic damage [12].

While the previously described mechanisms induced ACLI by causing liver hypoxia, it has been postulated that re-oxygenation is also required [7, 12]. Several observations support this role of ischemia/reperfusion injury in ACLI: (1) it has been described that liver cell necrosis occurs at the time of reperfusion not ischemia [7]; (2) the incidence and severity of CLN correlate with the duration of shock. In fulminant and refractory cardiogenic shock (median duration of shock was 3 hours), CLN was only observed in a minority of patients and was mild [21, 29], whereas earlier studies showed how the longer the period of shock the greater the severity and frequency of CLN [36, 37]. One explanation of these findings is that long-lasting shocks probably harbor transient periods of hemodynamic stability and re-oxygenation that can cause ischemia/reperfusion injury and subsequently induce ACLI. (3) In a minority of ACLI cases, liver necrosis is limited to the mediolobular zone and spares the centrilobular zone [38–40]. Henrion et al. postulated that this atypical histological pattern could be due to an incomplete liver reperfusion prior to death that only reached periportal and mediolobular liver cells. Hence, periportal and centrilobular cells would have survived, the former because of oxygen delivery remained sufficient, and the latter because of the absence of reperfusion injury. Mediolobular hepatocytes, on the other hand, would have been destroyed due to ischemia/reperfusion injury [7].

3.3 Clinical presentation and diagnosis

The majority of ACLI cases occur in elderly men (i.e., 65–70 years) with congestive HF that has deteriorated over the past few days. It must be highlighted that a shock state is far from being a constant feature as is observed in around half of the cases. Moreover, the cardiac component may not be apparent at first evaluation as usual signs of HF, such as painful hepatomegaly, ankle edema, or hepatojugular reflux, are frequently lacking. Therefore, the diagnosis of ACLI cannot be rejected because of the absence of shock and of signs of HF, and in case of uncertainty, a cardiac evaluation is warranted [6, 7]. Symptoms due to ACLI are often absent or resemble those from acute viral hepatitis [24], and more commonly, the clinical picture is dominated by symptoms of the underlying conditions. Overt jaundice is absent at admission, and encephalopathy can develop but is usually the result of hemodynamic instability and hypoxia, rather than liver failure [7, 12].

Laboratory tests show a substantial and rapid increase in aminotransferases and lactate dehydrogenase (LDH) levels to 10–20 times the upper limit of normal, usually 1–3 days after hemodynamic deterioration. These elevations generally return to normal within 7–10 days if hemodynamic stability is restored [3, 41]. A progressive increase in bilirubin is usually seen but is seldom severe [3, 7, 12]. The higher values reported by recent series may be explained by the inclusion of more patients with septic shock. Nonetheless, the mean bilirubin value in these studies was lower than 6 mg/dL [27, 28]. Higher values may suggest progression to acute liver failure [6]. Unlike in children where hypoglycemia has been regarded as a distinct feature of ACLI, in adults both hypoglycemia and hyperglycemia have been reported [7, 12]. Although no analytical alteration is pathognomonic of ACLI, there are some findings that suggest its diagnosis [7]: (1) an alanine aminotransferase (ALT)-to-LDH ratio <1.5 is of great help in the differential diagnosis as it is rarely seen in other etiologies of hepatitis [42]; (2) the aspartate aminotransferase (AST) generally peaks earlier and higher than ALT [41]. The rational behind this finding lays on the concentration of aminotransferases throughout the hepatic acinus. ALT reaches the highest concentration at the level of periportal hepatocytes (Rappaport liver zone 1) and the lowest concentration at the level of pericentral hepatocytes (Rappaport liver zone 3), while AST maintains a stable concentration throughout the entire acinus. Hence, after the hypoxic insult, the initial concentrations of AST are higher than those of ALT, since the lower oxygen concentration of pericentral hepatocytes makes them more susceptible to hypoxic damage [43]. Once the cause of liver damage is resolved, the concentration of ALT exceeds that of AST in subsequent days, due to its longer half-life (47 ± 10 hours versus 17 ± 5 hours, respectively) [44]. Aboelsoud et al. [41] universally observed this pattern, but it was only described in 75% of the cases in Henrion's study [22]. The rapid decline and reversal of the AST-ALT ratio may explain these differences, and therefore, an ALT higher than AST should not discard ACLI; (3) an early and sharp deterioration in prothrombin activity and renal function also supports ACLI. Such abnormalities are unusual at presentation in patients with viral or drug-induced hepatitis, unless ALF is already established [7]. **Figure 1** shows a typical biochemical profile of ACLI in a patient treated in our hospital.

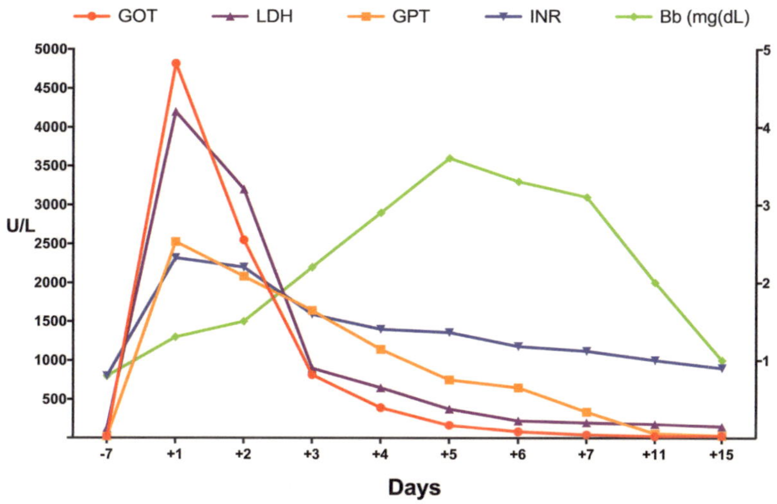

Figure 1.
Laboratory parameters during the course of ACLI in a patient with respiratory failure due to drug overdose. Abbreviations: AST: Aspartate aminotransferase; ALT: Alanine aminotransferase; LDH: Lactate dehydrogenase; Bb; bilirubin; INR: International normalized ratio.

In accordance with the above, diagnosis of ACLI is usually made when the following criteria are met [12, 22, 26]: (1) an appropriate clinical setting of cardiac, respiratory, or circulatory failure; (2) a severe increase in aminotransferase levels; and (3) exclusion of other causes of acute liver damage. The differential diagnosis for severe elevations of transaminases is relatively limited and includes ACLI, acute viral hepatitis, toxin- or drug-induced liver injury, autoimmune hepatitis, Wilson's disease, acute bile duct obstruction, and acute Budd-Chiari syndrome [44]. Imaging techniques are essential to rule out some of these etiologies and can also support the diagnosis by finding a dilation of inferior vena cava and suprahepatic veins due to passive congestion [7]. Liver biopsy is rarely necessary and only when the underlying cause remains unclear. It will show features of coagulative necrosis of centrilobular hepatocytes without significant inflammation (**Figure 2A–C**). In biopsies delayed several days, however, there may be neutrophils infiltrating the affected regions [25]. As already stated, necrosis rarely occurs predominantly in the middle zone [38–40].

3.4 Prognosis and treatment

The prognosis of ACLI is poor with an overall hospital mortality of 51% [26] and 1-year survival rate of approximately 25% [7]. The cause of death is usually the underlying condition, as it is an uncommon cause of ALF. In a study from the Acute Liver Failure Study Group, only 4.4% of the ALF cases had ACLI as their final diagnosis [45]. Nevertheless, there is some indirect evidence that suggests that ACLI influences outcome in this setting. Hence, prolonged international normalized ratio (INR) and jaundice have been identified as independent risk factors for ACLI mortality [27, 28, 41, 46]. Other factors that have been associated with increased risk of in-hospital mortality include a baseline liver disease [30], higher elevations of transaminases [27, 45], LDH [27, 41], serum phosphate [45], concomitant renal failure [28, 41], septic shock [27, 28], and more advanced encephalopathy [45].

The management of the underlying diseases remains the only established treatment for ACLI. Although data are limited, some experts recommend using N-acetylcysteine, avoiding excessive vascular filling to minimize passive congestion of the liver, and favoring the use of dobutamine in patients with low cardiac index given its inotropic and vasodilating effects [2, 3, 7, 12].

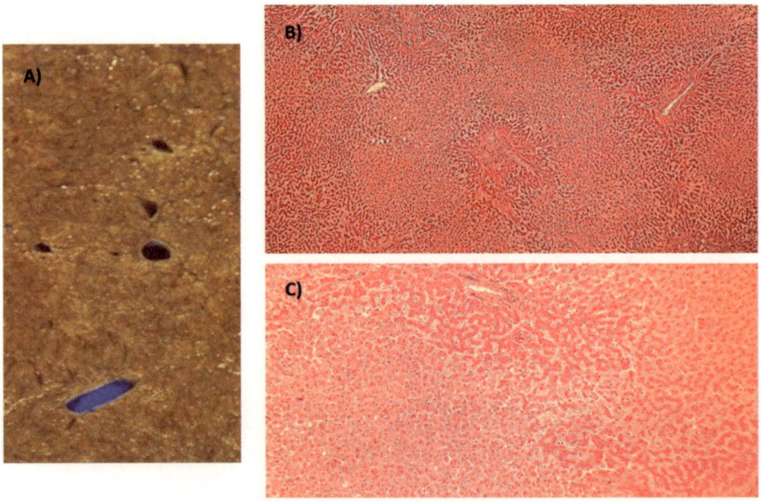

Figure 2.
(A) Postmortem example of a liver with ischemic zones around centrilobular veins. (B) Centrilobular regions show congestion and coagulative necrosis (hematoxylin-eosin). (C) Same findings than 2.B with greater magnification.

4. Congestive hepatopathy (CH)

Liver disease as a consequence of HF has been known for a long time. The histological description of the "nutmeg," congestive liver is attributed to Kiernan in 1833 [25, 47]. Earlier studies from the beginning of the twentieth century started providing data on the structural and functional changes that develop in the liver in the setting of HF [47, 48]. The classic work from Sheila Sherlock, published in 1951, stood for decades as the standard reference on this entity. In this article, the renowned author correlated liver tests, systemic hemodynamic parameters, and histology [47]. Progress has been made since then, but there are still important gaps concerning its pathophysiology, assessment of liver fibrosis, and clinical impact on overall HF prognosis [2, 6].

4.1 Epidemiology

CH occurs in the setting of any cause of right ventricular failure such as constrictive pericarditis, mitral stenosis, severe tricuspid regurgitation, cor pulmonale, or end-stage cardiomyopathies [8, 49]. The current spectrum of CH differs from earlier reports due to several reasons [3, 4, 6, 50]: (1) the etiology of HF has changed over the years with ischemic cardiomyopathy surpassing rheumatic valvular disease; (2) after major advances in medical treatment and the widespread use of heart transplantation, the prognosis of HF has greatly improved, and as a result, cardiac cirrhosis is declining; (3) these same medical advances are responsible for the improved survival of patients with a variety of congenital heart diseases that lead to right HF. The most illustrative example is the Fontan procedure to palliate single-ventricle physiology. Unlike patients with acquired heart disease, these patients may develop "cardiac cirrhosis" in early adulthood.

This heterogeneous cause of CH together with the limited validated techniques available to diagnose and, specially, stage the disease may explain that the burden of CH has not yet been adequately described [51]. Non-congenital HF studies using liver blood tests to determine the prevalence of CH have described figures ranging from 15 to 80%, depending on the severity of heart disease [24, 52–57]. However, liver blood tests neither accurately diagnose CH nor reflect the stage of liver disease [51]. Future studies should use a more comprehensive approach to overcome these biases and to provide solid data on this issue.

4.2 Pathophysiology

Congestion produces liver damage through several pathogenic mechanisms: (1) increased sinusoidal pressure leads to hepatic stellate cell activation and decreases nitric oxide production by endothelial cells through shear stress, all of which induce sinusoidal ischemia and promote fibrogenesis [51, 58]; (2) decreased hepatic blood flow further aggravates liver ischemia. Portal venous inflow is reduced as a result of the transmission of the elevated central venous pressure to the sinusoidal network, while arterial flow can also be compromised in patients who also harbor a left-sided HF [8, 51]; (3) Accumulation of exudate into the space of Disse due to the existing congestion impairs diffusion of oxygen and nutrients to hepatocytes and accelerates fibrosis pathways [8]; (4) Sinusoidal stasis and congestion promote sinusoidal thrombosis, which in turn contributes to liver fibrosis by causing parenchymal extinction and by activating hepatic stellate cells via protease-activated receptors [59, 60]. The former refers to a hypothesis based on retrospective observations of ex-vivo human liver specimens of patients with CH. In this autopsy study, Wanless et al. demonstrated sinusoidal thrombi confined to areas of fibrosis, thereby suggesting that intrahepatic thrombosis is involved in liver fibrosis progression [61]. A recent experimental study provided evidence of the mechanistic link between CH and liver fibrosis through this mechanism [58]. These findings settle the rational basis for testing anticoagulant drugs in patients with CH, but so far, no clinical trial has addressed this issue. In comparison, research in this area in primary liver cirrhosis is more advanced. Hence, several experimental studies have shown that anticoagulant therapy improves liver fibrosis and reduces portal hypertension [62–73], and a clinical trial demonstrated that anticoagulation led to a reduction in portal thrombosis and other complications of liver disease and to increase in survival [74]. New clinical trials are needed in order to confirm these preliminary results and to establish whether the stage of liver disease may influence its efficacy [75].

It must be highlighted that contrary to primary liver diseases, in CH inflammation seems to play no role in the progression of liver fibrosis. Indeed, several studies of patients with Fontan circulation demonstrated minimal inflammatory changes in liver biopsy specimens, despite accentuated hepatic fibrosis [76–78].

4.3 Clinical presentation and diagnosis

CH may be asymptomatic for a long time, and frequently, its presence is suspected through abnormalities in liver tests [8]. Symptoms attributed to CH may include dull right upper quadrant pain, nausea, vomiting, anorexia, early satiety, malaise, and mild jaundice [3]. The abdominal symptoms respond to the stretching of the liver capsule due to hepatic congestion and may occur in the absence of overt ascites or lower extremity edema. These symptoms, however, are usually masked by those related to right-sided HF [2].

Physical examination may often show hepatomegaly and signs of HF, including hepatojugular reflux and peripheral edema. A pulsatile liver may also be seen, and its loss suggests progression to cardiac cirrhosis [49]. Overt ascites is also a frequent finding, although it is rarely refractory. In a series of 83 patients with CH of whom only one had established cardiac cirrhosis, up to 57% had ascites. Moreover, ascites and edema had no relation to the extent of liver fibrosis, and therefore, they are due to elevated right-sided cardiac pressure hitting the sinusoidal network [50]. The differentiation of cardiac ascites from cirrhotic ascites can be cumbersome. In these conditions, the serum-ascites albumin gradient is ≥1.1 g/dL since they both respond to hepatic sinusoidal hypertension [79]. There are, however, some ascites findings that are useful to make a differential diagnosis. Cardiac ascites has higher protein levels (>2.5 g/dL). This is due to preserved liver synthetic function and absence of capillarization of the liver sinusoidal endothelial cells [3, 8, 80]. The latter refers to the lost of fenestrae and development of a basement membrane by these cells as a consequence of liver fibrosis. In cirrhosis, these features make hepatic sinusoids less leaky and prevent the passage of proteins to the space of Disse and from here to the peritoneal fluid [81]. Other less reliable findings in cardiac ascites are higher LDH levels and higher red blood cell counts due to leaking of red blood cells into the ascites via lymph tissue, with resulting lysis [80]. Despite these differences, a significant number of cases are still misclassified. Measurement of serum B-type natriuretic peptide (BNP) or of its inactive pro-hormone (N-terminal-proBNP) in serum and ascites has been recently suggested as an aid tool in uncertain cases. Thus, Sheer et al. reported that both serum and ascites NT-proBNP levels had high sensitivity and specificity in predicting HF as the cause of ascites [82]. More recently, Farias et al. found serum BNP to be superior to the total ascitic fluid protein concentration with regard to discriminating cardiac ascites from cirrhotic ascites. A serum BNP cutoff of >364 pg/mL had 98% sensitivity, 99% specificity, 99% diagnostic accuracy, and a positive likelihood ratio of 168.1 for the diagnosis of cardiac ascites. Conversely, a serum BNP cutoff of ≤182 pg/mL was excellent for ruling out ascites due to heart failure [79].

The differentiation of cardiac cirrhotic ascites from cardiac ascites without cirrhosis is especially challenging and of great clinical importance. On the one hand, the diagnosis of cardiac cirrhosis warrants further evaluations such as bi-annual surveillance ultrasonography or endoscopic screening for esophageal varices. On the other hand, its presence may preclude a heart transplant or require a combined heart-liver transplant. Apart from some diagnostic tools such as liver biopsy and hepatic venous pressure gradient (HVPG) that will be later discussed, there are some clinical clues that help in the differential diagnosis. In patients with cardiac ascites without cirrhosis, splenomegaly and spider angiomata are absent, and varices are rarely identified on upper endoscopy [3, 49]. This can be explained by the fact that varices represent collateral vessels from the high-pressure portal system to the low-pressure systemic circulation, and in CH without cirrhosis, no pressure gradient exists because pressure remains high along the entire path of venous return to the right atrium [50]. Complications of cirrhosis may occur in the late stages of cardiac cirrhosis. Although in the past the traditional patient with cardiac cirrhosis died from his cardiac disease before progressing to decompensated cirrhosis, advances in medical and surgical treatments are responsible for the increased number of liver complications in this setting [3]. The risk of hepatocarcinoma after the Fontan procedure is probably the best example. The success of this surgery to palliate right-sided congenital heart lesions permits long-term survival in the setting of elevated right-sided heart pressures. Eventually, the liver disease could become as clinically important as the cardiac disease and further complicate its management [51].

Besides the presence of right-sided HF (or other cause of high central pressures) and the aforementioned clinical findings, the diagnosis of CH should be further supported on compatible results of diagnostic tools and exclusion of other possible causes of liver disease [49, 50].

4.3.1 Biochemical profile

Elevation of serum cholestasis markers (alkaline phosphatase, GGT, and bilirubin) is characteristic of CH. Total bilirubin levels rarely exceed 3 mg/dL, and indirect bilirubin usually predominates over direct bilirubin [3]. The degree of cholestasis is related to the severity of both the elevation of right atrial pressure and tricuspid regurgitation [55, 83]. These data suggest that elevated right-sided filling pressures may contribute more to LFT elevation than reduced cardiac output [2]. The mechanism of cholestasis in this setting is thought to be due to the compression of the bile canaliculi and small ductules by centrally congested sinusoids [25]. Other laboratory findings include mild elevations of serum aminotransferases to two to three times the upper limit of normal and mild hypoalbuminemia. The latter may also be secondary to malnutrition or protein-losing enteropathy [8]. As liver disease progresses, liver function tests (i.e., bilirubin, INR, and albumin) may continue to worsen. Importantly, liver enzymes are often normal, and in the presence of other findings suggestive of CH, this diagnosis cannot be ruled out based on these normal values [3]. As already discussed, CH predisposes the liver to ACLI in the face of hemodynamic instability, instigating the aforementioned marked elevation of liver enzymes [8].

4.3.2 Imaging tests

Imaging tests help both to support the diagnosis of CH and to identify complications. Characteristic conventional imaging findings include dilation of inferior vena cava and hepatic veins, loss of normal triphasic hepatic venous wave-form, and abnormal kinetics of intravenous contrast enhancement (e.g., delayed bolus arrival to the liver suggesting slow systemic circulation, diffusion of extracellular contrast media into the periportal lymphatic space in the delayed phase, retrograde hepatic venous opacification during the early phase of intravenous contrast material injection into the upper extremities, and a predominantly peripheral heterogeneous pattern of hepatic enhancement due to stagnant blood flow) [84] (**Figure 3A**, **B**). Importantly, the appearance of a nodular or heterogeneous liver on standard imaging is not sufficient to diagnosis cirrhosis in CH [51].

CH may lead to the generation of benign regenerative nodules or focal nodular hyperplasia (FNH)-like lesions and hepatocarcinoma. The former is referred to as "FNH-like" despite having characteristic pathological findings of FNH due to the presence of abnormal background liver parenchyma. Although they most commonly demonstrate typical imaging findings (i.e., well-circumscribed, homogeneous nodule with late arterial hyperenhancement that fades to isointensity/isoattenuation on delayed phase imaging), they sometimes have a washout appearance that could be mistaken for hepatocarcinoma due to abnormally increased background parenchymal enhancement in the delayed phase [84] (**Figure 4**). Indeed, distinguishing hepatocarcinoma from these atypical imaging represents an unmet need, and biopsy is frequently required for accurate diagnosis. Radiological findings that support the diagnosis of hepatocarcinoma include the following: significant change in appearance of a nodule, venous invasion, a heterogeneous-appearing mass, and elevated alpha-fetoprotein [51, 84]. There are currently no screening guidelines for hepatocarcinoma in CH. In post-Fontan patients, some experts recommend to begin screening at 15–20 years after the operation [51], while the newly released guidelines from the American Heart Association recommend a much more comprehensive surveillance (**Table 1**) [85]. In patients with CH due to other conditions, it seems reasonable to perform bi-annual screening once cardiac cirrhosis is established.

4.3.3 Histology

The congestive liver explant has been characterized as a "nutmeg liver" due to the presence of dark centrilobular zones that reflect sinusoidal congestion alternating with pale periportal zones with normal or fatty liver tissue [84] (**Figure 5A**). Characteristic histological findings include sinusoidal dilatation and congestion, hepatocyte atrophy most prominent in zone 3, extravasation of red blood cells into the space of Disse, regenerative hyperplasia emerging from periportal regions, and

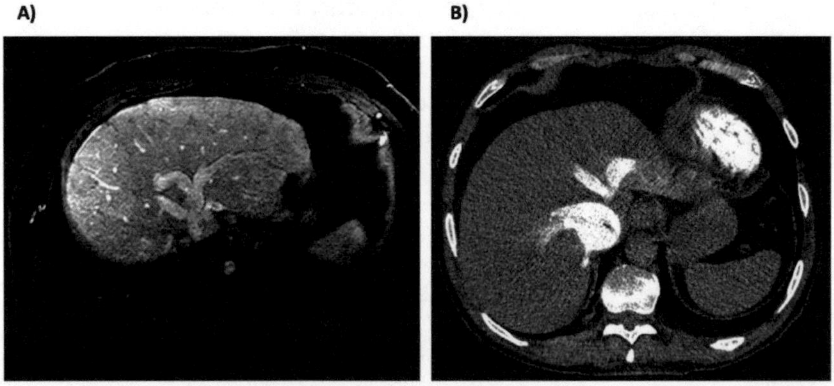

Figure 3.
(A) Idiopathic membranous inferior vena cava obstruction in a 44-year-old man. MRI shows a mildly nodular liver with altered parenchymal perfusion and dilatation of hepatic veins. (B) Severe tricuspid regurgitation in a 49-year-old man. CT scan shows dilatation of hepatic veins and reflux of contrast into the inferior vena cava and hepatic veins.

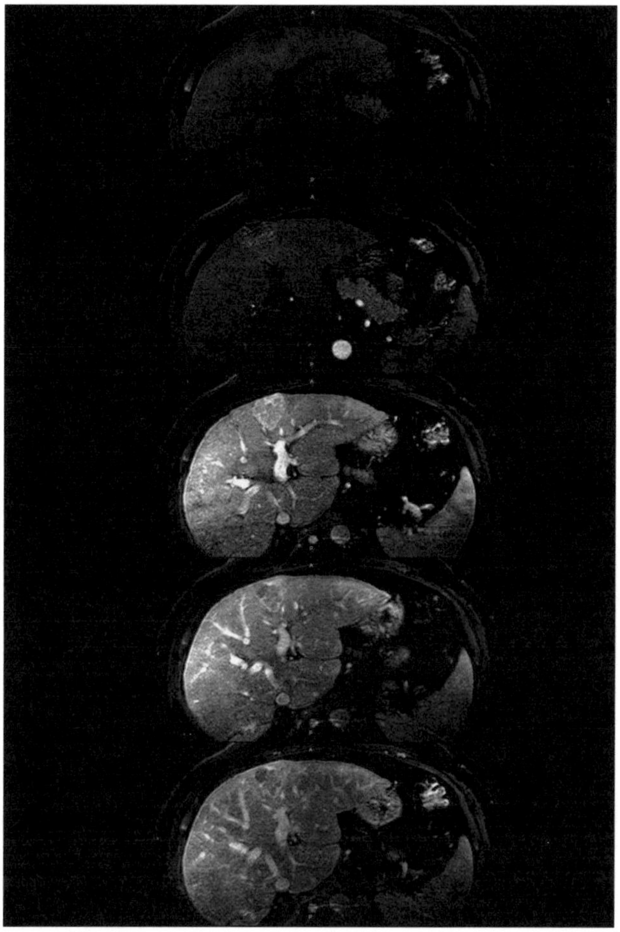

Figure 4.
Idiopathic membranous inferior vena cava obstruction in a 44-year-old man. The image shows the dynamic phase of MRI. Besides the significant hypertrophy of segment I, MRI shows a mass (3.8 cm × 4.2 cm) that after administration of intravenous contrast presents a heterogeneous enhancement in the arterial phase with washout in the portal phase. Liver biopsy showed histological changes compatible with focal nodular hyperplasia.

centrilobular fibrosis (**Figure 5B**, **C**) [25]. The degree of sinusoidal dilatation is positively correlated with the degree of elevation of right atrial pressure. As liver disease progresses, bridging fibrosis typically extends between central veins to produce a pattern that has been name "reversed lobulation" since it contrasts to the typical fibrosis pattern found in most primary liver diseases where bridging fibrosis occurs between portal triads (i.e., zone 1) [3]. As far as the correlation between fibrosis extension and systemic hemodynamic parameters is concerned, there are discordant results with most studies finding no correlation [50, 54, 86–89].

It must be highlighted that the distribution of fibrosis throughout the liver is extremely heterogeneous in patients with CH [86, 90], and it may be explained by the fibrogenic effects of intrahepatic thrombosis caused by static blood flow [61]. This variability raises concern about sampling error and about the role of liver biopsy as the gold standard tool for fibrosis assessment. Moreover, liver biopsies may not predict post-heart transplant outcomes. In a retrospective study, Louie et al. found that the presence of bridging fibrosis was not significantly associated with post-operative survival or post-operative liver failure, based on which they concluded that patients with bridging fibrosis may still be considered viable

	Basic*	In-Depth*	Investigational*
Childhood (every 3–4 years)	• CMP • Platelet count • Serum GGT	• PT/INR • Serum FibroSure biomarkers • Serum α-fetoprotein • Abdominal ultrasound • Total serum cholesterol	• Liver imaging via CT or MRI • Liver elastography (ultrasound or MRI) • Liver biopsy
Adolescence (every 1–3 years)	• CMP • Platelet count • Serum GGT • PT/INR	• Serum FibroSure biomarkers • Serum α-fetoprotein • Abdominal ultrasound • Total serum cholesterol • Liver imaging via CT or MRI • Liver elastography (ultrasound or MRI)	• Liver biopsy
Adulthood (every 1–2 years)	• CMP • Platelet count • Serum GGT • PT/INR • Total serum cholesterol • Abdominal ultrasound	• Serum FibroSure biomarkers • Serum α-fetoprotein • Liver imaging via CT or MRI • Liver elastography (ultrasound or MRI)	• Liver biopsy

**Tests are stratified as basic (fundamental and rudimentary level of assessment), in-depth (more detailed level of characterization), and investigational (possible or likely of value; however, greater experience and study may be necessary before widespread use can be suggested).*
Abbreviations: CMP: comprehensive metabolic panel; CT: computed tomography; GGT: γ-glutamyl transferase; INR: international normalized ratio; MRI: magnetic resonance imaging; PT: prothrombin time.

Table 1.
Tests recommended by the American Heart Association for surveillance of liver disease in post-Fontan patients.

candidates for isolated heart transplantation [90]. Similar results were described by Dhall et al. [86]. Regardless of these limitations, liver biopsy still plays an important role in the assessment of the stage of liver disease, in ruling out hepatocarcinoma and alternative etiologies of liver disease and in determining candidacy for isolated heart transplantation or combined heart-liver transplantation. Its findings, however, should be correlated with the clinical presentation and results of other diagnostic tools [51, 86].

4.3.4 Non-invasive assessment of liver fibrosis

Non-invasive diagnostic tests of liver fibrosis have been extensively studied and have excellent predictive value for advanced fibrosis in patients with viral hepatitis and non-alcoholic fatty liver disease [91]. Nevertheless, the performance of these tests in assessing the severity of fibrosis in CH is poor. A detail description of each of these tests in this setting is beyond the scope of this chapter and can be found elsewhere [51, 92, 93].

Briefly, among serological markers, the Model for End-Stage Liver Disease (MELD)-XI score has been suggested to be potentially useful as some studies have

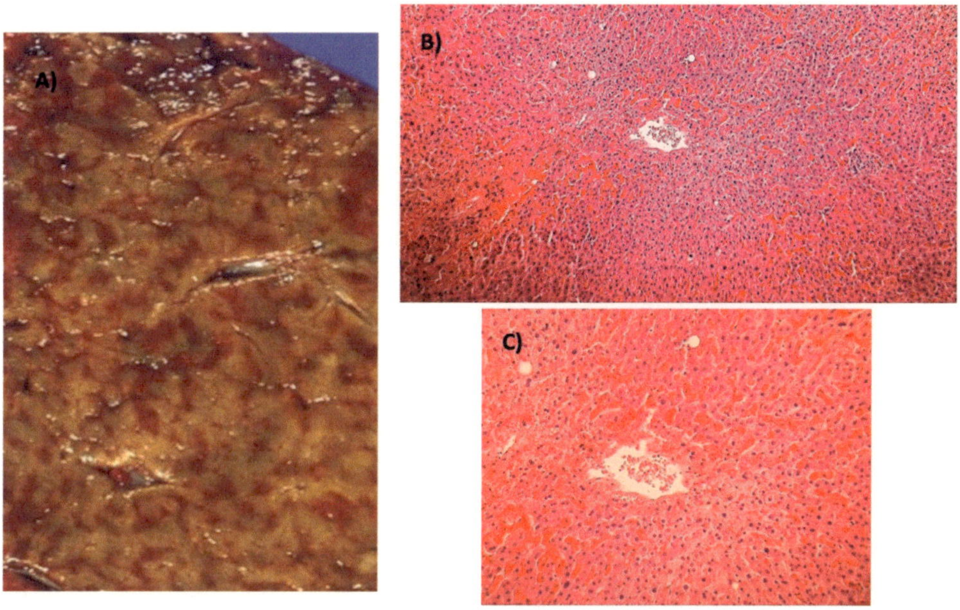

Figure 5.
(A) Postmortem example of the classical "nutmeg" liver with centrilobular congestion in CH. (B) Centrilobular regions show congestion and extravasation of red blood cells. (C) Same findings than 5.B with greater magnification.

shown a moderate correlation with the stage of fibrosis in post-Fontan patients [94, 95]. This score excludes INR given the high prevalence of anticoagulation use in CH. Despite these results, further studies are needed as other studies have described opposite results [78, 90]. The remaining tests (i.e., standard serum markers, FibroSure testing, hyaluronic acid levels, and most clinical risk calculators) are inaccurate at staging liver fibrosis [51]. The use of liver stiffness tools is hampered by the fact that congestion increases liver stiffness values [91]. Hence, in CH, it provides unreliable information regarding the grade of fibrosis, although some evidence suggests that liver and spleen stiffness calculated by magnetic resonance elastography may be more accurate. Finally, new advances in imaging techniques, such as magnetic resonance imaging with diffusion-weighted imaging, may potentially differentiate fibrosis from congestion but require validation [51].

4.3.5 Hepatic hemodynamic study

Hepatic vein catheterization with measurement of the HVPG is currently the gold standard technique for determining portal pressure. It represents the difference between the wedged hepatic venous pressure (WHVP) and the free hepatic venous pressure (FHVP). The WHVP is usually measured by occluding the right hepatic vein through the inflation of a balloon, whereas the FHVP is measured without occluding it. The occlusion of the vein forms a continuous static column of blood between the catheter and the hepatic sinusoids. Thus, WHVP measures sinusoidal pressure. Due to the scarce connections between sinusoids existing in cirrhosis, pressure cannot be decompressed through the sinusoidal network, and therefore, WHVP reflects portal pressure in this setting. FHVP, on the other hand, is a surrogate for inferior vena cava pressure. Normal values of HVPG are <5 mmHg. The HVPG is a strong and independent predictor of outcomes in compensated and decompensated cirrhosis due to primary liver diseases [96–98].

The diagnostic and prognostic value of HVPG measurement in CH has not been adequately assessed. In this context, both FHVP and WHPV are elevated, and the HVPG is within the normal range (**Figure 6**). Once cardiac cirrhosis is established, the HVPG is expected to increase beyond 6 mmHg (**Figure** 7) [51]. Hence, HVPG could theoretically provide relevant information about the stage of CH. The few clinical studies that have provided hemodynamic data in this regard have described inconsistent results. For instance, in the study of Myers et al., esophageal varices were seen in some patients despite having a HVPG below 6 mmHg. As previously explained, the high pressures along the entire path of venous return to the right atrium prevent the formation of varices unless the establishment of cirrhosis creates a pressure gradient between the portal and systemic circulation. In order to explain these discordant results, the same authors argued that it was possible that the varices observed in a few patients represented either false-positive endoscopies or undetected concomitant disease such as portal vein thrombosis [50]. Moreover, it has not yet been demonstrated that the HVPG correlates with the stage of fibrosis in CH [50, 86]. These findings probably respond to several confounders: the inclusion of few patients with advanced fibrosis, the variable distribution of fibrosis throughout the liver, and the absence of a full and reliable characterization of the liver disease. As far as its prognostic utility is concerned, no study has evaluated the HVPG for predicting hepatic decompensation events and survival after isolated heart transplantation [51]. Despite this, many academic centers, including our own, measure the HVPG to assist in the transplant decision-making process. Finally, it must be reminded that the hepatic vein catheterization also allows performing a transjugular liver biopsy. This technique is safer than the percutaneous biopsy and can be performed even under anticoagulation or ascites [99].

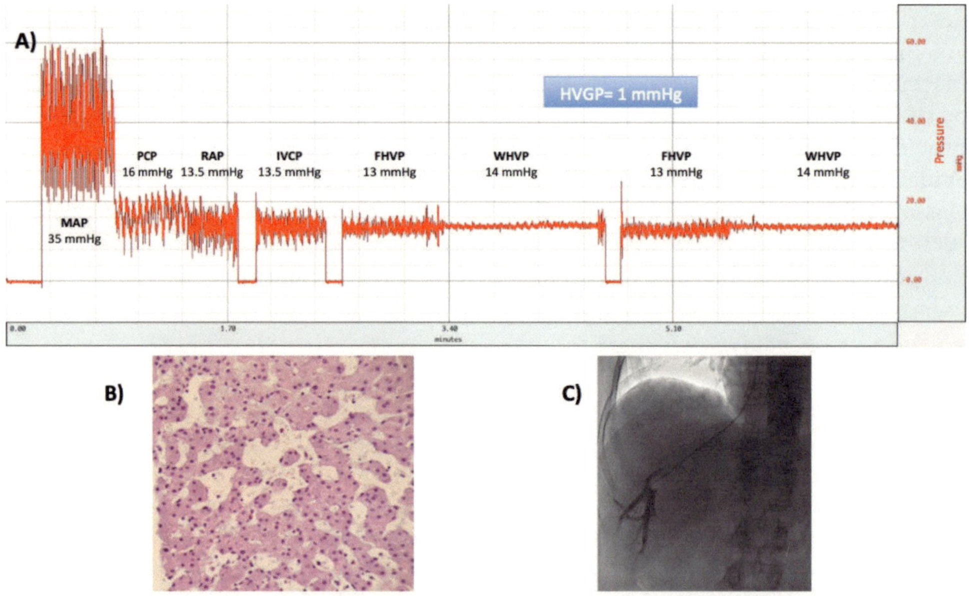

Figure 6.
(A) A typical hemodynamic tracing of a patient with congestive hepatopathy due to cor pulmonale. The HVPG is calculated as the difference between WHVP and FHVP. Both of them are elevated, but the HVPG is within the normal range. (B) Transjugular liver biopsy was performed and showed sinusoidal dilatation without significant fibrosis (hematoxylin-eosin stain; the image of Masson stain is not shown). (C) Occlusion of the hepatic vein with the balloon catheter. Abbreviations: MAP: Mean pulmonary arterial pressure; PCP: Pulmonary capillary pressure; RAP: Right atrial pressure; IVCP: Inferior vena cava pressure; FHVP: Free hepatic venous pressure; WHVP: Wedged hepatic venous pressure; HVPG: Hepatic venous pressure gradient.

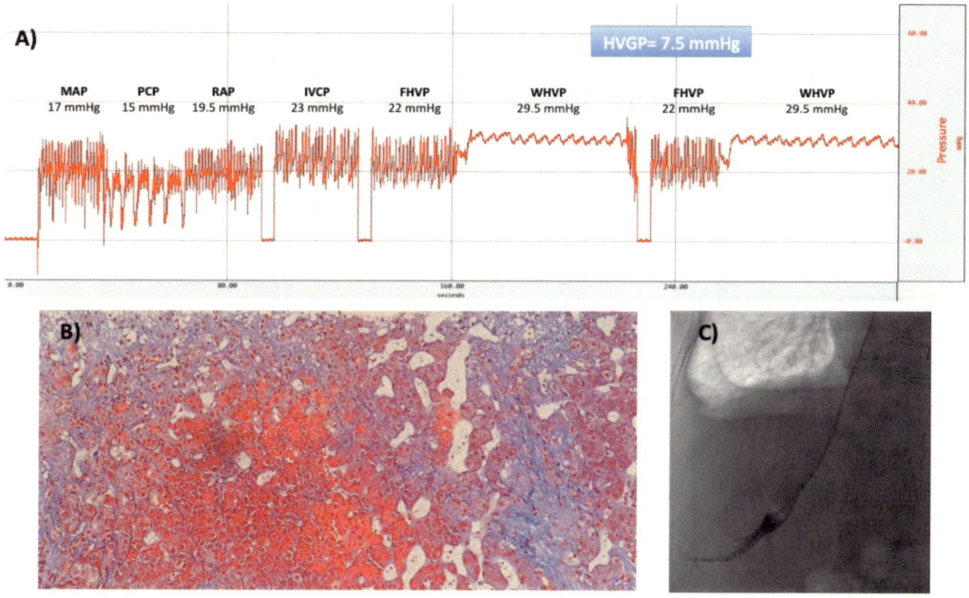

Figure 7.
(A) A typical hemodynamic tracing of a patient with severe tricuspid regurgitation and concomitant hepatitis C. The HVPG is calculated as the difference between WHVP and FHVP. Both of them are elevated, and the HVPG is slightly elevated. (B) Transjugular liver biopsy was performed and showed significant fibrosis forming nodules (Masson stain). (C) Occlusion of the hepatic vein with the balloon catheter. Abbreviations: MAP: Mean pulmonary arterial pressure; PCP: Pulmonary capillary pressure; RAP: Right atrial pressure; IVCP: Inferior vena cava pressure; FHVP: Free hepatic venous pressure; WHVP: Wedged hepatic venous pressure; HVPG: Hepatic venous pressure gradient.

4.4 Prognosis and treatment

The underlying cardiac disease generally determines prognosis in CH. Liver enzymes (i.e., bilirubin, alkaline phosphatase, GGT, and albumin) and scores such as the MELD and MELD-XI have been associated with prognosis in HF patients [53, 56, 100–103]. Based on these findings, both the American College of Cardiology and the European Society of Cardiology Heart Failure Guidelines recommend the inclusion of liver function tests in the diagnostic workup of all patients presenting with HF [1, 104]. However, it must be pointed out that they predict cardiac or overall mortality, not liver-related mortality. Therefore, they seem to act as indirect markers of the severity of cardiac disease rather than reflecting the effect of liver disease on outcomes. Indeed, the effect of cardiac cirrhosis on overall prognosis has not been clearly established [6].

Management of the underlying cardiac disease is the mainstay of treatment. There is no specific therapy of CH [8]. Concerns about modification of drug dosage have been raised, although there are no solid rules in this regard. This is partially explained by the lack of correlation of available diagnostic tools with the hepatic function [5]. Theoretically more relevant are the detrimental effects that some of the medical therapies used to treat HF may have on the physiopathology of cirrhosis. For instance, vasodilators such as angiotensin-converting-enzyme inhibitors are contraindicated in decompensated cirrhosis, and doses of diuretics in HF are often higher than in cirrhosis and may precipitate hepatorenal syndrome [3]. Again, no solid recommendations are available, and treatment modifications should be patient-specific. Eventually, some patients will require a heart transplant, and this poses the question of whether the liver is "in shape" to tolerate a heart transplant.

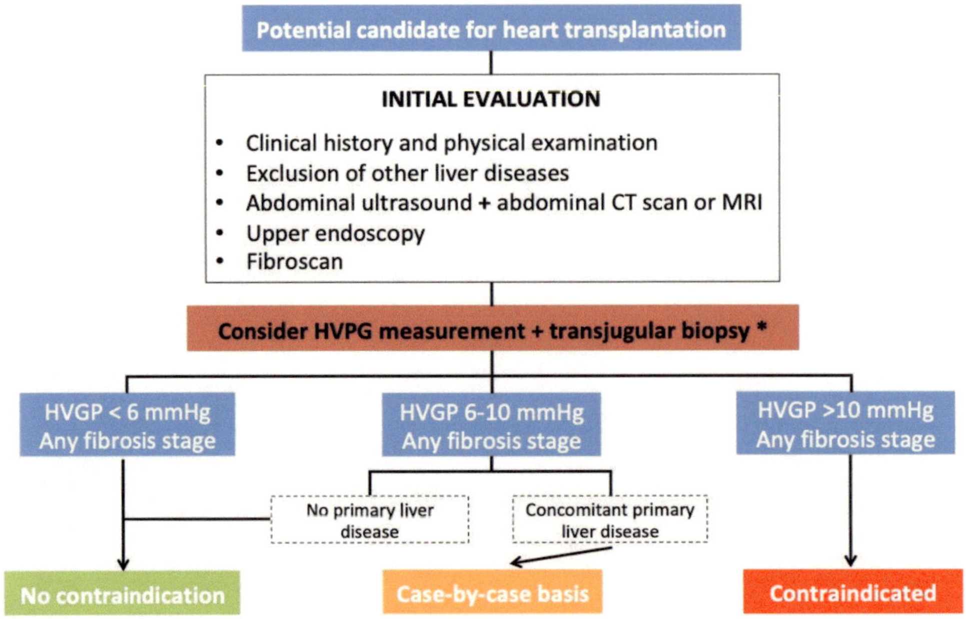

Figure 8.
Protocol to determine the recommendation regarding liver disease in a potential candidate for a heart transplant when CH is suspected. We proceed to HVPG measurement and transjugular biopsy in those patients in whom advanced liver disease cannot be ruled out after the initial evaluation (e.g., nodular appearance of the liver). Our recommendation is hemodynamic-dependent, regardless of the fibrosis stage. In cases with a HVPG below 5 mmHg, there is no contraindication to perform an isolated heart transplant, whereas a HVPG >10 mmHg discards it (no combined heart-liver transplantation has been performed so far in our hospital). In patients with a concomitant primary liver disease and a HVPG between 6 and 10 mmHg, the decision is patient-specific and relies mainly on the type of disease. If it is treatable (e.g., hepatitis C or B), we recommend proceeding with the heart transplant. Same recommendation is given in the absence of a primary liver disease and a HVPG between 6 and 10 mmHg. Abbreviations: CT: Computed tomography; MRI: Magnetic resonance imaging; HVPG: Hepatic venous pressure gradient.

4.5 Determining candidacy for heart transplantation

Given the aforementioned limitations of available invasive and non-invasive tests to assess hepatic fibrosis and function, determining whether a patient with CH is a candidate for isolated heart transplantation or may require a combined heart-liver transplantation is especially challenging. Not surprisingly, there are no official guidelines, evaluation is institution dependent, and the decision is often taken on a case-by-case basis. It must be highlighted that cardiac cirrhosis may be reversed after heart transplantation. Based on this premise, some centers use an HVPG value of <12 mmHg as a cutoff for offering isolated heart transplantation instead of combined heart-liver transplantation. Nevertheless, this protocol requires validation before its widespread use in clinical practice. **Figure 8** shows our protocol for determining our recommendation regarding liver disease in a potential candidate for a heart transplant when CH is suspected.

5. Take-home messages and pitfalls facing management

- The diagnosis of ACLI cannot be rejected because of the absence of shock and of signs of HF, and in case of uncertainty, a cardiac evaluation is warranted.

- CH is frequently observed in patients suffering ACLI since it predisposes the liver to hypoxic damage.

- Diagnosis of ACLI can be suspected based on the following analytical alterations: ALT-to-LDH ratio <1.5, AST higher than ALT at initial phase, and an early and sharp deterioration in prothrombin activity and renal function.

- The current spectrum of CH differs from earlier reports with HF due to ischemic cardiomyopathy and congenital heart disease having surpassed rheumatic valvular disease.

- Contrary to primary liver diseases, inflammation seems to play no role in the progression of liver fibrosis in CH.

- The clinical picture of CH is usually masked by symptoms and signs related to right-sided HF.

- There are some ascites findings that help differentiate cardiac ascites from cirrhotic ascites: higher protein (>2.5 g/dL) and LDH levels, and higher red blood cell counts. Serum BNP also seems to be a useful tool in this regard.

- The diagnosis of cardiac cirrhosis warrants further evaluations such as bi-annual surveillance ultrasonography or endoscopic screening for esophageal varices.

- CH may lead to the generation of benign regenerative nodules and hepatocarcinoma. Distinguishing one from the other frequently requires a liver biopsy due to the abnormal background liver parenchyma.

- In contrast to most primary liver diseases where bridging fibrosis occurs between portal triads, in CH it typically extends between central veins to produce a "reversed lobulation" pattern.

- The distribution of fibrosis throughout the liver is extremely heterogeneous in CH leading to sampling error. Moreover, fibrosis stage determined by liver biopsies does not seem to predict post-heart transplant outcomes.

- The performance of non-invasive diagnostic tests of liver fibrosis in CH is poor.

- HVPG measurement might be a useful tool for assessing the stage of CH and helps in the decision-making process of transplant candidacy. However, no evidence in this regard has been published so far.

- In both ACLI and CH, the prognosis is dependent on the underlying condition, and treatment is focused on the latter.

Conflict of interest

The authors declare no conflict of interest.

Author details

Jose Ignacio Fortea[1,2,3], Ángela Puente[1,2,3], Antonio Cuadrado[1,2,3], Patricia Huelin[1,2,3], Inés García[1], Marta Mayorga[4], Raul Pellon[5], Javier Crespo[1,2,3] and Emilio Fábrega[1,2,3]*

1 Gastroenterology and Hepatology Department, Marqués de Valdecilla University Hospital, Santander, Spain

2 Infection, Immunity and Digestive Pathology Group, Research Institute Marqués de Valdecilla (IDIVAL), Santander, Spain

3 Network Center for Biomedical Research in Hepatic and Digestive Diseases (CIBERehd), Madrid, Spain

4 Pathological Anatomy Service, Marqués de Valdecilla University Hospital, Santander, Spain

5 Radiology Department, Marqués de Valdecilla University Hospital, Santander, Spain

*Address all correspondence to: digfge@humv.es

References

[1] Ponikowski P, Voors AA, Anker SD, Bueno H, Cleland JG, Coats AJ, et al. 2016 ESC guidelines for the diagnosis and treatment of acute and chronic heart failure: The task force for the diagnosis and treatment of acute and chronic heart failure of the European Society of Cardiology (ESC). Developed with the special contribution of the heart failure association (HFA) of the ESC. European Journal of Heart Failure. 2016;**18**:891-975

[2] Samsky MD, Patel CB, DeWald TA, Smith AD, Felker GM, Rogers JG, et al. Cardiohepatic interactions in heart failure: An overview and clinical implications. Journal of the American College of Cardiology. 2013;**61**:2397-2405

[3] Ford RM, Book W, Spivey JR. Liver disease related to the heart. Transplantation Reviews. 2015;**29**:33-37

[4] Fouad YM, Yehia R. Hepato-cardiac disorders. World Journal of Hepatology. 2014;**6**:41-54

[5] Cagli K, Basar FN, Tok D, Turak O, Basar O. How to interpret liver function tests in heart failure patients? Turkish Journal of Gastroenterology. 2015;**26**:197-203

[6] Moller S, Bernardi M. Interactions of the heart and the liver. European Heart Journal. 2013;**34**:2804-2811

[7] Henrion J. Hypoxic hepatitis. Liver International. 2012;**32**:1039-1052

[8] Hilscher M, Sanchez W. Congestive hepatopathy. Clinical Liver Disease. 2016;**8**:68-71

[9] Zipprich A, Mehal WZ, Ripoll C, Groszmann RJ. A distinct nitric oxide and adenosine A1 receptor dependent hepatic artery vasodilatatory response in the CCl-cirrhotic liver. Liver International. 2010;**30**:988-994

[10] Lautt WW. Hepatic vasculature: A conceptual review. Gastroenterology. 1977;**73**:1163-1169

[11] Jacobsen KR, Ranek L, Tygstrup N. Liver function and blood flow in normal man during infusion of vasopressin. Scandinavian Journal of Clinical and Laboratory Investigation. 1969;**24**:279-284

[12] Waseem N, Chen PH. Hypoxic hepatitis: A review and clinical update. Journal of Clinical and Translational Hepatology. 2016;**4**:263-268

[13] Mallory FB. Necroses of the liver. The Journal of Medical Research. 1901;**6**:264-80.7

[14] Lambert RA, Allison BR. Types of lesion in chronic passive congestion of the liver. Bulletin of the Johns Hopkins Hospital. 1916;**27**:350-356

[15] Chinsky M, Sherry S. Serum transaminase as a diagnostic aid. A.M.A. Archives of Internal Medicine. 1957;**99**:556-568

[16] Fragge RG, Kopel FB, Iglauer A. Serum glutamic oxalacetic transaminase (SGO-T) in conngestive heart failure: Clinical study and review of the literature. Annals of Internal Medicine. 1960;**52**:1042-1050

[17] Killip T 3rd, Payne MA. High serum transaminase activity in heart disease. Circulatory failure and hepatic necrosis. Circulation. 1960;**21**:646-660

[18] Arcidi JM Jr, Moore GW, Hutchins GM. Hepatic morphology in cardiac dysfunction: A clinicopathologic study of 1000 subjects at autopsy. The American Journal of Pathology. 1981;**104**:159-166

[19] Birgens HS, Henriksen J, Matzen P, Poulsen H. The shock liver. Clinical and biochemical findings in patients with centrilobular liver necrosis following cardiogenic shock. Acta Medica Scandinavica. 1978;**204**:417-421

[20] Bynum TE, Boitnott JK, Maddrey WC. Ischemic hepatitis. Digestive Diseases and Sciences. 1979;**24**:129-135

[21] Henrion J, Luwaert R, Colin L, Schmitz A, Schapira M, Heller FR. Hypoxic hepatitis. Prospective, clinical and hemodynamic study of 45 cases. Gastroentérologie Clinique et Biologique. 1990;**14**:836-841

[22] Henrion J, Schapira M, Luwaert R, Colin L, Delannoy A, Heller FR. Hypoxic hepatitis: Clinical and hemodynamic study in 142 consecutive cases. Medicine. 2003;**82**:392-406

[23] Birrer R, Takuda Y, Takara T. Hypoxic hepatopathy: Pathophysiology and prognosis. Internal Medicine. 2007;**46**:1063-1070

[24] Xanthopoulos A, Starling RC, Kitai T, Triposkiadis F. Heart failure and liver disease: Cardiohepatic interactions. JACC Heart Failure. 2019;**7**:87-97

[25] Koehne de Gonzalez AK, Lefkowitch JH. Heart disease and the liver: Pathologic evaluation. Gastroenterology Clinics of North America. 2017;**46**:421-435

[26] Tapper EB, Sengupta N, Bonder A. The incidence and outcomes of ischemic hepatitis: A systematic review with meta-analysis. The American Journal of Medicine. 2015;**128**:1314-1321

[27] Fuhrmann V, Kneidinger N, Herkner H, Heinz G, Nikfardjam M, Bojic A, et al. Hypoxic hepatitis: Underlying conditions and risk factors for mortality in critically ill patients. Intensive Care Medicine. 2009;**35**:1397-1405

[28] Raurich JM, Llompart-Pou JA, Ferreruela M, Colomar A, Molina M, Royo C, et al. Hypoxic hepatitis in critically ill patients: Incidence, etiology and risk factors for mortality. Journal of Anesthesia. 2011;**25**:50-56

[29] Henrion J, Descamps O, Luwaert R, Schapira M, Parfonry A, Heller F. Hypoxic hepatitis in patients with cardiac failure: Incidence in a coronary care unit and measurement of hepatic blood flow. Journal of Hepatology. 1994;**21**:696-703

[30] Waseem N, Limketkai BN, Kim B, Woreta T, Gurakar A, Chen PH. Risk and prognosis of acute liver injury among hospitalized patients with hemodynamic instability: A Nationwide analysis. Annals of Hepatology. 2018;**17**:119-124

[31] Weemhoff JL, Woolbright BL, Jenkins RE, McGill MR, Sharpe MR, Olson JC, et al. Plasma biomarkers to study mechanisms of liver injury in patients with hypoxic hepatitis. Liver International. 2017;**37**:377-384

[32] Richman SM, Delman AJ, Grob D. Alterations in indices of liver function in congestive heart failure with particular reference to serum enzymes. The American Journal of Medicine. 1961;**30**:211-225

[33] Seeto RK, Fenn B, Rockey DC. Ischemic hepatitis: Clinical presentation and pathogenesis. The American Journal of Medicine. 2000;**109**:109-113

[34] Zhang H, Vincent JL. Oxygen extraction is altered by endotoxin during tamponade-induced stagnant hypoxia in the dog. Circulatory Shock. 1993;**40**:168-176

[35] Nelson DP, Samsel RW, Wood LD, Schumacker PT. Pathological supply

dependence of systemic and intestinal O2 uptake during endotoxemia. Journal of Applied Physiology. 1988;**64**:2410-2419

[36] Wilson WC, Macgregor AR, Stewart CP. The clinical course and pathology of burns and scalds under modern methods of treatment. British Journal of Surgery. 1938;**25**:826-865

[37] Ellenberg M, Osserman KE. The role of shock in the production of central liver cell necrosis. The American Journal of Medicine. 1951;**11**:170-178

[38] Mallory TB, Sullivan ER, Burnett CH, Simeone FA, Shapiro SL, Beecher HK. VII. The general pathology of traumatic shock. Surgery. 1950;**27**:629-644

[39] Brunson JG, Eckman PL, Campbell JB. Increasing prevalence of unexplained liver necrosis. The New England Journal of Medicine. 1957;**257**:52-56

[40] de la Monte SM, Arcidi JM, Moore GW, Hutchins GM. Midzonal necrosis as a pattern of hepatocellular injury after shock. Gastroenterology. 1984;**86**:627-631

[41] Aboelsoud MM, Javaid AI, Al-Qadi MO, Lewis JH. Hypoxic hepatitis—Its biochemical profile, causes and risk factors of mortality in critically-ill patients: A cohort study of 565 patients. Journal of Critical Care. 2017;**41**:9-15

[42] Cassidy WM, Reynolds TB. Serum lactic dehydrogenase in the differential diagnosis of acute hepatocellular injury. Journal of Clinical Gastroenterology. 1994;**19**:118-121

[43] Woreta TA, Alqahtani SA. Evaluation of abnormal liver tests. The Medical Clinics of North America. 2014;**98**:1-16

[44] Green RM, Flamm S. AGA technical review on the evaluation of liver chemistry tests. Gastroenterology. 2002;**123**:1367-1384

[45] Taylor RM, Tujios S, Jinjuvadia K, Davern T, Shaikh OS, Han S, et al. Short and long-term outcomes in patients with acute liver failure due to ischemic hepatitis. Digestive Diseases and Sciences. 2012;**57**:777-785

[46] Jager B, Drolz A, Michl B, Schellongowski P, Bojic A, Nikfardjam M, et al. Jaundice increases the rate of complications and one-year mortality in patients with hypoxic hepatitis. Hepatology. 2012;**56**:2297-2304

[47] Sherlock S. The liver IN heart failure relation of anatomical, functional, and circulatory changes. British Heart Journal. 1951;**13**:273-293

[48] Boland E, Willius F. Changes in the liver produced by chronic passive congestion with special reference to the problem of cardiac cirrhosis. Archives of Internal Medicine. 1938;**62**:723-739

[49] Kavoliuniene A, Vaitiekiene A, Cesnaite G. Congestive hepatopathy and hypoxic hepatitis in heart failure: A cardiologist's point of view. International Journal of Cardiology. 2013;**166**:554-558

[50] Myers RP, Cerini R, Sayegh R, Moreau R, Degott C, Lebrec D, et al. Cardiac hepatopathy: Clinical, hemodynamic, and histologic characteristics and correlations. Hepatology. 2003;**37**:393-400

[51] Lemmer A, VanWagner LB, Ganger D. Assessment of advanced liver fibrosis and the risk for hepatic decompensation in patients with congestive hepatopathy. Hepatology. 2018;**68**:1633-1641

[52] Kubo SH, Walter BA, John DH, Clark M, Cody RJ. Liver function abnormalities in chronic heart failure.

Influence of systemic hemodynamics. Archives of Internal Medicine. 1987;**147**:1227-1230

[53] Allen LA, Felker GM, Pocock S, McMurray JJ, Pfeffer MA, Swedberg K, et al. Liver function abnormalities and outcome in patients with chronic heart failure: Data from the candesartan in heart failure: Assessment of reduction in mortality and morbidity (CHARM) program. European Journal of Heart Failure. 2009;**11**:170-177

[54] Gelow JM, Desai AS, Hochberg CP, Glickman JN, Givertz MM, Fang JC. Clinical predictors of hepatic fibrosis in chronic advanced heart failure. Circulation. Heart Failure. 2010;**3**:59-64

[55] van Deursen VM, Damman K, Hillege HL, van Beek AP, van Veldhuisen DJ, Voors AA. Abnormal liver function in relation to hemodynamic profile in heart failure patients. Journal of Cardiac Failure. 2010;**16**:84-90

[56] Poelzl G, Ess M, Mussner-Seeber C, Pachinger O, Frick M, Ulmer H. Liver dysfunction in chronic heart failure: Prevalence, characteristics and prognostic significance. European Journal of Clinical Investigation. 2012;**42**:153-163

[57] Megalla S, Holtzman D, Aronow WS, Nazari R, Korenfeld S, Schwarcz A, et al. Predictors of cardiac hepatopathy in patients with right heart failure. Medical Science Monitor. 2011;**17**:Cr537-Cr541

[58] Simonetto DA, Yang HY, Yin M, de Assuncao TM, Kwon JH, Hilscher M, et al. Chronic passive venous congestion drives hepatic fibrogenesis via sinusoidal thrombosis and mechanical forces. Hepatology. 2015;**61**:648-659

[59] Marra F, DeFranco R, Grappone C, Milani S, Pinzani M, Pellegrini G, et al. Expression of the thrombin receptor in human liver: Up-regulation during acute and chronic injury. Hepatology. 1998;**27**:462-471

[60] Marra F, Grandaliano G, Valente AJ, Abboud HE. Thrombin stimulates proliferation of liver fat-storing cells and expression of monocyte chemotactic protein-1: Potential role in liver injury. Hepatology. 1995;**22**:780-787

[61] Wanless IR, Liu JJ, Butany J. Role of thrombosis in the pathogenesis of congestive hepatic fibrosis (cardiac cirrhosis). Hepatology. 1995;**21**:1232-1237

[62] Cerini F, Vilaseca M, Lafoz E, Garcia-Irigoyen O, Garcia-Caldero H, Tripathi DM, et al. Enoxaparin reduces hepatic vascular resistance and portal pressure in cirrhotic rats. Journal of Hepatology. 2016;**64**:834-842

[63] Nakao T, Arii S, Kaido T, Mori A, Murata T, Matsumori A, et al. Heparin accelerates liver regeneration following portal branch ligation in normal and cirrhotic rats with increased plasma hepatocyte growth factor levels. Journal of Hepatology. 2002;**37**:87-92

[64] Abdel-Salam OM, Baiuomy AR, Ameen A, Hassan NS. A study of unfractionated and low molecular weight heparins in a model of cholestatic liver injury in the rat. Pharmacological Research. 2005;**51**:59-67

[65] Li W, Zhang J, Huang Q, Zhu H, Zhang X. Long-term administering low anticoagulant activity heparin can lessen rat hepatic fibrosis induced by either CCl(4) or porcine serum injection. Hepatology Research. 2006;**36**:115-123

[66] Abe W, Ikejima K, Lang T, Okumura K, Enomoto N, Kitamura T, et al. Low molecular weight heparin prevents hepatic fibrogenesis caused by carbon tetrachloride in the rat. Journal of Hepatology. 2007;**46**:286-294

[67] Assy N, Hussein O, Khalil A, Luder A, Szvalb S, Paizi M, et al. The beneficial effect of aspirin and enoxaparin on fibrosis progression and regenerative activity in a rat model of cirrhosis. Digestive Diseases and Sciences. 2007;**52**:1187-1193

[68] Kukner A, Tore F, Firat T, Terzi EH, Oner H, Balaban YH, et al. The preventive effect of low molecular weight heparin on CCL(4)-induced necrosis and apoptosis in rat liver. Annals of Hepatology. 2010;**9**:445-454

[69] Lee JH, Lee H, Joung YK, Jung KH, Choi JH, Lee DH, et al. The use of low molecular weight heparin-pluronic nanogels to impede liver fibrosis by inhibition the TGF-beta/Smad signaling pathway. Biomaterials. 2011;**32**:1438-1445

[70] Shah B, Shah G. Antifibrotic effect of heparin on liver fibrosis model in rats. World Journal of Gastrointestinal Pharmacology and Therapeutics. 2012;**3**:86-92

[71] Anstee QM, Goldin RD, Wright M, Martinelli A, Cox R, Thursz MR. Coagulation status modulates murine hepatic fibrogenesis: Implications for the development of novel therapies. Journal of Thrombosis and Haemostasis. 2008;**6**:1336-1343

[72] Lee KC, Hsu WF, Hsieh YC, Chan CC, Yang YY, Huang YH, et al. Dabigatran reduces liver fibrosis in thioacetamide-injured rats. Digestive Diseases and Sciences. 2019;**64**:102-112

[73] Vilaseca M, Garcia-Caldero H, Lafoz E, Garcia-Irigoyen O, Avila MA, Reverter JC, et al. The anticoagulant rivaroxaban lowers portal hypertension in cirrhotic rats mainly by deactivating hepatic stellate cells. Hepatology. 2017;**65**:2031-2044

[74] Villa E, Camma C, Marietta M, Luongo M, Critelli R, Colopi S, et al. Enoxaparin prevents portal vein thrombosis and liver decompensation in patients with advanced cirrhosis. Gastroenterology. 2012;**143**: 1253-1260. e1-4

[75] Fortea JI, Zipprich A, Fernandez-Mena C, Puerto M, Bosoi CR, Almagro J, et al. Enoxaparin does not ameliorate liver fibrosis or portal hypertension in rats with advanced cirrhosis. Liver International. 2018;**38**:102-112

[76] Kiesewetter CH, Sheron N, Vettukattill JJ, Hacking N, Stedman B, Millward-Sadler H, et al. Hepatic changes in the failing Fontan circulation. Heart. 2007;**93**:579-584

[77] Kendall TJ, Stedman B, Hacking N, Haw M, Vettukattill JJ, Salmon AP, et al. Hepatic fibrosis and cirrhosis in the Fontan circulation: A detailed morphological study. Journal of Clinical Pathology. 2008;**61**:504-508

[78] Wu FM, Kogon B, Earing MG, Aboulhosn JA, Broberg CS, John AS, et al. Liver health in adults with Fontan circulation: A multicenter cross-sectional study. The Journal of Thoracic and Cardiovascular Surgery. 2017;**153**:656-664

[79] Farias AQ, Silvestre OM, Garcia-Tsao G, da Costa Seguro LF, de Campos Mazo DF, Bacal F, et al. Serum B-type natriuretic peptide in the initial workup of patients with new onset ascites: A diagnostic accuracy study. Hepatology. 2014;**59**:1043-1051

[80] Runyon BA. Cardiac ascites: A characterization. Journal of Clinical Gastroenterology. 1988;**10**:410-412

[81] McConnell M, Iwakiri Y. Biology of portal hypertension. Hepatology International. 2018;**12**:11-23

[82] Sheer TA, Joo E, Runyon BA. Usefulness of serum N-terminal-ProBNP

in distinguishing ascites due to cirrhosis from ascites due to heart failure. Journal of Clinical Gastroenterology. 2010;**44**:e23-e26

[83] Lau GT, Tan HC, Kritharides L. Type of liver dysfunction in heart failure and its relation to the severity of tricuspid regurgitation. The American Journal of Cardiology. 2002;**90**:1405-1409

[84] Wells ML, Venkatesh SK. Congestive hepatopathy. Abdominal Radiology. 2018;**43**:2037-2051

[85] Rychik J, Atz AM, Celermajer DS, Deal BJ, Gatzoulis MA, Gewillig MH, et al. Evaluation and management of the child and adult with Fontan circulation: A scientific statement from the American Heart Association. Circulation. 2019:Cir0000000000000696

[86] Dhall D, Kim SA, Mc Phaul C, Kransdorf EP, Kobashigawa JA, Sundaram V, et al. Heterogeneity of fibrosis in liver biopsies of patients with heart failure undergoing heart transplant evaluation. The American Journal of Surgical Pathology. 2018;**42**:1617-1624

[87] Dai DF, Swanson PE, Krieger EV, Liou IW, Carithers RL, Yeh MM. Congestive hepatic fibrosis score: A novel histologic assessment of clinical severity. Modern Pathology. 2014;**27**:1552-1558

[88] Bosch DE, Koro K, Richards E, Hoch BL, Jalikis F, Koch LK, et al. Validation of a congestive hepatic fibrosis scoring system. The American Journal of Surgical Pathology. 2019;**43**:766-772

[89] Surrey LF, Russo P, Rychik J, Goldberg DJ, Dodds K, O'Byrne ML, et al. Prevalence and characterization of fibrosis in surveillance liver biopsies of patients with Fontan circulation. Human Pathology. 2016;**57**:106-115

[90] Louie CY, Pham MX, Daugherty TJ, Kambham N, Higgins JP. The liver in heart failure: A biopsy and explant series of the histopathologic and laboratory findings with a particular focus on pre-cardiac transplant evaluation. Modern Pathology. 2015;**28**:932-943

[91] European Association for Study of L, Asociacion Latinoamericana para el Estudio del H. EASL-ALEH clinical practice guidelines: Non-invasive tests for evaluation of liver disease severity and prognosis. Journal of Hepatology. 2015;**63**:237-264

[92] Lemmer A, VanWagner L, Ganger D. Congestive hepatopathy: Differentiating congestion from fibrosis. Clinical Liver Disease. 2017;**10**:139-143

[93] Diamond T, Ovchinsky N. Fontan-associated liver disease: Monitoring progression of liver fibrosis. Clinical Liver Disease. 2018;**11**:1-5

[94] Evans WN, Acherman RJ, Ciccolo ML, Carrillo SA, Galindo A, Rothman A, et al. MELD-XI scores correlate with post-Fontan hepatic biopsy fibrosis scores. Pediatric Cardiology. 2016;**37**:1274-1277

[95] Friedrich-Rust M, Koch C, Rentzsch A, Sarrazin C, Schwarz P, Herrmann E, et al. Noninvasive assessment of liver fibrosis in patients with Fontan circulation using transient elastography and biochemical fibrosis markers. The Journal of Thoracic and Cardiovascular Surgery. 2008;**135**:560-567

[96] Bosch J, Abraldes JG, Berzigotti A, Garcia-Pagan JC. The clinical use of HVPG measurements in chronic liver disease. Nature Reviews. Gastroenterology & Hepatology. 2009;**6**:573-582

[97] Burroughs AK, Thalheimer U. Hepatic venous pressure gradient in 2010: Optimal measurement is key. Hepatology. 2010;**51**:1894-1896

[98] Abraldes JG, Sarlieve P, Tandon P. Measurement of portal pressure. Clinics in Liver Disease. 2014;**18**:779-792

[99] Dohan A, Guerrache Y, Boudiaf M, Gavini JP, Kaci R, Soyer P. Transjugular liver biopsy: Indications, technique and results. Diagnostic and Interventional Imaging. 2014;**95**:11-15

[100] Ruttmann E, Brant LJ, Concin H, Diem G, Rapp K, Ulmer H. Gamma-glutamyltransferase as a risk factor for cardiovascular disease mortality: An epidemiological investigation in a cohort of 163,944 Austrian adults. Circulation. 2005;**112**:2130-2137

[101] Assenza GE, Graham DA, Landzberg MJ, Valente AM, Singh MN, Bashir A, et al. MELD-XI score and cardiac mortality or transplantation in patients after Fontan surgery. Heart. 2013;**99**:491-496

[102] Kim MS, Kato TS, Farr M, Wu C, Givens RC, Collado E, et al. Hepatic dysfunction in ambulatory patients with heart failure: Application of the MELD scoring system for outcome prediction. Journal of the American College of Cardiology. 2013;**61**:2253-2261

[103] Deo SV, Al-Kindi SG, Altarabsheh SE, Hang D, Kumar S, Ginwalla MB, et al. Model for end-stage liver disease excluding international normalized ratio (MELD-XI) score predicts heart transplant outcomes: Evidence from the registry of the united network for organ sharing. The Journal of Heart and Lung Transplantation. 2016;**35**:222-227

[104] Yancy CW, Jessup M, Bozkurt B, Butler J, Casey DE Jr, Drazner MH, et al. 2013 ACCF/AHA guideline for the management of heart failure: A report of the American College of Cardiology Foundation/American Heart Association task force on practice guidelines. Circulation. 2013;**128**:e240-e327

Chapter 5

Hepatocellular Carcinoma: A Pharmacological Aspect

Mani Sharma, Neeraj Kumar Chouhan and Sandeep Vaidya

Abstract

Hepatocellular carcinoma (HCC) is the fifth most common cancer worldwide, deteriorating approximately 1000,000 lives. Annually rising HCC to the third most common cause of cancer mortality. Liver cancer varies geographically depending on multimodality treatments available for this heterogeneous malignancy. Conglomeration of treatments has been exercised to manage this type of cancer across distinct geographic regions. Unprecedented rise of scientific knowledge mining from the published literature is a boon to develop novel treatment modalities. We aim to focus such pharmacological aspects in HCC treatment that could effectively display the improved therapies. Extrapolating the details of liver cancer (classification, diagnosis, adequate treatments, therapeutic engineering involved in the therapy, causes, epidemiology, and survival ratio) and the result obtained through this research could be a magnificent approach in the advancement of drug delivery systems that could assist in clinical trials and further betterment of survival rate and improved therapy from this deadly cancer.

Keywords: category, symptoms, prognosis, pathophysiology, remedies, therapeutic engineering

1. Introduction

As per the current study performed by the international agency for research on cancer (World Health Organization), the number of liver cancer cases reported all over the globe was 841,080, i.e., 4.7% of the total cancer cases in year 2018. As per the reports of the American Cancer Society, there is an estimation of 42,030 new cases of liver cancer diagnosed in the United States alone for the year 2019. Three-fourths of those cases are of hepatocellular carcinoma (HCC) that is unquestionably the most serious and dreaded complication of chronic liver disease. The development of HCC is generally the terminal event of a long-standing, typically asymptomatic chronic liver disease, which originated decades earlier. Regardless of the etiology, the process begins with a frequently unrecognized acute or subacute liver insult that slowly advances to the development of cirrhosis, a potentially preneoplastic condition. Less commonly, HCC arises directly without antecedent cirrhosis. The average life expectancy after diagnosis of clinically apparent HCC is less than 12 months [1].

People with chronic liver diseases, such as cirrhosis caused by hepatitis B or hepatitis C infection, are most often prone to hepatocellular carcinoma. Hepatocellular carcinoma is traditionally related to liver cirrhosis and also with the ongoing process of liver necrosis or regeneration, where liver cirrhosis may be due to hepatitis B and C.

In regions of Africa, Asia, and China, intake of food contaminated with aflatoxins may be later associated with HCC, while in Europe only 30% of pediatric HCC cases are linked to liver cirrhosis, while others are de novo cases [2] . As per the report of the American Cancer Society, 31,780 liver cancer deaths occurred in the United States alone for the year 2019. Incidence rates (%) in total population the disease is approximately 2.5 per 100,000 population [3]. It is one of the most common malignancies in adults and is more common in men than women (2–4:1) and blacks than whites. All over the world, millions of deaths per year (about 10% of all deaths in the adult age range) can be attributed to hepatocellular carcinoma. Depending on geographic location, the occurrence of hepatocellular carcinoma varies. While incidence in the Western world is less than 2 per 100,000 males, it is currently 40–60 per 100,000 in Africa and parts of the Far East. People of East Asian origin suffers the most from Hepatocellular carcinoma in United States. In the future, the prevalence of hepatocellular carcinoma may increase in the United States.

People with long-term liver diseases are most vulnerable to the risk of hepatocellular carcinoma. As people who already have signs and symptoms of chronic liver disease are majorly suffering from HCC. Prolonged yellow skin, easy bruising from blood clotting abnormalities, abdominal swelling, appetite loss, weight loss, pain in the abdominal cavity, nausea, feeling tired, or vomiting may be directly associated with HCC [4]. The mortality rate of the patients (both sexes) suffering from liver around the world in 2018 is 781,631. Among which 72.4% of the total mortality cases were recorded in Asia. As per the current statistics, a comprehensive approach is urgently required that involves primary and secondary prevention and increased access to treatment, and more funding for liver-related research is needed to address the high death rates associated with chronic liver disease and liver cancer to decrease the average mortality rate by giving adequate treatments.

1.1 Risk factors

Cirrhosis of the liver mostly causes HCC, whereas other factors also majorly influence the risk of HCC among which 60–70% of cirrhosis is estimated to cause by heavy alcohol consumption (**Figure 1**).

Recognized risk factors include:

- Toxins: alcohol abuse, aflatoxin, iron overload state (hemochromatosis)
- Metabolic: nonalcoholic steatohepatitis, type 2 diabetes (probably aided by obesity)

There is a variable significance of these risk factors globally [5]. In regions where hepatitis B infection is endemic, such as southeast China, this is the predominant cause. In populations largely protected by hepatitis B vaccination, such as the United States, HCC is most often linked to causes of cirrhosis such as chronic hepatitis C, alcohol abuse, and obesity. The chance of developing HCC in children and adolescents increases if they suffer from congenital liver disorders.

1.2 Symptoms

Patients with hepatocellular carcinoma are frequently asymptomatic especially if the disease is diagnosed at an early stage. The major symptoms include abnormal weight loss, mild to high fever, diarrhea, fatigue, and anorexia [6].

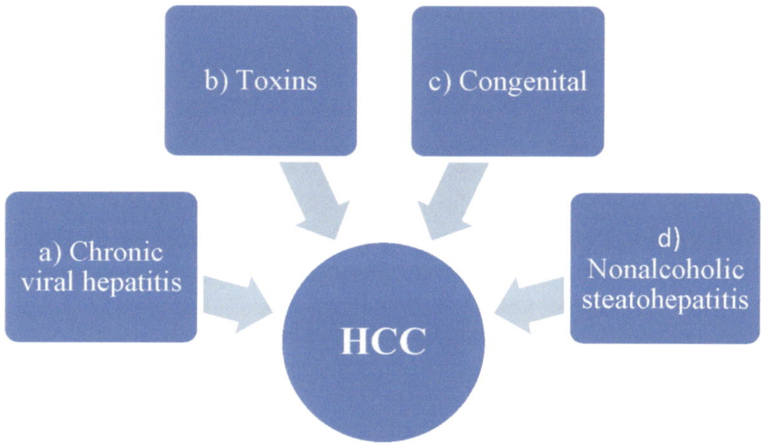

Figure 1.
Risk factors leading to the cause of HCC: (a) estimated cause of 80% cases globally, (b) alcohol abuse, aflatoxin; iron overload state (hemochromatosis); (c) alpha 1-antitrypsin deficiency; Wilson's disease.

Symptomatic patients—Patients with advanced lesions may present with mild to moderate upper abdominal pain, weight loss, early satiety, or a palpable mass in the upper abdomen [7]. Paraneoplastic syndrome may occasionally develop in a patient with HCC [8].

Hypoglycemia—Hypoglycemia, which usually occurs in advanced HCC, is thought to result from the tumor's high metabolic needs.Erythrocytosis—Tumor secretion of erythropoietin (EPO) majorly leads to erythrocytosis in HCC [9].

Hypercalcemia— Hypercalcemia can be present in association with osteolytic metastases, but it may also be seen in the absence of bony metastasis due to secretion of parathyroid hormone-related protein [10].

Diarrhea—Patients with HCC may infrequently present with intractable diarrhea and associated electrolyte disturbances (e.g., hyponatremia, hypokalemia, metabolic alkalosis). The underlying mechanism is not fully understood, but it may be related to secretion of peptides that cause intestinal secretion. These include vasoactive intestinal polypeptide, gastrin, and peptides with prostaglandin-like immunoreactivity [11]. Cutaneous features—Although skin changes are rare in patients with HCC, several cutaneous manifestations have been described; however, none is specific for the diagnosis [12].

It involves the following:

- Dermatomyositis may present with a variety of cutaneous findings (e.g., scaly, violaceous papules overlying bony prominences of the hands) and is associated with solid organ malignancies.

- Pemphigus foliaceus is a superficial blistering disease similar to pemphigus vulgaris, except it rarely involves the mucous membranes. Blisters often appear as shallow erosions associated with erythema, scale, and crust formation, and the appearance may resemble severe seborrheic dermatitis.

- Sudden appearance of multiple seborrheic keratosis is the sign of Leser-Trélat, with acanthosis nigricans and skin tags.

- Multiple, round, or oval, sharply demarcated scaling patches have been reported in South African black patients with HCC characterized as Pityriasis rotunda [13].

Other clinical presentations that may be seen in symptomatic patients with HCC are as follows.

A. Intraperitoneal bleeding due to tumor rupture. Tumor rupture is often associated with sudden onset of severe abdominal pain with distension and an acute drop in the hemoglobin and hypotension and is most commonly diagnosed by imaging the abdominal parts. A liver mass and free intraperitoneal blood can be demonstrated by doing computed tomography of the abdominal part [14]. Emergency angiography and embolization is required in case of bleeding as it can become a life-threatening complication [15]. If feasible, delayed resection may be considered although the risk of peritoneal dissemination is high [16].

B. Obstructive jaundice majorly caused by invasion of the biliary tree or due to compression of the intrahepatic duct.

C. Fever developing in association with central tumor necrosis.

D. Pyogenic liver abscess (very rare) [17].

1.3 Diagnosis

Early diagnosis of HCC is through screening or surveillance and is in treatable stage. Typically ultrasonography is performed every 6 months in screening and surveillance for abdominal imaging. A cross-sectional imaging of a detected nodule through ultrasonography using triple-phase CT or contrast-enhanced MRI is performed frequently. Increased tumor vascularity is observed in the arterial phase by radiographic features of HCC. Tumor invasion of the portal vein or lymph node enhancement identification is an additional imaging feature. Liver Imaging Reporting and Data System (LIRADS) systematically characterize these imaging findings diagnostic criteria that also incorporates tumor growth [18]. The resemblance of to normal hepatocytes to neoplastic cells assesses the degree of differentiation of HCC [19].

The possibility of tumor seeding during the biopsy, and the patients with chronic kidney disease represent a particular challenge since MRI contrast agents are contraindicated in end-stage renal disease given the risk of renal toxicity [20].

The evaluation after HCC diagnosis is done through different techniques.

A multidisciplinary setting is required to select therapy after the diagnosis of HCC is made for further evaluations. History and physical examination and serologic and imaging tests are obtained to assess the patient's liver reserve, performance status, comorbidities, extent of tumor spread, and potential eligibility for liver transplantation. "Staging and prognostic factors in hepatocellular carcinoma" are the Multidisciplinary evaluations [21].

1. Surgical resection

2. Liver transplantation

3. Locoregional therapies

4. Ablative therapies (radiofrequency ablation, microwave ablation, cryoablation)

5. Percutaneous ethanol or acetic acid ablation

6. Irreversible electroporation

7. Transarterial embolization (bland embolization, chemoembolization, radio-embolization)

8. External beam radiotherapy

9. Systemic chemotherapy and immunotherapy

10. Laboratory tests—Complete blood count, platelets, renal function tests, prothrombin time, albumin

11. Liver biochemical and function tests (i.e., bilirubin, aminotransferases, alkaline phosphatase)

12. Imaging—Extent of tumor spread may be evaluated with the following imaging exams:

    a. Contrast-enhanced abdominopelvic computed tomography (CT) or magnetic resonance imaging (MRI) tailored for liver lesion evaluation (see "Modalities for HCC diagnosis" above)

    b. Chest CT without or with intravenous contrast.

    c. Whole body technetium-99m bone scan, if clinically indicated

2. Pathophysiology of HCC

2.1 Anatomy of the liver

The liver is one of the most complex and largest organs in the abdominal cavity. Lobules are the major microscopic functional units of the liver. Removal of endogenous and exogenous materials from the blood, carbohydrate homeostasis, complex metabolic processes including bile production, lipid metabolism, urea formation, and immune functions are some of the major functions performed by the liver. The upper posterior surface of the liver is outside of mesogastrium, a structure through which liver arises. The liver is connected to the anterior body wall by the ligamentum teres and falciform ligament. It connects to the stomach by the lesser omentum and the coronary and triangular ligaments to the diaphragm. The liver is the largest internal organ. The position of the liver is just beneath your right lung and under your right ribs. It has two lobes (sections) involving the right lobe and the left lobe. Women are in more risk to develop hepatic cancer and FNH tumors than men [22] (**Figure 2**).

Another type of cells in the liver called as bile ducts are the cells that line small tubes in the liver. The bile ducts carry bile from the liver to the gallbladder or directly to the intestines. It has many important functions: it breaks down and stores many of the nutrients absorbed from the intestine that your body needs to function. It delivers bile into the intestines to help absorb nutrients (especially fats). It breaks down alcohol, drugs, and toxic wastes in the blood, which then pass from the body through urine and stool. Several types of malignant (cancerous) and

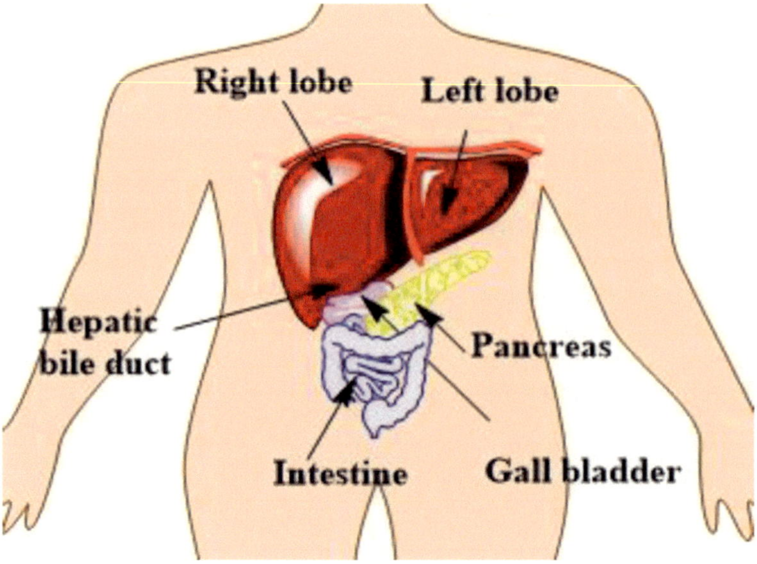

Figure 2.
Anatomy of the liver.

benign (noncancerous) tumors can be formed through different types of cells in the liver. These tumors generated via different cell origins have different root causes, different modes of treatments, and have a different outlook. Hepatitis infection was linked to HCC by Beasley in 1981 [23].

2.2 Category of liver cancer

2.2.1 Primary liver cancer

A cancer that starts in the liver is called primary liver cancer that can be more than one type.

2.2.1.1 Intrahepatic cholangiocarcinoma (bile duct cancer)

Intrahepatic cholangiocarcinomas covers 10–20% of cancers that start in the liver. This type of cancer mostly starts in the bile duct where carcinogenic conditions can be facilitated by the repetitions of inflammation [24].

2.2.1.2 Angiosarcoma and hemangiosarcoma

Cells lining the blood vessels of the liver are the rare causes of liver cancer. Exposure to vinyl chloride or to thorium dioxide (Thorotrast) may develop these cancers (see Liver cancer risk factors). Some other cases are thought to be caused by exposure to arsenic or radium or to an inherited condition known as hereditary hemochromatosis. It is difficult to investigate the exact cause for the development of cancer cells. These tumors grow quickly and are usually too widespread to be removed surgically by the time they are found. The pathogenesis of such HCC is made up of different genetic/epigenetic aberrations and alterations with many signaling pathways that lead to a known heterogeneity of the diseases' biologic and clinical behavior [25].

2.2.1.3 Hepatoblastoma

Children with the age of below 4 years develops this rare form of cancer, that usually seen in the younger age. Fetal liver cells are similar to the cells of hepatoblastoma. It is harder to treat such tumors if they spread outside the liver, where surgery and chemotherapy are the successful therapies in treating two out of three children suffering from such a tumor. The genetic pathways that are affecting hepablastoma have to be further studied and analyzed [26].

2.2.2 Secondary liver cancer (metastatic liver cancer)

Most of the time when cancer is found in the liver, it did not start there but has spread (metastasized) from somewhere else in the body, such as the pancreas, colon, stomach, breast, or lung. As this cancer spreads from its original site, it is called a secondary liver cancer.

2.2.2.1 Benign liver tumors

Sometimes larger growth of benign tumors causes problems, though they do not grow into nearby tissues or do not spread to other distant parts of the body. Surgery can be the best therapy for such a kind of cancer.

2.2.2.2 Hemangioma

Hemangiomas start in the blood vessels and are considered another most common type of liver cancer. They generally do not show any symptoms but need to operate in chronic cases Multidetector-row computed tomography (MDCT) [27].

2.2.2.3 Hepatic adenoma

This tumor starts from hepatocytes (the main type of liver cell) with symptoms like pain in the abdomen, lump in the stomach area, or blood loss. In such cases there is always a risk of tumor rapture or further growth into a vigorous liver cancer. Thus, surgery is the most effective treatment advised by the experts. Fibrolamellar, pseudoglandular (adenoid), pleomorphic (giant cell), and clear cell are microscopically, the four architectural and cytological types (patterns) of hepatocellular carcinoma [28].

2.3 Remedies and treatment (staging)

Patients with cirrhosis and varying degrees of hepatic dysfunction are majorly prone to HCC. A careful assessment of hepatic function in addition to tumor parameters is thus required for the adequate treatment of HCC. Patients are often managed by multidisciplinary teams at tertiary referral medical centers (**Figure 3**).

2.3.1 Drugs in market and drugs under clinical trial

Various chemotherapeutic potent drugs for the treatment of HCC have been efficiently developed, and many are in the pipeline under different phases of clinical trials. A brief enlisting of such drugs approved by the FDA and under clinical trials is depicted in **Tables 1** and **2** [29].

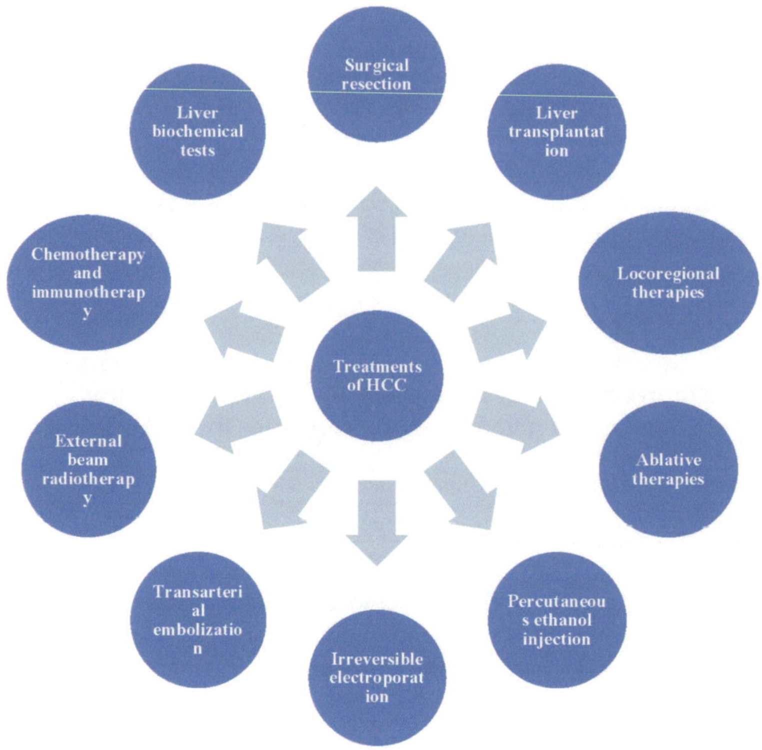

Figure 3.
Potential treatment options for HCC.

S. no.	Drugs	Company	Approved year
1	Sorafenib (Nexavar)	Bayer and Onyx	2007 in the United States
2	Regorafenib (Stivarga)	Bayer	2017 in the United States
3	Nivolumab (Opdivo)	Bristol-Myers Squibb	2017 in the United States
4	Lenvatinib (Lenvima)	Eisai Co.	2018 in the United States
5	Cabozantinib (Cabometyx)	Exelixis Inc.	2018 in Europe
6	Pembrolizumab (Keytruda)	Merck	2018 in the United States
7	Pembrolizumab	Merck	2018 in the United States
8	Rozlytrek (entrectinib)	Roche	2019 in the United States
9	Cabozantinib (Cabometyx)	Exelixis	2019 in the United States
10	Ramucirumab (Cyramza)	Eli Lilly	2019 in the United States
11	Atezolizumab	TECENTRIQ®	2019 in the United States

Table 1.
Recently approved drugs for the treatment of HCC [29].

2.4 Therapeutic engineering

The following therapeutic treatment engineering options are available to patients with hepatocellular carcinoma (**Figure 4**).

S. no.	Drugs	Developed by	Drugs in clinical trials
1	Milciclib (PHA-848125)	Tiziana Life Sciences	II Phase
2	Galunisertib (LY2157299)	Eli Lilly	II Phase
3	Ipafricept (OMP-54F28)	OncoMed	I Phase
4	Ipilimumab (Yervoy)	Bristol-Myers Squibb	II Phase
5	Brivanib	Bristol-Myers Squibb	III Phase

Table 2.
Drug candidates in the pipeline under different phases of clinical trials [30].

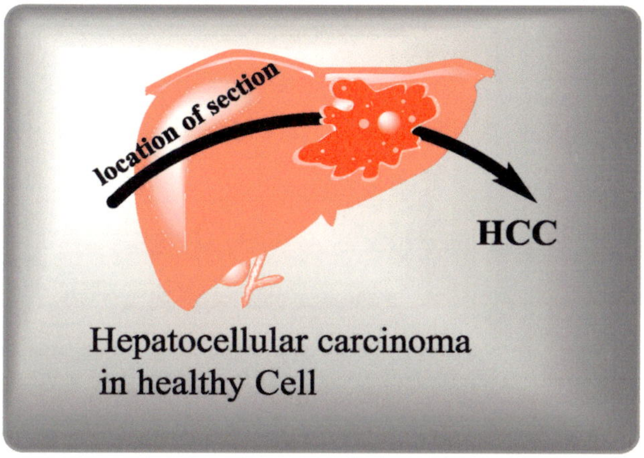

Figure 4.
Hepatocellular carcinoma in healthy cells.

2.4.1 Surgical therapy

Surgery is the treatment of choice for noncirrhotic patients suffering from HCC. However, only 20% of patients are potentially resectable at the time of presentation. In noncirrhotic patients, surgical mortality is less than 3% in experienced hands, but increases to 8% in patients with cirrhosis [3].

2.4.2 Liver resection

Surgery provides the best possibility for a cure. For that reason, every patient should be evaluated first and foremost for the possibility of resection. Organ removal can result in cure in early diagnosis states and overspreading of cancer in other organs.

Unfortunately, not all patients are eligible for liver resection. Resection is not indicated when (1) the tumor has spread to other parts of the liver or the body, (2) the size or location of the tumor resists the part of liver removal without compromising the total functionality of the organ, (3) the associated cirrhosis or disease limits the ability to safely operate upon or remove part of the liver, and (4) other medical conditions make surgery unsafe [3].

2.4.3 Cryosurgery

Cryosurgery is a technique utilizing subzero temperatures to destroy tumors. In most cases, the tumor is destroyed but not removed. The placement of one or more probes (cryoprobe) into the tumor site using ultrasound to guide the placement is adopted in such a technique [3] (**Figure 5**).

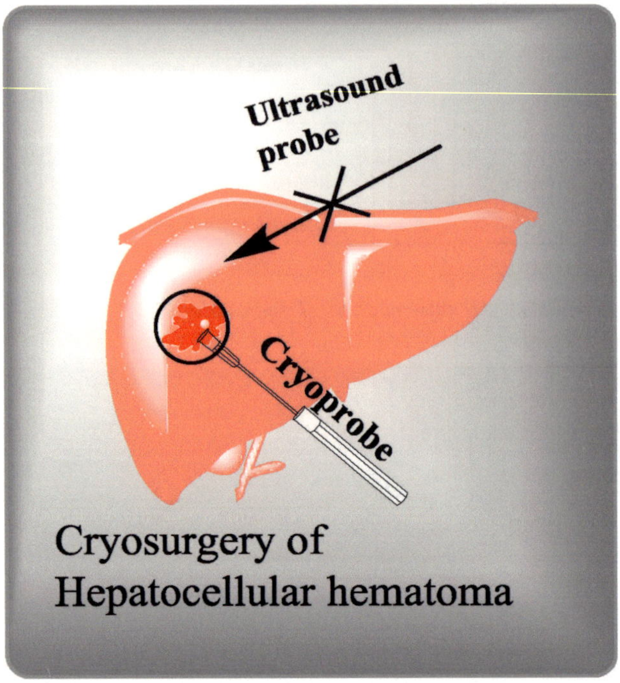

Figure 5.
Cryosurgery of hepatocellular carcinoma.

2.4.4 Radiofrequency ablation

Radiofrequency ablation (RFA) is a new technique that makes use of a "heating" probe to destroy tumors within the liver. A probe with thin tip is put into a tumor site. After deploying the tip array, an electrical current is applied, generating heat (80–100°C) that destroys the tumor (**Figure 6**).

This kind of technique can be done in an operating room or with a laparoscopic approach. RFA is used to treat the tumor, whereas the remaining parts of the tumor are removed by surgery.

2.4.5 Liver transplantation

In patients with small tumors and advanced cirrhosis (Child B or Child C) the treatment of choice is liver transplantation.

Patients who are not candidates for surgical resection or transplantation should be considered for other forms of treatment including cryosurgery, chemoembolization, ethanol or cisplatin infusion, or radiofrequency ablation (**Figure 7**).

2.4.6 Interventional radiological therapy

The most commonly performed procedures in the treatment of unresectable liver tumors (i.e., those that are inoperable) are hepatic artery chemoembolization and hepatic artery chemoradiation. Most hepatic tumors are supplied by the hepatic arterial system, as opposed to normal liver tissue, in which most of the blood supply comes from the portal venous system. Chemoembolization is considered superior over intravenous pump infusion therapy because it delivers drug with more target specification. System toxicity is reduced as 85% of the total drug administered in the body is trapped in the liver itself [3] (**Figure 8**).

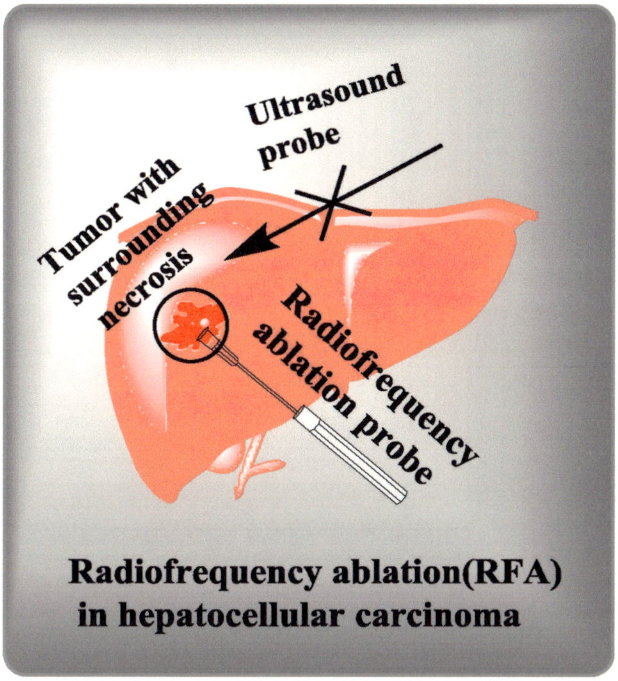

Figure 6.
Radiofrequency ablation in hepatocellular carcinoma.

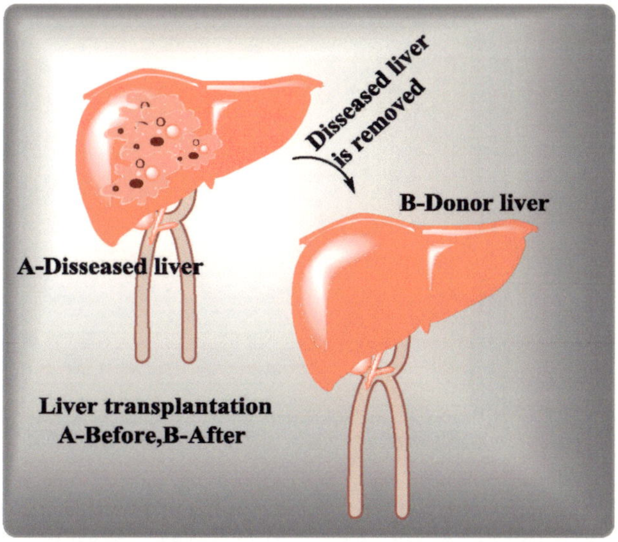

Figure 7.
Transplantation of the liver.

2.4.7 Ethanol injection by percutaneous method

Tumors less than 5 cm in diameter and patients with less than three lesions can be treated with percutaneous ethanol injection. It has been demonstrated that ethanol injection is more effective against hepatoma lesions than against metastatic lesions [3] (**Figure 9**).

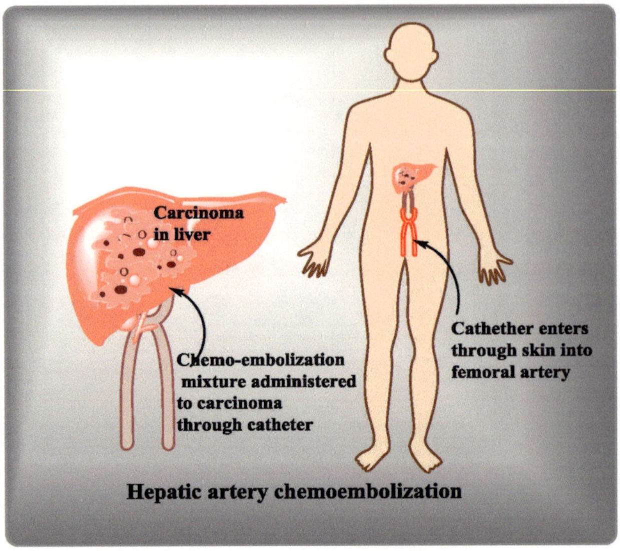

Figure 8.
Hepatic artery chemoembolization.

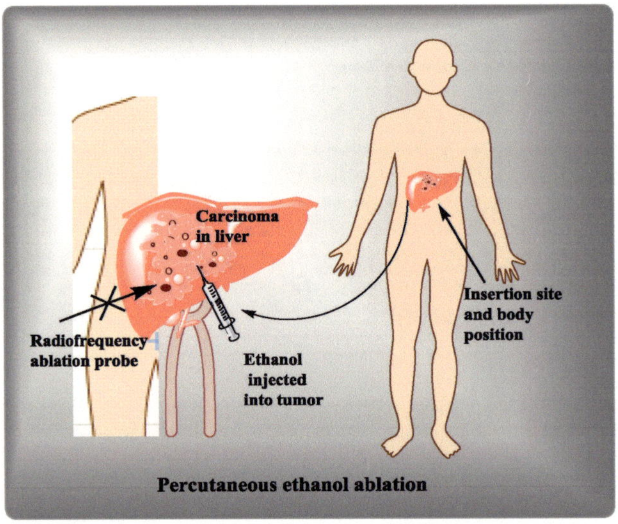

Figure 9.
Percutaneous ethanol injection in hepatic tumors.

Ultrasound vibrations are used to perform such a procedure. Ethanol is injected slowly into a lesion through a small needle that is inserted into the posterior aspect of the tumor. Patients may receive one or two sessions per week until the tumor is completely saturated. Post-procedural imaging, including CT and MRI, is typically conducted after 1 month and then every 4 months thereafter [3].

2.4.8 Percutaneous radiofrequency ablation

Frictional heat produced during percutaneous radiofrequency ablation causes destruction to the local tissues. This procedure is also performed under ultrasound guidance. A radiofrequency needle is inserted deep into the lesion, and multiple electrodes are deployed. The duration of the treatment varies from 6 to 15 minutes.

Only limited data are available regarding the use of this technique to treat unresectable liver tumors, but preliminary studies have shown a trend toward prolonged survival [3] (**Figure 10**).

2.4.8.1 Cisplatin gel infusion percutaneous

Unresectable liver tumors can be treated by cisplatin gel infusion technique that is a new and promising therapeutic option [3] (**Figure 11**).

Clinical trials of this technique are undergoing in the United States as it has been recently developed. It is almost similar to percutaneous ethanol injection method. This technique is also performed in ultrasound vibrations like the percutaneous method. Cisplatin gel is infused into the deepest part of the tumor through a small

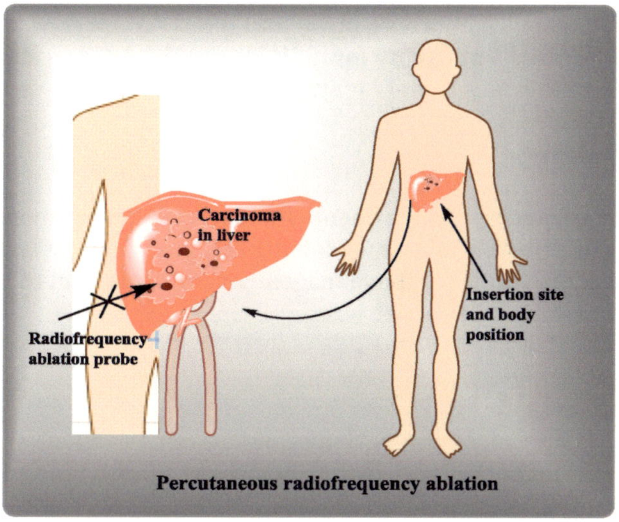

Figure 10.
Percutaneous radiofrequency ablation in hepatic tumors.

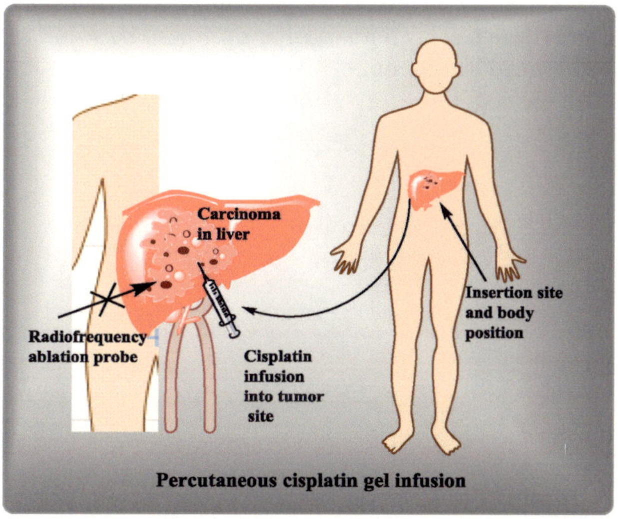

Figure 11.
Percutaneous cisplatin infusion in hepatic tumors.

needle. The chemotherapeutic drug is carried slowly by this gel into the tumor site. The gel slowly diffuses throughout the tumor and acts as a carrier of the chemotherapeutic drug [3].

3. Conclusion

These explanations and findings show that the etiology of HCC is extremely complex, with many confounding factors affecting disease course and patient prognosis. Excessive intake of alcohol, aflatoxin-contaminated food, obesity, and diabetes are the major risk factors for the development of HCC. A better understanding of HCC may offer us the best chance of achieving earlier diagnosis and intervention, which would ultimately improve the outlook for those at risk for developing HCC. These findings may support future studies in investigating the possibilities, developing adequate treatments with intra- and inter-variances of patients in mind, and aiming to improve the mortality for individuals with hepatocellular carcinoma.

4. Future directions

Despite many advances, the treatment of hepatocellular carcinoma is unsatisfactory. As per the current clinical data we can expect, gene therapy and immunotherapy may become more viable for the management and treatment of hepatocellular carcinoma in more safe and effective ways.

Acknowledgements

I thank all my coauthors who are listed, and the work was not funded by any institute or person.

Conflict of interest

We wish to declare that there are no known conflicts of interest associated with this publication, and there has been no significant financial support for this work that could have influenced its outcome.

Author details

Mani Sharma*, Neeraj Kumar Chouhan and Sandeep Vaidya
Council for Scientific and Industrial Research, Indian Institute of Chemical Technology, Hyderabad, India

*Address all correspondence to: mninup2015@gmail.com

References

[1] Seeff LB. Introduction: The burden of hepatocellular carcinoma. Gastroenterology. 2004;**127**(5):S1-S4

[2] Jung HJ, Kim HY, Jung SE, Park KW, Kim WK. Primary hepatic tumors in children. Journal of the Korean Association of Pediatric Surgeons. 2005;**11**(2):107-114

[3] Gurakar A, Hamilton JP, Koteish A, Li Z, Mezey E. Hepatocellular Carcinoma (Liver Cancer): Introduction. 2001

[4] Blumgart LH, Fong Y, Jarnagin WR. Hepatobiliary Cancer. PMPH USA; 2000

[5] White DL, Kanwal F, El-Serag HB. Association between nonalcoholic fatty liver disease and risk for hepatocellular cancer, based on systematic review. Clinical Gastroenterology and Hepatology. 2012;**10**(12):1342-1359.e2

[6] Spagnolo P, du Bois RM, Cottin V. Rare lung disease and orphan drug development. The Lancet Respiratory Medicine. 2013;**1**(6):479-487

[7] Kew M, Dos Santos H, Sherlock S. Diagnosis of primary cancer of the liver. British Medical Journal. 1971;**4**(5784):408-411

[8] Luo J-C, Hwang S-J, Wu J-C, Lai C-R, Li C-P, Chang F-Y, et al. Clinical characteristics and prognosis of hepatocellular carcinoma patients with paraneoplastic syndromes. Hepato-Gastroenterology. 2002;**49**(47):1315-1319

[9] Tefferi A, Schrier SL. Diagnostic Approach to the Patient with Polycythemia. 2014

[10] Yen TC, Hwang SJ, Wang CC, et al. Hypercalcemia and parathyroid hormone-related protein in hepatocellular carcinoma. Liver. 1993;**13**:311

[11] Steiner E, Velt P, Gutierrez O, et al. Hepatocellular carcinoma presenting with intractable diarrhea. A radiologic-pathologic correlation. Archives of Surgery. 1986;**121**:849

[12] Dogra S, Jindal R. Cutaneous manifestations of common liver diseases. Journal of Clinical and Experimental Hepatology. 2011;**1**:177

[13] DiBisceglie AM, Hodkinson HJ, Berkowitz I, Kew MC. Pityriasis rotunda. A cutaneous marker of hepatocellular carcinoma in South African blacks. Archives of Dermatology. 1986;**122**:802

[14] Choi BG, Park SH, Byun JY, et al. The findings of ruptured hepatocellular carcinoma on helical CT. The British Journal of Radiology. 2001;**74**:142

[15] Chearanai O, Plengvanit U, Asavanich C, Damrongsak D, Sindhvananda K, Boonyapisit S. Spontaneousruptureofprimaryhepatoma: Report of 63 cases with particular reference to the pathogenesis and rationale treatment by hepatic artery ligation. Cancer. 1983;**51**(8):1532-1536

[16] Curley SA, Barnett Jr CC, Abdalla EK, Singal AG. Management of potentially resectable hepatocellular carcinoma: Prognosis, role of neoadjuvant and adjuvant therapy, and posttreatment surveillance.

[17] Lin YT, Liu CJ, Chen TJ, et al. Pyogenic liver abscess as the initial manifestation of underlying hepatocellular carcinoma. The American Journal of Medicine. 2011;**124**:1158

[18] Mitchell DG, Bruix J, Sherman M, Sirlin CB. LI-RADS (liver imaging reporting and data system): Summary, discussion, and consensus of the LI-RADS Management working group and future directions. Hepatology. 2015;**61**(3):1056-1065

[19] Goodman ZD. Neoplasms of the liver. Modern Pathology. 2007;**20** (Suppl 1):S49-S60

[20] Swaminathan S, Horn TD, Pellowski D, Abul-Ezz S, Bornhorst JA, Viswamitra S, et al. Nephrogenic systemic fibrosis, gadolinium, and iron mobilization. The New England Journal of Medicine. 2007;**357**(7):720-722

[21] Schwartz JM, Carithers Jr RL, Sirlin CB, Kressel HY, Savarese DM. Clinical features and diagnosis of hepatocellular carcinoma.

[22] Mikołajczyk A. Invited brief commentary on the article "breast cancer association with Cytomegalo virus—A tertiary center case-control study" is Cytomegalo virus a breast cancer etiologic risk factor. Journal of Investigative Surgery. 2017;**30**:1-2

[23] Dongiovanni P, Romeo S, Valenti L. Hepatocellular carcinoma in nonalcoholic fatty liver: Role of environmental and genetic factors. World Journal of Gastroenterology. 2014;**20**:1294

[24] Block TM, Mehta AS, Fimmel CJ, Jordan R. Molecular viral oncology of hepatocellular carcinoma. Oncogene. 2003;**22**:5093-5107

[25] Bertino G, Demma S, Ardiri A, Proiti M, Gruttadauria S, Toro A, et al. Hepatocellular carcinoma: Novel molecular targets in carcinogenesis for future therapies. BioMed Research International. 2014;**2014**:203693

[26] McKillop IH, Moran DM, Jin X, Koniaris LG. Molecular pathogenesis of hepatocellular carcinoma. The Journal of Surgical Research. 2006;**136**:125-135

[27] Utsunomiya D, Oda S, Funama Y, Awai K, Nakaura T, Yanaga Y, et al. Comparison of standard-and low-tube voltage MDCT angiography in patients with peripheral arterial disease. European Radiology. 2010;**20**(11):2758-2765

[28] Chan AW, Zhang Z, Chong CC, Tin EK, Chow C, Wong N. Genomic landscape of lymphoepithelioma-like hepatocellular carcinoma. The Journal of Pathology. 2019

[29] Available from: https://www.cancer.gov/about-cancer/treatment/drugs/liver

[30] María R, Leonardo GDF, Sandrine F. New trials and results in systemic treatment of HCC. Journal of Hepatology. 2018

Chapter 6

Acute on Chronic Liver Failure: Role of the Bacterial Infections

Mauro Borzio and Elena Dionigi

Abstract

Acute-on-chronic liver failure (ACLF) refers to a syndrome characterized by acute deterioration of liver function of a pre-existing chronic liver disease with increased short-term mortality at 3 months due to multiorgan failure. Definition of ACLF has been refined, but differences between western and eastern areas still exist. Diagnosis of ACLF as recommended by the EASL-CLIF consortium is based on the assessment of organ dysfunction. The pathogenesis of this syndrome is attributable to an exaggerated host response to inflammation, responsible for the severe haemodynamic derangement leading to multiorgan failure. ACLF is triggered by precipitating events like acute hepatitis either viral, drug-induced, toxic, or alcoholic, variceal bleeding and sepsis. Bacterial infection is currently considered the most frequent trigger of ACLF in Western countries. Cirrhotic patients, particularly if decompensated are prone to develop bacterial infection because loss of integrity of the intestinal mucosal barrier and translocation of pathogen-associated molecular patterns (PAMPs). Bacterial translocation may develop into overt infection at different sites, along with sepsis and septic shock that may lead to ACLF. Epidemiology of bacterial infection in cirrhosis has been changing and this accounts for new antibiotic regimens as empirical therapy in critically ill cirrhotic patients with bacterial infection. In this chapter, we will discuss on definition, pathogenesis, clinical aspects and therapy of bacterial infection-related ACLF.

Keywords: acute-on-chronic liver failure (ACLF), bacterial infection, multi-drug-resistant bacteria, cirrhosis, sepsis, septic shock

1. Introduction

Acute-on-chronic liver failure (ACLF) is a recently recognized syndrome characterized by acute function deterioration on an underlying liver cirrhosis or chronic liver disease associated with a high short-term mortality and an immense health care expenditure. There is a worldwide agreement that ACLF represents an acute deterioration of pre-existing chronic liver disease, usually triggered by a precipitating event.

Although the pathogenesis of this syndrome is still under investigation, it seems to be largely attributable to an exaggerate host response to inflammation with release of circulatory proinflammatory cytokines and mediators which lead to hemodynamic and cellular dysfunction (cytokine storm). Bacterial infection represents the most important and frequent trigger cause of ACLF even though other trigger events like HBV reactivation or alcohol play a relevant role.

The prognosis of this syndrome remains dismal mainly because available therapeutic strategies, beside OLT, are ineffective and novel approaches are still lacking.

2. Acute-on-chronic liver failure

2.1 Definition

Definition of ACLF differs worldwide [1]. Three widely used definitions of ACLF are currently available from different geographic areas: the definition proposed by European ACLF consortium (EASL-CLIF) [2] and the North American Consortium (North American Consortium for the Study of End-Stage Liver Disease NACSELD) [3] mostly adopted in western countries and definition proposed by the APASL consortium (ACLF research Consortium: AARC) which is largely employed in eastern countries [4, 5]. All these definitions are derived from analysis of data obtained in large series of patients prospectively recruited in different centers [2, 3, 5]. These definitions share some common items such as high mortality, but also significant differences including precipitating events, underlying liver disease, diagnostic and prognostic criteria. In the western areas, bacterial infection plays the most important pathogenetic role [6, 7] followed by alcohol abuse [8], whereas in the East, both hepatitis B and alcoholic hepatitis are considered the most frequent precipitating events [5]. In the CANONIC study the following factors were considered as precipitating events for ACLF: infection, current alcohol drinking, acute reactivation of chronic viral hepatitis, gastrointestinal bleeding or a recent medical procedure like paracentesis or transjugular intrahepatic portosystemic shunt positioning [6]. It is important to note that others clinical conditions have joined the list of precipitating causes of ACLF as DILI-related injury (mainly antitubercular drugs, herbal medicine, anti-retroviral drugs and methotrexate) [9, 10], autoimmune hepatitis reactivation [11] and more recently NASH [12].

The definition of organ failures is also variable among different definitions suggesting that ACLF is not the same worldwide. Moreover, ACLF can occur not only in association with advanced cirrhosis but, as recently reported, even in chronic liver disease without cirrhosis and this issue is differently addressed in ACLF definitions [1]. However, ACLF should be distinguished from an acute liver failure in a preexisting perfectly normal liver. The definition of short-term mortality is not uniform as well. For example, in APASL definition this time frame is settled at 28 days whereas in EASL definition is settled at 3 months. All these differences account for the difficulty in assessing the true prevalence of ACLF. In order to merge the different ACLF definitions, the World Gastroenterology Organization (WGO) tentatively proposed the following one: "ACLF is a syndrome in patients with chronic liver disease with or without previously diagnosed cirrhosis, characterized by acute hepatic decompensation resulting in liver failure (jaundice and prolongation of the international normalized ratio or INR) and one or more extrahepatic organ failures, associated with increased mortality up to 3 months [13]."

According to EASL-CLIF the definition of ACLF necessitates of extrahepatic organ failures (renal, brain, respiratory, and circulatory systems), being the sole liver failure insufficient for the diagnosis [3, 5, 6]. This specification is crucial to avoid to classify as ACLF an acute decompensation of an end-stage liver disease. Unfortunately, the definition of organ failure is not homogeneous among different regions being the agreement only on the definition of brain failure which should be graded as 3–4. Main issues showing agreement/disagreement among different definitions of ACLF are listed in **Table 1**.

	APASL	EASL-CLIF	NACSELD
Definition	Acute hepatic insult manifesting as jaundice (serum bilirubin ≥5 mg/dL) and coagulopathy (INR ≥ 1.5 or prothrombin activity <40%) and complicated within 4 weeks by ascites and/or hepatic encephalopathy in a patient with previously diagnosed or undiagnosed chronic liver disease associated with high mortality	An acute deterioration of a preexisting chronic liver disease usually related to a precipitating event and associated with increased mortality at 3 months due to multisystem organ failure	A syndrome characterized by acute deterioration in a patient of cirrhosis due to infection presenting with two or more extrahepatic organ failure
Definition of liver failure	Bilirubin≥5 mg/dL, INR ≥ 1.5	Bilirubin >12 mg/dL	Not specified
Source of definition	Prospective cohort of 3300 patients	Prospective cohort of 1343 patients	Prospective cohort of 507 patients
Inclusion criteria	Compensated cirrhosis CLD without cirrhosis Acute insult to liver	Cirrhosis (compensated or decompensated) Renal failure (mandatory) Presentation not necessarily by liver failure Repeated episode of ACLF admitted	Cirrhosis (compensated or decompensated) Two extrahepatic organ failure Presentation not necessarily by liver failure Repeated episode of ACLF admitted
Exclusion criteria	Prior decompensation	HCC	Patients with infection but did not require hospitalization
	HCC		Cirrhosis without infection
			HIV
			Prior OLT
			Disseminated malignancies
Time frame	4 weeks	4–12 weeks (variable)	Not defined
Acute insult	Hepatic	Hepatic or systemic	Infection
Sepsis	Consequence/complication	Cause/precipitant	Cause/precipitant
Organ failure	Hepatic first, extrahepatic subsequently	Systemic inflammation leading to kidney failure as the primary with or without other organ failure	Systemic inflammation leading to extrahepatic organ failure
Disease severity score	AARC-score	CLIF-C OF	MELD
			NACSELD-ACLF
Syndrome reversibility	Yes	Not described	Not described

Table 1.
Agreement/disagreement among different ACLF definition.

In summary, the most important differences between east and west definition of ACLF is the time frame of syndrome recognition. The western paradigm of organ failure as a prerequisite for the diagnosis of ACLF delays de facto of 7–14 days the presentation/diagnosis of the syndrome as compared to the eastern paradigm which indeed put the acute hepatic insult and liver failure as the starting point. According to AACR consortium, organ failure should not be used for definition of the syndrome, but only for prognostication [14].

2.2 Pathogenesis of ACLF

AS previously stated, ACLF is characterized by an excessive inflammatory response to different insults leading to a severe circulatory dysfunction involving several organs and ending to multiorgan failure. Bacterial infection is a well-recognized cause of ACLF worldwide and it is the prevalent precipitating event according to the western definitions. Gut bacterial translocation is the initiating pathogenic mechanism. Infection by viable bacteria can induce inflammation through two classes of molecules: pathogen-associated molecular patterns (PAMPs) and virulence-related factors [15]. Both PAMPS and virulence-related factors interact with the innate immunity through innate pattern recognition receptors (PRRs), and this results in production of several proinflammatory cytokines. If this response becomes excessive, the inflamed organism is exposed to a sort of "cytokine storm" responsible for tissue damage, which, in turn, causes the release of additional molecules: the damage-associated molecular patterns (DAMPs) which accentuate and perpetuate inflammation [15]. This inflammatory cascade is the driven force leading to a full-blown ACLF.

However, not all cirrhotic patients exposed to bacterial infection will develop an ACLF. This would suggest that an individual susceptibility to inflammation does exist, the explaining mechanisms of which are still poorly understood. Furthermore, many patients developing ACLF do not have any identifiable precipitating event [6]. In these cases, it is hypothesized that ACLF might be initiated and sustained by undetected bacterial or fungal infection with subclinical intestinal translocation of bacterial PAMPs and succeeding increase of DAMP release. Targets of the "cytokine storm" are circulatory system, heart, lung, kidney, adrenal glands and brain [16]. The severity of dysfunction and the number of organ/systems involved are the main determinants of ACLF prognosis [13]. Circulatory dysfunction is characterized by a progressive peripheral arteriolar vasodilation (PAV) due to reduced vascular resistance responsible of reduced effective volemia and organ hypo-perfusion with consequent tissue damage. Heart failure is another hallmark of ACLF. Cardiac dysfunction is typically found in advanced cirrhosis and contributes to the reduction of effective volemia since the hyperdynamic state as a compensatory response to hypovolemia, becomes no longer able to compensate arterial vasodilation [17, 18]. By worsening of inflammation, hyper-dynamic state becomes even more pronounced and may shift into the so called "cirrhotic cardiomyopathy" found in 40–50% of cirrhotic patients [19]. Damaged heart becomes no longer responsive to vasoactive compounds and this causes further tissue damage perpetuating the vicious circle.

Renal failure is particularly frequent in ACLF. Acute kidney injury (AKI) defined as an increase in serum creatinine by ≥0.3 mg/dL in <48 hours or a 50% increase from a stable baseline within the past 3 months, occurs in about 20% of all hospitalized patients with cirrhosis [20]. AKI represents the most frequent organ failure in ACLF patients with a worse prognosis, hepatorenal syndrome type 1 being the most frequent prototype [21]. Hemodynamic instability and systemic inflammation both concur to renal failure. AKI in ACLF is frequently associated with organic damage of kidney which should be ruled out as soon as possible in order to set the proper therapeutic approach (plasma volume expansion with albumin plus vasoconstriction therapy or renal replacement) [22].

Brain failure, defined as grade 3 or 4 hepatic encephalopaty (HE), is part for the EASL-CLIF definition of ACLF and it is a strong prognostic predictor. In a large North American study, HE predicted short-term mortality independently of other organ failure [23, 24].

Relative adrenal insufficiency (RAI) is another complication detectable in almost half of cirrhotic patient with acute liver decompensation and should be regarded as part of multiorgan failure. It has been found to be associated with poor in-hospital survival, refractory shock, and renal failure [25]. In a prospective observational study, Piano et al. reported that cirrhotic patients with RAI have a high risk of developing sepsis, septic shock, organ failure, and death within 90 days. The authors concluded that RAI has similar prognostic value as non-renal organ failures and it should be included in the EASL-CLIF classification of ACLF [26].

2.3 Prognostic scores

The prognosis of ACLF is universally considered dismal with a mortality at 4 weeks as high as 39%. Quantitation of short- and long-term mortality risk is of paramount importance to correctly planning therapeutic measures. This quantitation is quite difficult owing to the fact that ACLF patients differ as to precipitating events, grade of cirrhosis decompensation, number of organs involved and comorbidities.

Among single easily available laboratory parameters as predictors of outcome, lactate seems to be the most accurate one. In a cooperative European study [27] serum lactate on admission was directly related to the number of organs failing and to 28-day mortality (AUROC 0.72). In addition, both baseline lactate ≥5 mmol/L and 12-hour lactate clearance emerged as independent predictors of 1-year mortality [27].

Multiple predictive scores have been proposed in the last few years. Classical scores as Child-Pugh score (CP), or the model for end-stage liver disease (MELD) and MELD-Na revealed to be inaccurate to correctly predict short-term mortality in ACLF patients. Therefore, several other multiparametric score systems have been proposed in the last few years, from western and eastern areas [14, 28, 29].

Recently, the EASL-CLIF consortium proposed the CLIF-SOFA score (Chronic Liver Failure-Sequential Organ Failure) [6] (**Table 2**). This score includes biochemical and clinical parameters indicative of organ function and stratifies ACLF patients into three grades of severity [6, 30–32]. This score was constructed over the assumption, borrowed from the point of view of intensivists, that with increasing number of organ dysfunction or failure, the mortality would cumulatively increase. The CLIF-SOFAs, however, is complex, based on consensus and expert opinion rather than data, and did not significantly improve the prediction accuracy of other scores

Organ system	Score = 1	Score = 2	Score = 3
Liver: bilirubin (mg/dL)	<6	6–12	>12
Kidney: creatinine(mg/dL)	<2	2–3.5	>3.5 or renal replacement therapy
Brain: grade (West Haven)	0	1–2	3–4
Coagulation: INR	<2.0	2.0 to <3.5	≥3.5
Circulation: MAP (mmHg)	≥70	<70	Vasopressors
Respiratory (PaO2/FiO2)	>300	≤300 to > 200	≤200
or SpO2/FiO2	>357	>214 to ≤ 357	≤214

Column 3 defines organ failure.

Table 2.
CLIF-C OF score and parameters to define organ failure.

like Child-Pugh and MELD. For these reasons, in 2014 the CLIF Consortium, using CANONIC database, developed a simplified score named CLIF-C OF score (Organ Failure) derived from CLIF-SOFA one. Patients are stratified into three-point range and scored 6–18. This score confirmed to perform better than CP and MELD. A further refinement was obtained by adding to CLIF-C OF score age and white blood cells count. This refined version, named CLIF-C ACLF, was the result of a mathematical model constructed by logistic analysis carried out upon CANONIC database and validated on a validation set of ACLF patients. Patients are scored 1–100 by a bedside easy-to-use tool which is now available at the CLIF Consortium website: http://www.clifconsortium.com/ [28]. Both CLIF-C OF and CLIF-C ACLF scores showed better prognostic performance than the conventional prognostic scores [2, 28, 33]. In a recent retrospective study carried out on a cohort of 343 consecutive cirrhotic patients with ACLF diagnosed according to the EASL-CLIF definition and aimed at comparing eight different prognostic scores, emerged that CLIF-SOFA and CLIF-C OF scores displayed the highest predictive accuracy [34]. In this study a CLIF-C OF score of 8 or lower had a 92.0% NPV and 97.8% sensitivity, while a score of 17 or higher allowed for a 95.0% PPV and 99.4% specificity for the prediction of 28-day mortality.

The North American Consortium for the Study of End-Stage Liver Disease (NACSELD) in 2014 built a predictive score of short-term mortality named NACSELD-score further refined in 2018 [3]. According to NACSELD-ACLF score the presence of at least two organ failures such as shock, grade 3 or 4 encephalopathy, renal failure requiring hemodialysis, or respiratory failure requiring mechanical ventilation, accurately predicted 30-day survival. This score has been further validated in a population-based study on over 100,000 patients included in a large, North America representative database of hospital discharges (NIS). In this study, NACSELD-ACLF predicted survival with an area under the ROC curve 0.77 [35].

APASL consortium proposed a prognostic score named AARC with an elevated accuracy to predict early and late mortality (AUROC >80%) in patients with ACLF. Variables included in AARC score are bilirubin, INR, lactate, ascites and HE [14] (**Table 3**). According to this score patients are stratified as Grade I for a score of 5–7, Grade II for 8–10 and Grade III for 11–15 with 28-day mortality of 12.7, 44.5 and 85.9%, respectively. The score also predicted well 28 and 90-day survival.

In summary, beyond which is the best available predictive score of ACLF to be adopted, early diagnosis and rapid prognostication are essential to positively impact on outcome of this severe complication.

2.4 Treatment

Treatment of ACLF demands for a multi-disciplinary approach involving hepatologist, intensivist, infection control team, nutritionist and transplant team. The target of treatment is to cure the precipitating event on one side and liver, kidney, heart and brain failure and circulatory dysfunction on the other.

Points	Total bilirubin (mg/dL)	HE grade	PT-INR	Lactate (mml/L)	Creatinine (mg/dL)
1	<15	0	<1.8	<1.5	<0.7
2	15–25	I–II	1.8–2.5	1.5–2.5	0.7–1.5
3	>25	III–IV	>2.5	>2.5	>1.5

Grade1: score 5–7, Grade 2: score 8–10, Grade 3: score 11–15.

Table 3.
AACR-ACLF score.

2.4.1 Treatment of liver failure

In the setting of ACLF, liver transplant (OLT) is the only potentially curative option. However survival benefit shows great variability ranging from 43 to 75% in European series [36–38] and above 90% in Asia-Pacific regions [39]. The decision whether or not to list a patient for OLT has to cope with two relevant issues: urgency and futility. Urgency is motivated by the finding of around 67% mortality on waiting list for ACLF patients. This high rate of mortality is mainly due to sepsis, respiratory failure with mechanical ventilation, high vasopressor requirement and need of renal replacement treatment (RRT).

On the other hands futile transplants must be avoided. Indeed, post-transplant course in too sick patients if often characterized by severe prognosis. Many authors agree that OLT should not be offered when cardiac or pulmonary support is needed or there is rapidly progressive organ failure since, in these instances, OLT is unlike to offer survival benefit [40]. A recent observational study by Sundaram et al. [41] revealed that in patients with impairment of ACLF-3 grade score at listing to a lower grade at transplantation, post-transplant mortality was significantly lower than in patients without this impairment (12% vs. 18%). Improvement in circulatory failure, brain failure, or removal from mechanical ventilation has the strongest impact on post-transplant survival. These data further reinforce the paradigm that early selection of good candidates for OLT (realistically within the first week from admission) is mandatory to avoid futility. To maximize survival benefit through a correct selection of good candidate to OLT, some algorithms have been proposed but they are still waiting an external validation [42, 43].

Besides OLT, other therapies for liver failure have been tempted in the last few years with discordant results. This is due, at least in part, to the different criteria employed to define ACLF from different geographic areas, making hard drawing definite conclusions. Based on the assumption that ACLF may result from an exaggerated response to inflammation with high levels of circulating pro- and antiinflammation substances, extracorporeal depurating devices such as molecular adsorbent recirculating system (MARS) [44] and the PROMETHEUS [45] could have a role as a bridging therapy to OLT. Unfortunately, data on efficacy of these instruments are disappointing. In a meta-analysis and systematic review by Kiaergard et al., no benefit of MARS treatment in reducing mortality as compared to standard medical therapy was noted [46]. These conclusions were further confirmed by two recently published European randomized multicentric controlled trials, that is, HELIOS (for Prometheus) [45] and RELIEF trial (for MARS) [44] showing no benefit with these modalities on short-term transplant-free survival. Hence, their use is currently not recommended by international guidelines. Bioartificial liver (BAL) support devices such as AMC-BAL Bioreactor, HepatAssist device (employing porcine hepatocytes attached to collagen-coated micro carriers and charcoal columns) and extracorporeal liver assist device (ELAD)-C3A employing human hepatoblastoma cells provided inconsistent results on survival [47].

Thus, besides OLT, treatment of liver failure still remains largely disappointing.

An interesting issue is the use of non-selective beta-blockers in ACLF patients. In a retrospective study by Mookerjee et al. carried out on a subgroup of patients enrolled in the CANONIC study, those patients on carvedilol treatment (47%) had lower 28-day mortality (24% vs. 34%, $p = 0.048$), a less severe ACLF and a slower progression of ACLF during the study period than those not on NSBB. Moreover, patients who discontinued NSBBs ($n = 78$) after development of ACLF had a higher mortality (37% vs. 13%) [48]. These data prompted a randomized controlled trial by Kumar et al. [49] on carvedilol administration to ACLF patients without esophageal varices and moderately increased HVPG. The authors reported that carvedilol leaded to improved survival and lowered the risk of developing AKI and SBP up to 28 days. However, these preliminary data need to be further confirmed, before carvedilol can enter the medical armamentarium of hepatologists to cure ACLF.

2.4.2 Treatment of renal failure

Acute kidney injury (AKI) is the most common organ failure in patients with ACLF, being type1 hepatorenal syndrome (HRS1) the more severe prototype. It has been demonstrated that AKI complicating ACLF is more severe than AKI complicating cirrhosis and lesser responsive to treatment [22]. The correct approach to AKI in cirrhosis has been specifically addressed in the last few years. Early diagnosis of AKI is crucial to adopt the correct treatment. A multidisciplinary panel of experts recently proposed a useful diagnostic algorithm based on serum creatinine (Scr) monitoring [50]. It should be remembered that serum creatinine tends to overestimate kidney function in cirrhotic patients. For hospitalized patients, the International Ascites Club suggests referring to the Scr determined in the last 3 months as a baseline value to monitor and stage AKI while GFR assessment is not recommended [20]. Oliguria is a useful tool for diagnostic purposes and even a useful clinical parameter in determining the severity of renal dysfunction as well. Worsening oliguria or development of anuria should be considered as AKI until proven otherwise, regardless of any rise in Scr [20]. Volume expansion is the mainstay step for management of AKI. Albumin should be preferred over crystalloids owing to its oncotic and non-oncotic properties and it must be the first choice plasmaexpander in case of bacterial infection, suspected type-1 HRS or when the cause of AKI is unclear. The recommend regimen is infusion of 25% albumin 1 g/kg day 1 followed by 20–40 g/day until renal function improves [20]. The goal of albumin infusion is to counteract the dramatic renal hypoperfusion and intrarenal vasoconstriction. Albumin plus vasoconstrictors infusion as terlipressin is the recommended combined therapy for HRS1 and it should be started as soon as possible. The earlier we start vasoconstrictor therapy the greater the chance of survival [51].

Renal replacement is the only reasonable approach when renal damage supervenes. RRT is recommended in case of worsening AKI, worsening fluid overload despite diuretic therapy or worsening acid-base status [52]. The role of dialysis however, is still under evaluation and in clinical practice; it is mostly reserved to patients candidate for OLT [50, 53].

2.4.3 Treatment of circulatory and cardiac dysfunction

As previously outlined, circulatory dysfunction due to vascular vasodilation and consequent hypotension is a severe complication of ACLF. Cirrhotic patients with hyperdynamic and hypodynamic circulatory state have a higher risk of fatal ACLF [54]. It has been shown that arterial hypotension is an independent risk factor for ACLF development [55]. In particular, cirrhotic patients with hyperdynamic state as expressed by increased cardiac index, (>CI4.2 L/min/m2) have increased levels of circulating IL-6/8 and PCR and are at major risk to develop fatal ACLF [54]. Pharmacologic support including the amine infusion, inotropic substances and fluid administration are the recommended approach [53]. In critically ill patients, a mean arterial pressure of 60 mmHg or more should be the target [56]. Repeated serum lactate determination is the best way to monitor circulatory dysfunction and repeated lactate determination is more informative than the absolute value due to the impaired lactate clearance in patients with cirrhosis [57].

Careful attention to fluid supplementation is mandatory since, in cirrhosis, an aggressive fluid administration may lead to tissue edema and to an increased total body water retention which may adversely affect the outcome [58–62]. It is well known that cirrhotic patients are particularly prone to develop extracellular edema, ascites and pulmonary edema as a consequence of too aggressive fluid administration. In volume depleted patients, normal 0.9% saline solution at an initial dose of 10–20 ml/kg or balanced salt solutions such as PlasmaLyte are recommended [63, 64]. Albumin infusion as plasmaexpander is highly recommended. The benefits of albumin infusion in patients with cirrhosis go beyond simple volume expansion and rely on its numerous biological properties [65, 66]. Albumin infusion is strongly recommended in three specific situations: SBP, large volume paracentesis and type-1 HRS [67–72]. In addition, albumin infusion prevents AKI in patients with infections other than SBP [73, 74]. As to the amine choice, norepinephrine should be the first line agent being associated to fewer adverse events [75]. Vasopressin and terlipressin may be used as second line agents able to achieve hemodynamic improvement [76–79]. Corticosteroids in critically ill patients may be beneficial in reducing vasopressor doses and increasing the rate of shock reversal [25, 80, 81]. The rationale of corticosteroids administration lies on the relative adrenal insufficiency (RAI) that commonly comes along with circulatory dysfunction in critically ill cirrhotic patients. Corticosteroids have demonstrated a survival benefit in some [25, 82] but not in all studies [80, 81]. Hydrocortisone 200–300 mg/day in divided doses should be administered to patients partially responsive to vasopressor agents [83, 84].

2.4.4 Treatment of neurologic dysfunction

Brain dysfunction is part of multiorgan failure complicating ACLF and HE grade 3 or 4 is required for diagnosis of ACLF according to EASL-CLIF definition. The correct interpretation and differential diagnosis of brain dysfunction is challenging since several conditions may be in cause. EEG changes are of limited value in the diagnosis of HE, even though EEG may help excluding other causes of altered mental status. Brain imaging could be useful to exclude other causes of altered mental status and, in particular, to exclude intra-cerebral hemorrhage in critically ill cirrhotic patients with coagulative disorders [85].

Measurement of fasting ammonia is routinely performed in clinical practice to differentiate HE from other conditions. Nevertheless, high ammonia levels alone are not recommended for diagnosis of HE since false positive results are frequent. West-Haven criteria (WHC) are useful for HE staging and managing [50] and advanced grade [3, 4] indicate those patients needing airways protection. Glasgow coma scale (GCS) is another simple clinical tool widely employed in HE patients and a threshold <8 is a useful parameter to decided airway protection [86].

Lactulose is the recommended initial therapy for HE. Other options such as rifaximine, LOLA, intravenous albumin, or other laxatives are currently not recommended for HE treatment [50].

3. Multidrug-resistant bacterial infections in patients with acute-on- chronic liver failure

3.1 Epidemiologic considerations

Cirrhotic patients are particularly prone to develop bacterial infection [87] and bacterial infection may trigger an ACLF in up to 50% of cases in western countries [3, 6, 88–90]. On the other hand, patients with ACLF are likely to develop spontaneous and secondary bacterial infections. [6, 88, 91]. Bacterial infections increase short-term mortality by 2–4 fold, [7, 91, 92] and it is the most important prognostic predictor of bad outcome [88, 93–95].

Epidemiologic characteristics of bacterial infection have changed in the last decades. Until the 90s, Gram-negative bacteria were by far the main organisms detected in patients with cirrhosis and spontaneous bacterial peritonitis (SBP) and pneumonia were the most frequent sites of infection [9, 96–98]. In the last two decades we witnessed a steady increase of gram-positive isolates. In a recent international cooperative study (Global Study) by Piano et al. including 1302 patients with bacterial infections (43% from Europe,32% from Asia and 25% from America), the prevalence of positive bacteria was up to 38% [99]. As to the site of infection, more recent studies, confirmed SBP, urinary tract infection, and pneumonia as the most frequent sites [99–106]. Fungal infection is an emerging problem as well, particularly in cirrhotic patients needing ICU stay [107]. Noticeably, in the multi-center study of Galbois et al. [108], including 31.251 patients in ICU for septic shock, the fungal infections were more frequent in cirrhotic than non-cirrhotic patients (9.9% vs. 6.3%, $P < 0.05$). Unfortunately, in most instances fungal infection is not recognized and this could cause delayed diagnosis, treatment failure and high mortality rates [109–111]. Thinking to prophylactic antifungal treatment in severely ill patients without improvement after 48 hours of antibiotics, or in those in dialysis, corticosteroid treatment or carrying central devices is highly warranted and could also help improving the otherwise poor outcome.

Experts agree that early diagnosis is critical in determining the course of infection in cirrhotic patients [88, 112]. The acute phase proteins, such as C-reactive protein and procalcitonin, were reliable and early biomarkers for bacterial infection and are currently recommended as screening tools for the presence of bacterial infections along with routine cultural examination. Biomarkers such as galactomannan or B–D glucan are recommended for supporting the diagnosis of invasive fungal infection.

In the last 20 years, however, we record an increasing rate of bacterial infections sustained by multidrug-resistant (MDR) bacteria, and resistance to antibiotics is becoming a major global public health problem [113–118]. Recurrent hospitalizations, invasive procedures and repeated exposures to prophylactic or therapeutic antibiotics constitute known risk factors for drug-resistant organisms, in patients with decompensated cirrhosis [115]. According to internationally accepted definition, resistant bacteria can be divided into three different groups, depending on susceptibility to different class of antibiotics. Multidrug resistant bacteria (MDR) are isolates non-susceptible to at least one agent in three or more antimicrobial categories, extensively-drug resistant (XDR) are those non-susceptible to at least one agent in all but 2 or fewer antimicrobial categories and pandrug-resistant (PDR) are those non-susceptible to all currently available agents [119].

Data on prevalence and type of MDR derive mainly from single-center studies [89, 90, 96–98, 120, 113, 115–117, 121, 122] or from multicenter studies performed in specific countries [102] or assessing specific infections [123]. Canonic Study database represents an important source of information on the prevalence of MDR bacterial infections in cirrhosis across Europe, potential epidemiological differences among regions and centers, the characteristics of these infections, their impact on prognosis, risk factors for MDR and type and efficacy of empirical antibiotic treatment employed [6, 106]. According to CANONIC data, prevalence of MDR bacterial infections in Europe varies in different countries being higher in Northern and Western Europe [106].

In the Global study [99], the overall prevalence of MDR bacterial infections varies among series from a minimum of 8% in Turkey to 27–46% in Italy peaking in Korea and India (87 and 69%, respectively). This high rate of MDR bacteria found in India may be, at least in part, explained by non-prescriptional access to antibiotics in this country [124].

In Europe and USA, the highest prevalence of MDR is registered in nosocomial and health-care associated infections [91, 100, 103, 104, 116, 117, 121, 122, 125–129].

All these data unequivocally confirm that the rate of MDR bacterial infections has increased almost 10%, in the last 10 years and it is becoming a problem of growing clinical relevance in decompensated cirrhosis and ACLF. As to the type of MDR, ESBL-producing Enterobacteriaceae, VSE and MRSA are those most frequently isolated [28, 89, 102, 122, 123, 130]. However, the type of resistant strain significantly differs across countries and centers [91, 99, 106]. The Canonic study revealed that ESBL and Amp-C producing Enterobacteriaceae were more frequently isolated in France, Italy, the UK and the Netherlands; VSE predominated in France and Austria and MRSA in infections occurring in the Netherlands, the UK and Ireland. This continuous change in isolated strains among countries demands to develop surveillance programs aimed at investigating the prevalence and epidemiological pattern of MDROs at each hospital [131].

XDR bacteria must be considered extremely dangerous in cirrhosis (as in other settings), and their prevalence is far from being negligible. In the study of Piano et al., the rate of XDR was 16% in Asia,4% in America and 5% in Europe [99].

The problem of multi-drug resistance is particularly evident in ACLF or acute liver decompensation. In a study by Fernandez et al., prevalence of overall infection and, in particular, of nosocomial infections (53% vs. 22%, $p < 0.001$) caused by MDRs (16% vs. 3%, $p = 0.01$) was significantly higher in ACLF than AD [91]. In CANONIC database [106], ESBL-producing *Escherichia coli*, VSE, MRSA and ESBL-producing *Klebsiella pneumoniae* were the most frequent strands. The overall prevalence of MDR bacterial infections was 14.8% and 29.2% in culture-positive episodes and were more frequently isolated in bacteremia (28.6%), pneumonia (23.5%), and UTI (20.7%). MDR bacteria were also more frequently isolated in the ICU (23.8% vs. 12.2%, $p = 0.005$) and in nosocomial infections (21.3% vs. 8.3% and 6.6% in CA and HCA infections, respectively, $p < 0.001$). Finally, MDRs were more prevalent in infections causing severe sepsis/shock (30.3% vs. 12.2%, $p < 0.001$) or ACLF (20.5% vs. 9.4%, $p < 0.001$).

3.2 Therapeutic considerations

Due to the urgency to treat suspected bacterial infection in critically ill cirrhotic patients before susceptibility tests are available, an empirical approach is the rule. Two types of empirical antibiotic strategies are usually employed: "classical" strategies based on third-generation cephalosporins, amoxicillin-clavulanic-acid/cloxacillin or quinolones and "MDR covering strategies" including piperacillin-tazobactam, carbapenems, ceftazidime/cefepime ± glycopeptides or linezolid/daptomycin. The latter is generally considered when we face to healthcare-associated (HCA) or nosocomial infections [91, 113].

The initial empirical antibiotic therapy is considered appropriate when the antibiotic has activity in vitro adequate for the isolated pathogen in culture positive infections or when it solves the infection without need for further escalation, in culture-negative infections. Otherwise, the initial therapy is considered inappropriate [91]. When the first-line empiric antibiotic therapy failed, patients experienced a higher rate of renal failure and death during hospitalization [102, 132] as confirmed by the study by Umgelter et al. [127] who found an association between failure of antibiotic first line regimen and mortality in SBP patients. Even, Fernandez et al. [113] reported a frequent inefficacy of the empiric antibiotic therapy in patients with high risk of death, especially in nosocomial infections. All these observations reinforce the relevance of an appropriate first line antibiotic administration in ACLF [88].

3.3 Type and efficacy of first line antibiotic strategies

The emergence of multidrug-resistant (MDR) and extensively drug-resistant (XDR) bacteria has led to a decrease in the efficacy of classical empirical strategies based on the administration of third-generation cephalosporins. The resistance to classical empirical antibiotic regimens is associated with a higher mortality rate, an increased duration of in-hospital stays and higher healthcare related costs when compared to infections caused by susceptible strains [89, 91, 98, 99, 116, 133, 134]. To date, it is recommended to treated nosocomial and HCA infections with empirical MDR covering strategies, whether a classical empirical approach is recommended for CA infections (**Table 4**). Empirical MDR covering strategies are usually more effective than empiric classical schemes in nosocomial infections (81.7% vs. 68%, respectively, $p = 0.01$) with a positive impact on short-term survival. A trend towards statistical significance is also observed in severe sepsis/shock (81.3% vs. 60.9%, $p = 0.06$). Inadequacy of first line antibiotic strategies increased 28-day mortality in both AD (33.3% vs. 7.7%, $p < 0.001$) and ACLF patients (50% vs. 25.8%, $p = 0.002$).

Thus, broad schemes covering all potential pathogens should be empirically used in the nosocomial setting and in severe sepsis/shock, followed by rapid de-escalation strategies to avoid a further spread of antibiotic resistance [88, 106, 114, 135]. In a recent retrospective study from Germany [136] the authors evaluated the efficacy of different first line empirical antibiotic therapies in ACLF patients with SBP. From this study emerged that meropenem-daptomycin (99.5%), meropenem-linezolid, (98.5%) and meropenem-vancomycin (96.8%) combination scheme had the highest antimicrobial susceptibility rates and piperacillin/tazobactam had the highest antimicrobial susceptibility rates among the monotherapies/fixed combinations considering all of the Gram-negative and Gram-positive bacteria. On the contrary, classical empiric therapy based on cefotaxime or ceftriaxone showed a sensibility as low as 60%. Susceptibility of bacteria to these combination regimens positively impacted on inpatient mortality and complications. However, some pharmacologic and pharmacokinetic properties of these antibiotics should be considered when empirical MDR covering therapy has to be started. Linezolid achieves rapid penetration in peritoneum and rapidly reaches high concentration in tissue [137]. However, in patients with concomitant sepsis, it might not be the best option because the effect is more towards the bacteriostatic side, and thus might be too weak to ideally treat the bacteremia component [137]. Contrarily to linezolid, vancomycin has a lower tissue concentration and weak penetrability [138]. It is therefore should be preferred for sepsis [138]. Daptomycin has a very low concentration in the peritoneal cavity (only 6% of that in serum) [139]. Thus, daptomycin should be the first-choice antibiotic to treat bacteremia and sepsis being safer than vancomycin. As to gram-negative infection, thanks to their moderate volume of distribution and excellent penetrability both piperacillin/tazobactam and meropenem could be used for infection of peritoneum as well as bacteremia/sepsis [140, 141].

As in other settings, there is a cogent need to evaluate new strategies for preventing the spread of antibiotic resistance in cirrhotic population. Many studies are investigating epidemiological surveillance through regular assessment of potential carriers of MDRs through rectal and nasal swabs during hospitalization [142, 143], rapid microbiological tests [144, 145] and antibiotic stewardship programs [112, 146, 147].

As previously stated, fungal infection is an emerging problem in cirrhotic patients, particularly in those with ACLF hospitalized in ICU. An early diagnosis of fungal infection and antifungal treatment is prognostically crucial and it has been associated with improved outcome [148]. Triazoles (fluconazole, itraconazole, voriconazole, and posaconazole) are the most frequently employed antifungal agents. However, due to reported emergence of azole resistant non-albicans spp., the first line treatment recommended in critically ill patients shifted toward a new antifungal class: the echinocandins (caspofungin, anidulafungin, and micafungin). Echinocandins are indeed, the recommended first-line treatment for patients with cirrhosis and nosocomial spontaneous fungal peritonitis. The usual intravenous

	Type of infection		Suspected MDR		
	Community acquired	**Nosocomial health-care associated**	**ESBL-P**	**MRSA VSE**	**VRE**
SBP	Cefotaxime or ceftriaxone	Piperacilline/tazobactam	Carbapenems/meropen em	Vancomicin or teicoplanin	Linezolid or Daptomycin
Spontaneous bacteremia	Cefotaxime or ceftriaxone	Piperacilline/tazobactam	Carbapenems/meropen em	Vancomicin or teicoplanin	Linezolid or Daptomycin
UTI Uncomplicated	ciprofloxacin	Nitrofurantoin or fosfomycin	Carbapenems/meropen em	Vancomicin or teicoplanin	Linezolid or Daptomycin
With sepsis	Cefotaxime or ceftriaxone	Piperacilline/tazobactam			
Pneumonia	Ciprofloxacin or moxifloxacin or	Ceftazidime	Carbapenems + ciprofloxacin	Vancomicin or teicoplanin	Linezolid or Daptomycin
	Cefotaxime or ceftriaxone		Meropenem + ciprofloxacin		

SBP, spontaneous bacterial peritonitis; UTI, urinary tract infection; ESBL-P, extended spectrum beta-lactamase producers; MRSA, methicillin-resistent Staphylococcus aureus; VSE, vancomycin susceptible; VRE, vancomycin resistant.

Table 4.
Empirical antibiotic treatment of infection in cirrhosis (adapted from Allaire et al.) [149].

dosing regimens for invasive candidiasis are as follows: caspofungin: loading dose 70 mg, then 50 mg daily. No dose adjustement are recommended in case of moderate and severe liver disease except for caspofungin (loading dose 70 mg, then 35 mg daily) [148, 150]. De-escalation from echinocandins to fluconazole is advised in those cirrhotic patients when their condition becomes stable.

4. Conclusions

Acute-on-chronic liver failure (ACLF) is a clinical independent entity capturing the interest of hepatologists from the East and the West in the past 2 decades. Although universal definition does not exist, there is a substantial agreement that this syndrome should refer to liver failure, usually after an acute event, in a patient with chronic liver disease and characterized by an elevated short-term mortality. It should be distinguished from an ordinary decompensation of chronic liver disease and from acute liver failure of a normal liver. Although the pathophysiological mechanisms leading to this syndrome are only partly understood, systemic inflammation seems to play a crucial role. Exaggerated inflammatory response, the so-called "cytokine storm" is the main driving event leading to multiorgan failure. In most cases, bacterial infection is the initiating event of ACLF and early identification and treatment is mandatory to stop SIRS-sepsis cascade and to prevent multiorgan failure. An emerging clinical problem is represented by infection sustained by of MDR bacteria. This new epidemiologic reality has completely changed antibiotic strategies for empirical approach in decompensated cirrhosis. Control and prevention of MDR infection widespread, in particular in the nosocomial setting, as well as to make available new treatment opportunities, beside OLT, to manage liver failure are the challenge of the near future.

Conflict of interest

None to be declared.

Author details

Mauro Borzio[1*] and Elena Dionigi[2]

1 Department of Gastroenterology, ASST Melegnano-Martesana, Milano, Italy

2 Department of Medicine, ASST Melegnano-Martesana, Milano, Italy

*Address all correspondence to: mauro.borzio@gmail.com

References

[1] Bajaj JS, Moreau R, Kamath PS, Vargas HE, Arroyo V, Reddy KR, et al. Acute-on-chronic liver failure: Getting ready for prime time? Hepatology. 2018;**68**:1621-1632

[2] Jalan R, Pavesi M, Saliba F, Amorós A, Fernandez J, Holland-Fischer P, et al. The CLIF consortium acute Decompensation score (CLIF-C ADs) for prognosis of hospitalised cirrhotic patients without acute-on-chronic liver failure. Journal of Hepatology. 2015;**62**:831-840

[3] O'Leary JG, Reddy KR, Garcia-Tsao G, Biggins SW, Wong F, Fallon MB, et al. NACSELD acute-on-chronic liver failure (NACSELD-ACLF) score predicts 30-day survival in hospitalized patients with cirrhosis. Hepatology. 2018;**67**:2367-2374

[4] Sarin SK, Chandan K, Zaigham A, Amarapurkar B, Bihari C, Chan AC, et al. Acute-on-chronic liver failure: Consensus recommendations of the Asian Pacific association for the study of the liver (APASL). Hepatology International. 2014;**8**:453-471

[5] Sarin SK, Choudhury A, Sharma MK, Maiwall MK, Mahtab M, Saigal RS, et al. Acute-on-chronic liver failure: Consensus recommendations of the Asian Pacific association for the study of the liver (APASL): An update. Hepatology International. 2019;**13**:353-390

[6] Moreau R, Jalan R, Ginès P, Pavesi M, Angeli P, Cordoba J, et al. Acute-on-chronic liver failure is a distinct syndrome developing in patients with acute decompensation of cirrhosis. Gastroenterology. 2013;**144**:1426-1437

[7] Gustot T, Felleiter P, Pickkers P, Sakr Y, Rello J, Velissaris D, et al. Impact of infection on the prognosis of critically ill cirrhotic patients: Results from a large worldwide study. Liver International. 2014;**34**:1496-1503

[8] Gustot T, Jalan R. Acute-on-chronic liver failure in patients with alcohol-related liver disease. Journal of Hepatology. 2019;**70**:319-327

[9] Chalasani N, Bonkovsky HL, Fontana R, Lee W, Stolz A, Talwalkar J, et al. Features and outcomes of 899 patients with drug-induced liver injury: The DILIN prospective study. Gastroenterology. 2015;**148**:1340-1352

[10] Qin G, Shao JG, Zhu YC, Xu AD, Yao JH, Wang XL, et al. Population-representative incidence of acute-on-chronic liver failure. A prospective cross-sectional study. Journal of Clinical Gastroenterology. 2016;**50**:670-675

[11] Anand L, Choudhury A, Bihari C, Sharma BC, Kumar M, Maiwall R, et al. APASL ACLF (APASL ACLF research consortium) Working party. Flare of autoimmune hepatitis causing acute on chronic liver failure (ACLF): Diagnosis and response to corticosteroid therapy. Hepatology. 2019;**70**:587-596

[12] Axley P, Ahmed Z, Arora S, Haas A, Kuo YF, Kamath PS, et al. NASH is the most rapidly growing etiology for acute-on-chronic liver failure-related hospitalization and disease burden in the United States: A population-based study. Liver Transplantation. 2019;**25**:695-705

[13] Jalan R, Yurdaydin C, Bajaj JS, Acharya SK, Arroyo V, Lin HC, et al. Toward an improved definition of acute-on-chronic liver failure. Gastroenterology. 2014;**147**:4-10

[14] Choudhury A, Jindal A, Maiwal R, Sarin SK, Sharma LK, Pamecha V, et al. Liver failure determines the outcome in patient of acute-on-chronic liver failure (ACLF)-comparison of APASL-ACLF

research consortium (AARC) and CLIF-SOFA model. Hepatology International. 2017;**11**:461-471

[15] Iwasaki A, Medzhitov R. Control of adaptive immunity by the innate immune system. Nature Immunology. 2015;**16**:343-353

[16] Bernardi M, Moreau R, Angeli P, Schnabl B, Arroyo V. Mechanisms of decompensation and organ failure in cirrhosis: From peripheral arterial vasodilation to systemic inflammation hypothesis. Journal of Hepatology. 2015;**63**:1272-1284

[17] Ruiz-del-Arbol L, Monescillo A, Arocena C, Valer P, Gines P, Moreira V, et al. Circulatory function and hepatorenal syndrome in cirrhosis. Hepatology. 2005;**42**:439-447

[18] Nazar A, Guevara M, Sitges M, Terra C, Solá E, Guigou C, et al. Left ventricular function assessed by echocardiography in cirrhosis: Relationship to systemic hemodynamics and renal dysfunction. Journal of Hepatology. 2013;**58**:51-57

[19] Moller S, Hove JD, Dixen U, Bendtsen F. New insights into cirrhotic cardiomyopathy. International Journal of Cardiology. 2013;**167**:1101-1108

[20] Angeli P, Gines P, Wong F, Bernardi M, Boyer TD, Gerbes A, et al. Diagnosis and management of acute kidney injury in patients with cirrhosis: Revised consensus recommendations of the International Club of Ascites. Gut. 2015;**64**:531-537

[21] Angeli P, Rodriguez E, Piano S, Ariza X, Morando F, Sola E, et al. Acute kidney injury and acute-on-chronic liver failure classifications in prognosis assessment of patients with acute decompensation of cirrhosis. Gut. 2015;**64**:1616-1622

[22] Maiwall R, Kumar S, Chandel SS, Kumar G, Rastogi A, Bihari C, et al. AKI in patients with acute on chronic liver failure is different from acute decompensation of cirrhosis. Hepatology International. 2015;**9**: 627-639

[23] Cordoba J, Ventura-Cots M, Simon-Talero M, Amoros A, Pavesi M, Vilstrup H, et al. Characteristics, risk factors, and mortality of cirrhotic patients hospitalized for hepatic encephalopathy with and without acute-on-chronic liver failure (ACLF). Journal of Hepatology. 2014;**60**:275-281

[24] Bajaj JS, O'Leary JG, Tandon P, Wong F, Garcia-Tsao G, Kamath PS, et al. Hepatic encephalopathy is associated with mortality in patients with cirrhosis independent of other extrahepatic organ failures. Clinical Gastroenterology and Hepatology. 2017;**15**:565-574

[25] Fernandez J, Escorsell A, Zabalza M, Felipe V, Navasa M, Mas A, et al. Adrenal insufficiency in patients with cirrhosis and septic shock: Effect of treatment with hydrocortisone on survival. Hepatology. 2006;**44**:1288-1295

[26] Piano S, Favaretto E, Tonon M, Antonelli G, Brocca A, Sticca A, et al. Including relative adrenal insufficiency in definition and classification of acute on chronic liver failure. Clinical Gastroenterology and Hepatology. 2020;**18**:1188-1196

[27] Drolz A, Horvatits T, Rutter K, Landahl F, Roald K, Meersseman P, et al. Lactate improves prediction of short-term mortality in critically ill patients with cirrhosis: A multinational study. Hepatology. 2019;**69**:258-269

[28] Jalan R, Saliba F, Pavesi M, Amoros A, Moreau R, Ginès P, et al. Development and validation of a prognostic score to predict mortality in patients with acute-on-chronic liver failure. Journal of Hepatology. 2014;**61**:1038-1047

[29] Lee M, Lee JH, Oh S, Jang Y, Lee W, Lee HJ, et al. CLIF-SOFA scoring system accurately predicts short-term mortality in acutely decompensated patients with alcoholic cirrhosis: A retrospective analysis. Liver International. 2015;**35**:46-57

[30] Wehler M, Kokoska J, Reulbach U, Hahn EG, Strauss R. Short-term prognosis in critically ill patients with cirrhosis assessed by prognostic scoring systems. Hepatology. 2001;**34**:255-261

[31] Das V, Boelle PY, Galbois A, Guidet B, Maury E, Carbonell N, et al. Cirrhotic patients in the medical intensive care unit: Early prognosis and long-term survival. Critical Care Medicine. 2010;**38**:2108-2116

[32] Levesque E, Hoti E, Azoulay D, Ichaï P, Habouchi H, Castaing D, et al. Prospective evaluation of the prognostic scores for cirrhotic patients admitted to an intensive care unit. Journal of Hepatology. 2012;**56**:95-102

[33] Perdigoto DN, Figueiredo P, Luís TL. The role of the CLIF-C OF and the 2016 MELD in prognosis of cirrhosis with and without acute-on-chronic liver failure. Annals of Hepatology. 2019;**18**:48-57

[34] Maipang K, Potranun P, Chainuvati S, Nimanong S, Chotiyaputta W, Tanwandee T, et al. Validation of the prognostic models in acute on-chronic liver failure precipitated by hepatic and extrahepatic insults. PLoS One. 2019;**14**(7):e0219516

[35] Rosenblatt R, Shen N, Tafesh Z, Cohen-Mekelburg S, Crawford CV, Kumar S, et al. The north American consortium for the study of end-stage liver disease-acute-on-chronic liver failure score accurately predicts survival: An external validation using a national cohort. Liver Transplantation. 2020;**26**:187-195

[36] Gustot T, Fernandez J, Garcia E, Morando F, Caraceni P, Alessandria C, et al. Clinical course of acute-on-chronic liver failure syndrome and effects on prognosis. Hepatology. 2015;**62**:243-252

[37] Artru F, Louvet A, Ruiz I, Levesque E, Labreuche J, Ursic-Bedoya J, et al. Liver transplantation in the most severely ill cirrhotic patients: A multicenter study in acute-on-chronic liver failure grade 3. Journal of Hepatology. 2017;**67**:708-715

[38] Finkenstedt A, Nachbaur K, Zoller H, Joannidis M, Pratschke J, Graziadei IW, et al. Acute-on-chronic liver failure: Excellent outcomes after liver transplantation but high mortality on the wait list. Liver Transplantation. 2013;**19**:879-886

[39] Jalan R, Gines P, Olson JC, Mookerjee RP, Moreau R, Garcia-Tsao G, et al. Acute-on chronic liver failure. Journal of Hepatology. 2012;**57**:1336-1348

[40] Bahirwani R, Shaked O, Bewtra M, Forde K, Reddy KR. Acute-on-chronic liver failure before liver transplantation: Impact on post-transplant outcomes. Transplantation. 2011;**92**:952-957

[41] Sundaram V, Kogachi S, Wong RJ, Karvellas CJ, Fortune BE, Mahmud N, et al. Effect of the clinical course of acute-on-chronic liver failure prior to liver transplantation on post-transplant survival. Journal of Hepatology. 2020;**72**:481-488

[42] Choudhury AK, Sharma M, Mehtab M, Sarin SK, for APASL ACLF Working party, et al. The decision for liver transplant in acute-on-chronic liver failure (ACLF)—First week is the crucial period-analysis of the APASL ACLF research consortium (AARC) prospective data of 1021 patients. Journal of Hepatology. 2016;**64**:S1-S51

[43] Pamecha V, Kumar S, Bharathy KG. Liver transplantation

in acute-on-chronic liver failure: Challenges and an algorithm for patient selection and management. Hepatology International. 2015;**9**:534-542

[44] Banares R, Nevens F, Larsen FS, Jalan R, Albillos A, Dollinger M, et al. Extracorporeal albumin dialysis with the molecular adsorbent recirculating system in acute-on-chronic liver failure: The RELIEF trial. Hepatology. 2013;**57**:1153-1162

[45] Kribben A, Gerken G, Haag S, Herget-Rosenthal S, Treichel U, Betz C, et al. Effects of fractionated plasma separation and adsorption on survival in patients with acute-on-chronic liver failure. Gastroenterology. 2012;**142**:782-789

[46] Kjaergard LL, Liu J, Als-Nielsen B, Gluud C. Artificial and bioartificial support systems for acute and acute-on-chronic liver failure: A systematic review. JAMA. 2003;**289**:217-222

[47] Zheng Z, Li X, Li Z, Ma X. Artificial and bioartificial liver support systems for acute and acute-on-chronic hepatic failure: Meta-analysis and meta-regression. Experimental and Therapeutic Medicine. 2013;**6**:929-936

[48] Mookerjee RP, Pavesi M, Thomsen KL, Mehta G, Macnaughtan J, Bendtsen F, et al. Treatment with non-selective beta-blockers associated with reduced severity of systemic inflammation and improved survival of patients with acute-on-chronic liver failure. Journal of Hepatology. 2016;**64**:574-582

[49] Kumar M, Kainth S, Choudhury A, Maiwall R, Mitra LG, Saluja V, et al. Treatment with carvedilol improves survival of patients with acute-on-chronic liver failure: A randomized controlled trial. Hepatology International. 2019;**13**:800-813

[50] Nadim MK, Durand F, Kellum JA, Levitsky J, O'Leary JG, Karvellas CJ, et al. Management of the critically ill patients with cirrhosis: A multidisciplinary perspective. Journal of Hepatology. 2016;**64**:717-735

[51] Krag A, Moller S, Henriksen JH, Holstein-Rathlou NH, Larsen FS, Bendtsen F. Terlipressin improves renal function in patients with cirrhosis and ascites without hepatorenal syndrome. Hepatology. 2007;**46**:1863-1871

[52] Saraiva IE, Ortiz-Soriano VM, Mei X, Gianella FG, Woc WS, Zamudio R, et al. Continuous renal replacement therapy in critically ill patients with acute on chronic liver failure and acute kidney injury: A retrospective cohort study. Clinical Nephrology. 2020;**93**:187-194

[53] Bajaj JS, O'Leary JG, Reddy KR, Wong F, Biggins SW, Patton H, et al. Survival in infection-related acute-on-chronic liver failure is defined by extrahepatic organ failures. Hepatology. 2014;**60**:250-256

[54] Praktiknjo M, Monteiro S, Grandt J, Kimer N, Madsen JL, Werge MP, et al. Cardiodynamic state is associated with systemic inflammation and fatal acute-on-chronic liver failure. Liver International. 2020. DOI: 10.1111/liv.14433

[55] Piano S, Tonon M, Vettore E, Stanco M, Pilutti C, Romano A, et al. Incidence, predictors and outcomes of acute-on-chronic liver failure in outpatients with cirrhosis. Journal of Hepatology. 2017;**67**:1177-1184

[56] LeDoux D, Astiz ME, Carpati CM, Rackow EC. Effects of perfusion pressure on tissue perfusion in septic shock. Critical Care Medicine. 2000;**28**:2729-2732

[57] Funk GC, Doberer D, Kneidinger N, Lindner G, Holzinger U, Schneeweiss B. Acid-base disturbances in critically

ill patients with cirrhosis. Liver International. 2007;**27**:901-909

[58] Rhodes A, Cusack RJ, Newman PJ, Grounds RM, Bennett ED. A randomised, controlled trial of the pulmonary artery catheter in critically ill patients. Intensive Care Medicine. 2002;**28**:256-264

[59] National Heart, Lung, and Blood Institute Acute Respiratory Distress Syndrome (ARDS) Clinical Trials Network, Wiedemann HP, Wheeler AP, Bernard GR, Thompson BT, Hayden D, et al. Comparison of two fluid management strategies in acute lung injury. The New England Journal of Medicine. 2006;**354**:2564-2575

[60] Brandstrup B, Tonnesen H, Beier-Holgersen R, Hjortso E, Ording H, Lindorff-Larsen K, et al. Effects of intravenous fluid restriction on postoperative complications: Comparison of two perioperative fluid regimens: A randomized assessor-blinded multicenter trial. Annals of Surgery. 2003;**238**:641-648

[61] Rosenberg AL, Dechert RE, Park PK, Bartlett RH. Review of a large clinical series: Association of cumulative fluid balance on outcome in acute lung injury: A retrospective review of the ARDSnet tidal volume study cohort. Journal of Intensive Care Medicine. 2009;**24**:35-46

[62] Humphrey H, Hall J, Sznajder I, Silverstein M, Wood L. Improved survival in ARDS patients associated with a reduction in pulmonary capillary wedge pressure. Chest. 1990;**97**:1176-1180

[63] Finfer S, Bellomo R, Boyce N, French J, Myburgh J, Norton R. A comparison of albumin and saline for fluid resuscitation in the intensive care unit. The New England Journal of Medicine. 2004;**350**:2247-2256

[64] Myburgh JA, Mythen MG. Resuscitation fluids. The New England Journal of Medicine. 2013;**369**:1243-1251

[65] Arroyo V, Garcia-Martinez R, Salvatella X. Human serum albumin, systemic inflammation, and cirrhosis. Journal of Hepatology. 2014;**61**:396-407

[66] Banares R, Bernardi M. Long-term albumin administration in patients with decompensated cirrhosis. It is time for a reappraisal. Liver International. 2019;**39**:45-48

[67] Ortega R, Gines P, Uriz J, Cardenas A, Calahorra B, De Las HD, et al. Terlipressin therapy with and without albumin for patients with hepatorenal syndrome: Results of a prospective, nonrandomized study. Hepatology. 2002;**36**:941-948

[68] Sort P, Navasa M, Arroyo V, Aldeguer X, Planas R, Ruiz-del-Arbol L, et al. Effect of intravenous albumin on renal impairment and mortality in patients with cirrhosis and spontaneous bacterial peritonitis. The New England Journal of Medicine. 1999;**341**:403-409

[69] Gluud LL, Christensen K, Christensen E, Krag A. Systematic review of randomized trials on vasoconstrictor drugs for hepatorenal syndrome. Hepatology. 2010;**51**:576-584

[70] Gines A, Fernandez-Esparrach G, Monescillo A, Vila C, Domenech E, Abecasis R, et al. Randomized trial comparing albumin, dextran 70, and polygeline in cirrhotic patients with ascites treated by paracentesis. Gastroenterology. 1996;**111**:1002-1010

[71] Moreau R, Valla DC, Durand-Zaleski I, Bronowicki JP, Durand F, Chaput JC, et al. Comparison of outcome in patients with cirrhosis and ascites following treatment with albumin or a synthetic colloid: A randomised controlled pilot trail. Liver International. 2006;**26**:46-54

[72] Sola-Vera J, Minana J, Ricart E, Planella M, Gonzalez B, Torras X, et al. Randomized trial comparing albumin and saline in the prevention of paracentesis-induced circulatory dysfunction in cirrhotic patients with ascites. Hepatology. 2003;**37**:1147-1153

[73] Guevara M, Terra C, Nazar A, Sola E, Fernandez J, Pavesi M, et al. Albumin for bacterial infections other than spontaneous bacterial peritonitis in cirrhosis. A randomized, controlled study. Journal of Hepatology. 2012;**57**:759-765

[74] Thevenot T, Bureau C, Oberti F, Anty R, Louvet A, Plessier A, et al. Effect of albumin in cirrhotic patients with infection other than spontaneous bacterial peritonitis. A randomized trial. Journal of Hepatology. 2015;**62**:822-830

[75] De Backer D, Biston P, Devriendt J, Madl C, Chochrad D, Aldecoa C, et al. Comparison of dopamine and norepinephrine in the treatment of shock. New England Journal of Medicine. 2010;**362**:779-789

[76] Albanese J, Leone M, Delmas A, Martin C. Terlipressin or norepinephrine in hyperdynamic septic shock: A prospective, randomized study. Critical Care Medicine. 2005;**33**:1897-1902

[77] O'Brien A, Clapp L, Singer M. Terlipressin for norepinephrine-resistant septic shock. Lancet. 2002;**359**:1209-1210

[78] Morelli A, Rocco M, Conti G, Orecchioni A, De Gaetano A, Cortese G, et al. Effects of terlipressin on systemic and regional haemodynamics in catecholamine-treated hyperkinetic septic shock. Intensive Care Medicine. 2004;**30**:597-604

[79] Delmas A, Leone M, Rousseau S, Albanese J, Martin C. Clinical review: Vasopressin and terlipressin in septic shock patients. Critical Care. 2005;**9**:212-222

[80] Arabi YM, Aljumah A, Dabbagh O, Tamim HM, Rishu AH, Al-Abdulkareem A, et al. Low-dose hydrocortisone in patients with cirrhosis and septic shock: A randomized controlled trial. CMAJ. 2010;**182**:1971-1977

[81] Harry R, Auzinger G, Wendon J. The effects of supraphysiological doses of corticosteroids in hypotensive liver failure. Liver International. 2003;**23**:71-77

[82] Harry R, Auzinger G, Wendon J. The clinical importance of adrenal insufficiency in acute hepatic dysfunction. Hepatology. 2002;**36**:395-402

[83] Annane D, Sebille V, Charpentier C, Bollaert PE, Francois B, Korach JM, et al. Effect of treatment with low doses of hydrocortisone and fludrocortisone on mortality in patients with septic shock. JAMA. 2002;**288**:862-871

[84] Tsai MH, Peng YS, Chen YC, Liu NJ, Ho YP, Fang JT, et al. Adrenal insufficiency in patients with cirrhosis, severe sepsis and septic shock. Hepatology. 2006;**43**:673-681

[85] Gronbaek H, Johnsen SP, Jepsen P, Gislum M, Vilstrup H, Tage-Jensen U, et al. Liver cirrhosis, other liver diseases, and risk of hospitalisation for intracerebral haemorrhage: A Danish population-based case-control study. BMC Gastroenterology. 2008;**8**:16

[86] Vilstrup H, Gluud C, Hardt F, Kristensen M, Kohler O, Melgaard B, et al. Branched chain enriched amino acid versus glucose treatment of hepatic encephalopathy. A double-blind study of 65 patients with cirrhosis. Journal of Hepatology. 1990;**10**:291-296

[87] Borzio M, Salerno F, Piantoni L, Cazzaniga M, Angeli P, Bissoli F, et al.

Bacterial infection in patients with advanced cirrhosis: A multicentre prospective study. Digestive and Liver Disease. 2001;**33**:41-48

[88] Jalan R, Fernández J, Wiest R, Schnabl B, Moreau R, Angeli P, et al. Bacterial infections in cirrhosis: A position statement based on the EASL special conference 2013. Journal of Hepatology. 2014;**60**:1310-1324

[89] Fernández J, Navasa M, Gómez J, Colmenero J, Vila J, Arroyo V, et al. Bacterial infections in cirrhosis: Epidemiological changes with invasive procedures and norfloxacin prophylaxis. Hepatology. 2002;**35**:140-148

[90] Merli M, Lucidi C, Giannelli V, Giusto M, Riggio O, Falcone M, et al. Cirrhotic patients are at risk for health care-associated bacterial infections. Clinical Gastroenterology and Hepatology. 2010;**8**:979-985

[91] Fernández J, Acevedo J, Wiest R, Gustot T, Amoros A, Deulofeu C, et al. Bacterial and fungal infections in acute-on-chronic liver failure: Prevalence, characteristics and impact on prognosis. Gut. 2018;**67**:1870-1880

[92] Arvaniti V, D'Amico G, Fede G, Manousou P, Tsochatzis E, Pleguezuelo M, et al. Infections in patients with cirrhosis increase mortality four-fold and should be used in determining prognosis. Gastroenterology. 2010;**139**:1246-1256

[93] Blasco-Algora S, Masegosa-Ataz J, Gutiérrez-García ML, Alonso-López S, Fernández-Rodríguez C. Acute-on-chronic liver failure: Pathogenesis, prognostic factors and management. World Journal of Gastroenterology. 2014;**21**:12125-12140

[94] Hernaez R, Solà E, Moreau R, Ginès P. Acute-on-chronic liver failure: An update. Gut. 2017;**66**:541-553

[95] Gupta T, Dhiman R, Rathi S, Agrawal S, Duseja A, Taneja S, et al. Impact of hepatic and extrahepatic insults on the outcome of acute-on-chronic liver failure. Journal of Clinical and Experimental Hepatology. 2017;7:9-15

[96] Chaulk J, Charbonneau M, Qamar H, Keough A, Chang HJ, Ma M, et al. Third-generation cephalosporin-resistant spontaneous bacterial peritonitis: A single-center experience and summary of existing studies. Canadian Journal of Gastroenterology & Hepatology. 2014;**28**:83-88

[97] Campillo B, Richardet JP, Kheo T, Dupeyron C. Nosocomial spontaneous bacterial peritonitis and bacteremia in cirrhotic patients: Impact of isolate type on prognosis and characteristics of patients. Clinical Infectious Diseases. 2002;**35**:1-10

[98] Tandon P, Delisle A, Topal JE, Garcia-Tsao G. High prevalence of antibiotic-resistant bacterial infections among patients with cirrhosis at a US liver center. Clinical Gastroenterology and Hepatology. 2012;**10**:1291-1298

[99] Piano S, Singh V, Caraceni P, Maiwall R, Alessandria C, Fernandez J, et al. Epidemiology and effects of bacterial infection in cirrhosis worldwide. Gastroenterology. 2019;**156**:1368-1380

[100] Nahon P, Lescat M, Layese R, Bourcier V, Talmat N, Allam S, et al. Bacterial infection compensated viral cirrhosis impairs 5-year survival (ANRS CO12 Cir Vir prospective cohort). Gut. 2017;**66**:330-341

[101] Dionigi E, Garcovich M, Borzio M, Leandro G, Majumdar A, Tsami A, et al. Bacterial infections change natural history of cirrhosis irrespective of liver disease severity. The American Journal of Gastroenterology. 2017;**112**:588-596

[102] Salerno F, Borzio M, Pedicino C, Simonetti R, Rossini A, Boccia S, et al. The impact of infection by multidrug-resistant agents in patients with cirrhosis: A multicenter prospective study. Liver International. 2017;**37**:71-79

[103] Park JK, Lee CH, Kim HI, Kim SM, Jang JW, Kim SH, et al. Clinical characteristics and prognostic impact of bacterial infections in hospitalized patients with alcoholic liver disease. Journal of Korean Medical Science. 2015;**30**:598-605

[104] Jain M, Varghese J, Michael T, Kedarishetty CKGB, Swaminathan S, Venkataraman J. An insight into antibiotic resistance to bacterial infection in chronic liver disease. Journal of Clinical and Experimental Hepatology. 2017;7:305-309

[105] Zhao R, Ma J, Li P, Fang H, Sun S, Wu W, et al. Multidrug-resistant bacterial infections in cirrhotic patients: An epidemiological study. Expert Review of Gastroenterology & Hepatology. 2018;**5**:1-8

[106] Fernández J, Prado V, Trebicka J, Amoros A, Gustot T, Wiest R, et al. Multidrug-resistant bacterial infections in patients with decompensated cirrhosis and with acute-on-chronic liver failure in Europe. Journal of Hepatology. 2019;**70**:398-411

[107] Verma N, Singh S, Taneja S, Duseja A, Singh V, Dhiman RK, et al. Invasive fungal infections amongst patients with acute-on-chronic liver failure at high risk for fungal infections. Liver International. 2019;**39**:503-513

[108] Galbois A, Aegerter P, Martel-Samb P, Housset C, Thabut D, Offenstadt G, et al. Improved prognosis of septic shock inpatients with cirrhosis: A multicenter study. Critical Care Medicine. 2014;**42**:1666-1675

[109] Gravito-Soares M, Gravito-Soares E, Lopes S, Ribeiro G, Figueiredo P. Spontaneous fungal peritonitis: A rare but severe complication of liver cirrhosis. European Journal of Gastroenterology & Hepatology. 2017;**29**:1010-1016

[110] Hwang SY, Yu SJ, Lee JH, Kim JS, Yoon JW, Kim YJ, et al. Spontaneous fungal peritonitis: A severe complication in patients with advanced liver cirrhosis. European Journal of Clinical Microbiology & Infectious Diseases. 2014;**33**:259-264

[111] Bassetti M, Peghin M, Carnelutti A, Righi E, Merelli M, Ansaldi F, et al. Clinical characteristics and predictors of mortality in cirrhotic patients with candidemia and intra-abdominal candidiasis: A multicenter study. Intensive Care Medicine. 2017;**43**:509-518

[112] Fernández J, Tandon P, Mensa J, Garcia-Tsao G. Antibiotic prophylaxis in cirrhosis: Good and bad. Hepatology. 2016;**63**:2019-2031

[113] Fernández J, Acevedo J, Castro M, Garcia O, Rodríguez de Lope C, Roca D, et al. Prevalence and risk factors of infections by multi resistant bacteria in cirrhosis: A prospective study. Hepatology. 2012;**55**:1551-1561

[114] Fernández J, Bert F, Nicolas-Chanoine MH. The challenges of multi- drug-resistance in hepatology. Journal of Hepatology. 2016;**65**:1043-1054

[115] Di Gregorio V, Lucidi C, Giannelli V, Lattanzi B, Giusto M, Iacovone G, et al. Bacterial infections in cirrhotic patients: Risk factors and rate of failure of the empirical antibiotic therapy. Journal of Hepatology. 2014;**60**:S227

[116] Merli M, Lucidi C, Di Gregorio V, Falcone M, Giannelli V, Lattanzi B, et al. The spread of multi drug resistant infections is leading to an increase in the

empirical antibiotic treatment failure in cirrhosis: A prospective survey. PLoS One. 2015;**10**:e0121448

[117] Ariza X, Castellote J, Lora-Tamayo J, Girbau A, Salord S, Rota R, et al. Risk factors for resistance to ceftriaxone and its impact on mortality in community, healthcare and nosocomial spontaneous bacterial peritoni tis. Journal of Hepatology. 2012;**56**:825-832

[118] Carlet J, Pulcini C, Piddock LJV. Antibiotic resistance: a geopolitical issue. Clinical Microbiology and Infection. 2014;**20**:949-953

[119] Magiorakos A-P, Srinivasan A, Carey RB, Carmeli Y, Falagas ME, Giske CG, et al. Multidrug-resistant, extensively drug-resistant and pandrug-resistant bacteria: An international expert proposal for interim standard definitions for acquired resistance. Clinical Microbiology and Infection. 2012;**18**:268-281

[120] Song KH, Jeon JH, Park WB, Park SW, Kim HB, Oh MD, et al. Clinical outcomes of spontaneous bacterial peritonitis due to extended-spectrum beta-lactamase-producing *Escherichia coli* and *Klebsiella* species: A retrospective matched case-control study. BMC Infectious Diseases. 2009;**9**:41-46

[121] Cheong HS, Kang CI, Lee JA, Moon SY, Joung MK, Chung DR, et al. Clinical significance and outcome of nosocomial acquisition of spontaneous bacterial peritonitis in patients with liver cirrhosis. Clinical Infectious Diseases. 2009;**48**:1230-1236

[122] Bartoletti M, Giannella M, Caraceni P, Domenicali M, Ambretti S, Tedeschi S, et al. Epidemiology and outcomes of bloodstream infection in patients with cirrosis. Journal of Hepatology. 2014;**61**:51-58

[123] Bartoletti M, Giannella M, Lewis R, Caraceni P, Tedeschi S, Paul M, et al. A prospective multicentre study of the epidemiology and outcomes of bloodstream infection in cirrhotic patients. Clinical Microbiology and Infection. 2018;**24**:546 e1-546 e8

[124] Laxminarayan R, Chaudhury RR. Antibiotic resistance in India: Drivers and opportunities for action. Plo S Med. 2016;**13**(3):e1001974

[125] Piroth L, Pechinot A, Minello A, Jaulhac B, Patry I, Hadou T, et al. Bacterial epidemiology and antimicrobial resistance in ascitic fluid: A 2-year retrospective study. Scandinavian Journal of Infectious Diseases. 2009;**37**:2-8

[126] Novovic S, Semb S, Olsen H, Moser C, Knudsen JD, Homann C. First-line treatment with cephalosporins in spontaneous bacterial peritonitis provides poor antibiotic coverage. Scandinavian Journal of Gastroenterology. 2012;**47**:212-216

[127] Umgelter A, Reindl W, Miedaner M, Schmid RM, Huber W. Failure of current antibiotic first-line regimens and mortality in hospitalized patients with spontaneous bacterial peritonitis. Infection. 2009;**37**:2-8

[128] Alexopoulou A, Vasilieva L, Agiasotelli D, Siranidi K, Pouriki S, Tsiriga A, et al. Extensively drug-resistant bacteria are an independent predictive factor of mortality in 130 patients with spontaneous bacterial peritonitis or spontaneous bacteremia. World Journal of Gastroenterology. 2016;**22**:4049-4055

[129] Sargenti K, Prytz H, Strand A, Nilsson E, Kalaitzakis E. Healthcare-associated and nosocomial bacterial infections in cirrhosis: Predictors and impact on outcome. Liver International. 2015;**35**:391-400

[130] Yang et al. Bacterial infections in acute-on-chronic liver failure. Seminars in Liver Disease. 2018;**38**:121-133

[131] European Center for Disease Prevention and Control. Antimicrobial Resistance Surveillance in Europe. 2013. Avaialble from: http://ecdc.europa.eu/en/publi-cations/Publications/antimicrobial-resistance-europe-2013.pdf

[132] Arabi YM, Dara SI, Memish Z, et al. Antimicrobial therapeutic determinants of outcomes from septic shock among patients with cirrhosis. Hepatology. 2012;**56**:2305-2315

[133] Acevedo J. Multiresistant bacterial infections in liver cirrhosis: Clinical impact and new empirical antibiotic treatment policies. World Journal of Hepatology. 2015;7(7):916

[134] Dupeyron C, Campillo B, Mangeney N, Bordes M, Richardet JP, Leluan G. Carriage of *Staphylococcus aureus* and gram-negative bacilli resistant to third generation cephalosporins in cirrhotic patients a prospective assessment of hospital-acquired infections. Infection Control and Hospital Epidemiology. 2001;**22**:427-432

[135] Bassetti M, Merelli M, Temperoni C, Astilean A. New antibiotics for bad bugs: Where are we? Annals of Clinical Microbiology and Antimicrobials. 2013;**12**:22

[136] Wieser A, Li H, Zhang J, Liss I, Markwardt D, Hornung R, et al. Evaluating the best empirical antibiotic therapy in patients with acute-on-chronic liver failure and spontaneous bacterial peritonitis. Digestive and Liver Disease. 2019;**51**:1300-1307

[137] Dryden M. Linezolid pharmacokinetics and pharmacodynamics in clinical treatment. The Journal of Antimicrobial Chemotherapy. 2011;**66**(Suppl. 4):iv7-iv15

[138] Marsot A, Boulamery A, Bruguerolle B, Simon N. Vancomycin: A review of population pharmacokinetic analyses. Clinical Pharmacokinetics. 2012;**51**:1-13

[139] Cardone KE, Lodise TP, Patel N, Hoy CD, Meola S, Manley HJ, et al. Pharmacokinetics and pharmacodynamics of intravenous daptomycin during continuous ambulatory peritoneal dialysis. Clinical Journal of the American Society of Nephrology. 2011;**6**:1081-1088

[140] Ulldemolins M, Vaquer S, Llauradó-Serra M, Pontes C, Calvo G, Soy D, et al. Beta-lactam dosing in critically ill patients with septic shock and continuous renal replacement therapy. Critical Care. 2014;**18**:227

[141] Karjagin J, Lefeuvre S, Oselin K, Kipper K, Marchand S, Tikkerberi A, et al. Phar-macokinetics of meropenem determined by microdialysis in the peritoneal fluid of patients with severe peritonitis associated with septic shock. Clinical Pharmacology and Therapeutics. 2008;**83**:452-459

[142] Bert F, Larroque B, Dondero F, Durand F, Paugam-Burtz C, Belghiti J, et al. Risk factors associated with preoperative fecal carriage of extended-spectrum b-lactamase-producing Enterobacteriaceae in liver transplant recipients. Transplant Infectious Disease. 2014;**16**:84-89

[143] Crum-Cianflone NF, Sullivan E, Ballon-Landa G. Fecal microbiota transplantation and successful resolution of multidrug-resistant-organism colonization. Journal of Clinical Microbiology. 2015;**53**:1986-1989

[144] Naas T, Cuzon G, Truong H, Bernabeu S, Nordmann P. Evaluation of a DNA microarray, the check-points ESBL/KPC array, for rapid detection of TEM, SHV, and CTX-M extended-spectrum b-lactamases and KPC carbapenemases. Antimicrobial Agents and Chemotherapy. 2010;**54**:3086-3092

[145] Mancini N, Infurnari L, Ghidoli N, Valzano G, Clementi N, Burioni R, et al. Potential impact of a microarray-based nucleic acid assay for rapid detection of Gram-negative bacteria and resistance markers in positive blood cultures. Journal of Clinical Microbiology. 2014;**52**:1242-1245

[146] Perez KK, Olsen RJ, Musick WL, Cernoch PL, Davis JR, Peterson LE, et al. Integrating rapid diagnostics and antimicrobial stewardship improves outcomes in patients with antibiotic-resistant Gram-negative bacteremia. The Journal of Infection. 2014;**69**:216-225

[147] Kaki R, Elligsen M, Walker S, Simor A, Palmay L, Daneman N. Impact of antimicrobial stewardship in critical care: A systematic review. The Journal of Antimicrobial Chemotherapy. 2011;**66**:1223-1230

[148] Kollef M, Micek S, Hampton N, Doherty JA, Kumar A. Septicshock attributed to Candida infection: Importance of empiric therapy and source control. Clinical Infectious Diseases. 2012;**54**:1739-1746

[149] Allaire M et al. Management of infections in patients with cirrhosis in the context of increasing therapeutic resistance: A systematic review. Clinics and Research in Hepatology and Gastroenterology. 2019. DOI: 10.1016/j.clinre

[150] Yeoh SF, Lee TJ, Chew KL, Lin S, Yeo D, Setia S. Echinocandins for management of invasive candidiasis in patients with liver disease and liver transplantation. Infection and Drug Resistance. 2018;**11**:805-819

Chapter 7

Left Side Gallbladder: Clinical and Anatomical Implication

Filippo Banchini and Patrizio Capelli

Abstract

Left side gallbladder is a rare anatomical anomaly reported in the literature. It is associated with various anatomical variations of the biliary way and intrahepatic portal supply. Most of the time, it is discovered as an incidental finding during intervention for cholecystectomy, exposing patients and surgeons to high risk of complication. To prevent this, we analyze the critical aspects that must be known to perform safe interventions either in the normal setting or in the emergency setting. Different theories are proposed to describe this anomaly, but a debate is still open. Reviewing the literature and analyzing the different processes of formation, we create a classification that can explain how this anomaly can occur, dividing into four variation types.

Keywords: left side, gallbladder, fusion of plans, liver resection, biliary, agenesis, abnormality, cholecystectomy, right umbilical vein, liver, hepatic

1. Introduction

The left side gallbladder (LSG) is a very rare alteration defined by the attachment of the gallbladder to the left lobe of the liver at the right side of the ligament tears.

Since Hochstetter's first description in 1886 [1], about 150 cases have been reported in the literature. The attempts to explain the cause of this anomaly have been different, but the numerous variations described do not allow a clear definition of its origin. Although this debate is still open, it is of considerable importance to know that LSG is frequently associated with alterations of both the portal branches and the intrahepatic biliary tree. The association of these anomalies, therefore, represents an important risk, especially if surgical treatment is necessary. There are two cases in which surgical treatment may be required: the first is gallbladder stones and in particular acute cholecystitis, and the second is the need for liver resection surgery. In the first case, the diagnosis of gallstones and cholecystitis is made only with ultrasound, but often this method does not describe the anomaly of the LSG. In fact, in most cases described, the diagnosis is made intraoperatively, making the surgical treatment problematic and risky due to the lack of correct anatomical knowledge. In the case of liver resection, the diagnosis is made before surgery, highlighting anatomical variations that require complex dissection strategies. Knowledge of the anomalies associated with a LSG can be of considerable help in preventing serious complications.

IntechOpen

2. Estimation incidence and diagnosis

The real estimation of this anomaly is very difficult because most of the published articles are case reports and only a few of them have high numbers of cases. The literature analysis revealed 114 articles concerning LSG: 89 authors describe 1 case only, 11 present 2 cases, 3 present 3 cases, 3 present 4 cases, 3 describe 6 cases, 1 describes 7 cases, 2 describe 9 cases, 1 describes 10 cases, and 1 describes 26 cases, with a total of 211 cases (**Table 1**).

The incidence is variable and remains always below 0.3%: Idu et al. [109] describe 5 cases of LSG on 1764 cases of cholecystectomy (0.3%), Nagai et al. [90] 3 cases out of 1621 (0.2%), Sadhu et al. [43] 1 out of 1258 (0.08%), and Rozsos et al. [37] 1 out of 2536 (0.04%).

Naganuma et al. [87], in a series of 67.994 patients studied with ultrasound, found 18 cases of abnormal gallbladder position with an incidence of 0.026%. These included retrohepatic, supraphrenic, and floating gallbladder, and only nine cases of LSG, with an incidence of 0.013%. However, ultrasound is not the main exam to make the diagnosis. Pereira et al. [115] show that ultrasound has a positive predictive value of only 2.7% and that in 81.1% LSG is initially detected at surgery. Also, Lee et al. [36], in his series of 10 cases operated on for cholecystic stones or acute cholecystitis symptoms, describes the discovery: intraoperative in 8 cases and as an incidental finding on abdominal computed tomography (CT) in 2 cases.

The CT scan is the main examination capable of making a correct diagnosis. However, as reported in the review of Pereira et al. [115], CT has a positive predictive value of only 60%. This can be explained by the simultaneous proximity of the two hepatic lobes to the gallbladder, simulating the contact and not the adhesion to the left lobe of the liver. Considering the position of the gallbladder, if it is in the normal site, its right margin generally appears free (**Figure 1A**). If the gallbladder is positioned on the left, its left margin may appear free (**Figure 1B**) or included in the left lobe with a space between the two hepatic lobes (**Figure 1C**), making diagnosis easy. If the gallbladder appears between the right and left hepatic lobes, the diagnosis may remain unknown (**Figure 1D**) mimicking hypertrophy of the left hepatic lobe as also reported by Banchini et al. [20] and Iskandar et al. [6].

However, the CT remains the main examination as it can provide the anatomical portal and arterial variations that, as we will see, frequently occur in association with this anomaly.

3. Theories and embryology

The embryological theories of LSG development are numerous and complex, but we can distinguish two main ones. The first theory concerns an alteration that only concerns the development of the gallbladder and a second one that concerns the development of the central portion of the liver and consequently the malpositioning of the gallbladder.

In the theory of gallbladder development proposed by Gross [116], there are two ways in which gallbladder can develop:

- The first modality suggests a normal growth of the gallbladder migrating from the right side of the liver to the left side and attaching to the left lobe. In this case, the cystic duct originates from the right side of the bile duct and moves anteriorly and to the left of the liver pedicle.

Reference	Author	Number of cases	Reference	Author	Number of cases	Reference	Author	Number of cases
[2]	Abe	1	[3]	Ishii	1	[4]	Noritomi	1
[5]	Abongwa	1	[6]	Iskandar	1	[7]	Ogawa	1
[8]	Alharthi	1	[9]	Jona	1	[10]	Ogino	1
[11]	Almodhaiberi	1	[12]	Jung	1	[13]	Oshima	1
[14]	Aoki	1	[15]	Kanazumi	2	[16]	Ozeki	26
[17]	Asonuma	4	[18]	Kawai	1	[19]	Pradeep	4
[20]	Banchini	1	[21]	Kehr	1	[22]	Quah	1
[23]	Banzo	1	[24]	Kelly	1	[25]	Qureshi	1
[26]	Bender	1	[27]	Kim	4	[28]	Rafailidis	1
[29]	Bonomo	1	[30]	Kinoshita	2	[31]	Reddy	1
[32]	Chrungoo	2	[33]	Kubo	1	[34]	Rocca	1
[35]	Chuang	1	[36]	Lee	10	[37]	Rozsos	1
[38]	Chung	1	[39]	Leone	1	[40]	Saafan	1
[41]	Cirla	1	[42]	Lin	1	[43]	Sadhu	1
[44]	Colovic	2	[45]	Maetani	1	[46]	Sakihara	1
[47]	Dhulkotia	1	[48]	Makni	1	[49]	Schiffino	1
[50]	Donthi	1	[51]	Masood	1	[52]	Seiberman	1
[53]	Ergun	1	[54]	Matsumoto	1	[55]	Shen	1
[56]	Etter	1	[57]	Matsumura	1	[58]	Shimizu	1
[59]	Feldman	1	[60]	Matsuoka	1	[61]	Shirono	1
[62]	Fujita	1	[63]	Mazzamurro	1	[64]	Siebermair	1
[65]	Fujita	1	[66]	McGowan	1	[67]	Si-Youn	3

Reference	Author	Number of cases	Reference	Author	Number of cases	Reference	Author	Number of cases
[68]	Fukuda	1	[69]	Mendoza-Calderon	2	[70]	Strong	1
[71]	Funakoshi	1	[72]	Mizray	1	[73]	Surjan	1
[74]	Futamura	1	[75]	Mohammed	6	[76]	Szanto	1
[77]	Gondra	1	[78]	Moo-Young	1	[79]	Tachibana	2
[80]	Gui	1	[81]	Moravik	1	[82]	Takemura	1
[83]	Hasbahceci	1	[84]	Moriyama	2	[85]	Takiguchi	1
[86]	Herrington	1	[87]	Naganuma	9	[88]	Tomiyama	1
[89]	Hirohata	1	[90]	Nagay	3	[91]	Uesaka	2
[1]	Hochstetter	1	[92]	Nagendram	1	[93]	Velimezis	7
[94]	Hopper	1	[95]	Nakakubo	1	[96]	Watanabe	1
[97]	Hsu	9	[98]	Namikawa	1	[99]	Wong	1
[100]	Huang	6	[101]	Nastos	2	[102]	Wu	2
[103]	Hwang	3	[104]	Nemours	1	[105]	Yamazaki	1
[106]	Iaccarino	1	[107]	Newcombe	1	[108]	Yu	2
[109]	Idu	6	[110]	Nguyena	1	[111]	Zografos	1
[112]	Ikoma	1	[113]	Nishio	1	[114]	Zoulamoglou	1

Table 1.
Number of cases reported in the literature for each author.

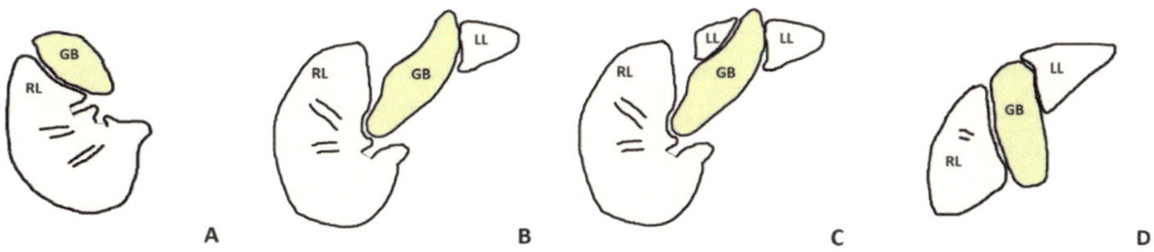

Figure 1.
CT scan visualization of the gallbladder. (A) Normal right side gallbladder attached to the right lobe; (B) left side gallbladder attached to left lobe with empty space between gallbladder fundus and right lobe; (C) left side gallbladder with fundus surrounded by left lobe and empty space between right lobe and left lobe; (D) left side gallbladder interposed between right lobe and left lobe, mimicking hypertrophy of right lobe. RL: right lobe; LL: left lobe; GB: gallbladder.

- The second modality hypothesizes the formation of the gallbladder directly on the left side of the bile duct with its positioning directly under the left hepatic lobe. In this case, the cystic duct originates in the left part of the bile duct.

The literature defines as a true LSG when it is located on the right side of the round ligament, and the cystic duct is inserted on the left side of the bile duct. The presence of true LSG, described in this way, represents a remarkably rare event, constituting 4.3% of the cases of left side gallbladder [18], and most of the cases described are therefore a different alteration.

The ways in which the cystic duct enters the biliary duct are numerous even in the absence of the left gallbladder, and as reported by Sarawagi et al. [117], the normal right conjunction is present in 51.1% of cases, while its medial (left) insertion can be presented in 16.1%. Pereira et al. [115], in his review, describe the insertion of the cystic duct on the right side 65.6%, on the left side of common hepatic duct 9.5%, left hepatic duct 9.5%, on the right hepatic duct 7.6%, and in a branch of the right hepatic duct 2.4%. Six patients had other minor biliary anomalies, and one had a duplicate common bile duct (CBD).

The second theory about the development of the central portion of the liver was first described by Ozeki in 1987 [16] and later defined by Nagai in 1997 [90] as "right side round ligament." This theory is associated with numerous alterations in intrahepatic anatomy and appears to account for over 95% of cases in which a left side gallbladder is present.

To understand this complex theory, it is necessary to investigate some moments of fetal evolution, in which the persistence of a right umbilical vein and/or hypertrophy of the left portion of the liver seem to be associated. According to the embryological studies of Arey [118] when the embryo measures 6 mm, there are at the same time two vitelline's veins, one on the right side and one on the left side, everyone having a branch that enters the liver. The two veins inside the liver have branches that join them together. When the embryo reaches the size of 7 mm, the right vein goes into atrophy leaving the left side predominant. It is assumed that, if the right side vein does not atrophy, there is a persistence of this umbilical vein either extrahepatic or intrahepatic. In this case, the opposite process to the previous one occurs, with atrophy of the left side and hypertrophy of the right side (Matsumoto's hypothesis) [119]. When this happens, we have the positioning of the gallbladder in the left portion of the liver.

Although this theory seems to be the most accreditable, there are cases in the literature of persistence of the right umbilical vein with the gallbladder positioned normally, showing how this theory does not always prove to be real [42].

Lucidarme et al. [120] describe this variation in portal anatomy as a defect in the evolution of the central portion of the liver, in which the right and left parts join together in a variable way, renaming this as "Fusion of hepatic plans." Considering these different descriptions, we can say that there is an anomaly in the mechanism of persistence or atrophy of the right umbilical vein and/or the liver surrounding it.

Based on these descriptions, we propose to combine the mechanism of atrophy of the central part of the liver with persistence of the right umbilical vein and the mechanism of fusion of the plans, trying to verify how these can give rise to different anatomical variations. In this way, we create a classification that can explain how this anomaly can occur.

As seen before, during fetal development, the right and left umbilical veins have a Y shape with one arm entering the liver and one passing laterally to it. At this stage, there is a set of vessels inside the liver that connect the two internal branches of the intrahepatic umbilical veins. This connection forms a venous conduit that we will call "intrahepatic right umbilical vein" (IRUV), which flows directly into the ligament of Arantius or enters the right umbilical vein at Rex's recess. The extrahepatic portion of the right umbilical vein can enter the liver in a variable position between segment 5 and segment 4b. Imagine looking at the liver from its lower face, corresponding to segments 5 and 4b, we can divide this area into four parts as shown in **Figure 2**: the superficial part, corresponding to the acute margin of the liver, in the portion of segment 5 (**Figure 2**: yellow segment 5), and the portion of segment 4b (**Figure 2**: blue segment 4b) and a deep part toward the hilum of the liver (**Figure 2**: red segment 5; green segment 4b).

The involution of the right umbilical vein may affect the surrounding hepatic parenchyma differently, depending on its extension and site, determining unusual alterations.

If atrophy affects the superficial parts (**Figure 2**: yellow and blue), the result is a volumetric reduction in the corresponding liver segments. If the atrophy affects the deep part toward the hilum (**Figure 2**: red and green), we can have alterations that cause variations of the portal vein and the biliary tract. Complete or partial atrophy can also explain in various ways incomplete forms of gallbladder malposition such as the medioposition described by Hsu et al. [97].

The different possibilities with which the right umbilical vein can evolve are four, and we describe them as follows (**Figure 3**):

Type A: complete atrophy of the right umbilical vein and normal left umbilical vein.

Type B: atrophy of the right external umbilical vein and persistence of the IRUV.

Type C: persistence of the IRUV and extrahepatic umbilical vein and atrophy of the left umbilical vein.

Type D: persistence of the right extrahepatic umbilical vein and atrophy of the left umbilical vein.

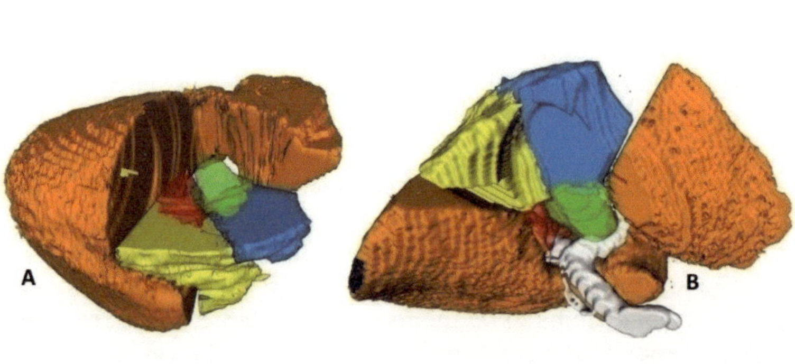

Figure 2.
Liver with the central portion divided into four parts: the superficial part of segment 5 in yellow; the lower part close to the hilum in red; the superficial part of segment 4 in blue; and the lower part of segment 4 close to the hilum in green. (A) Superior view and (B) inferior view.

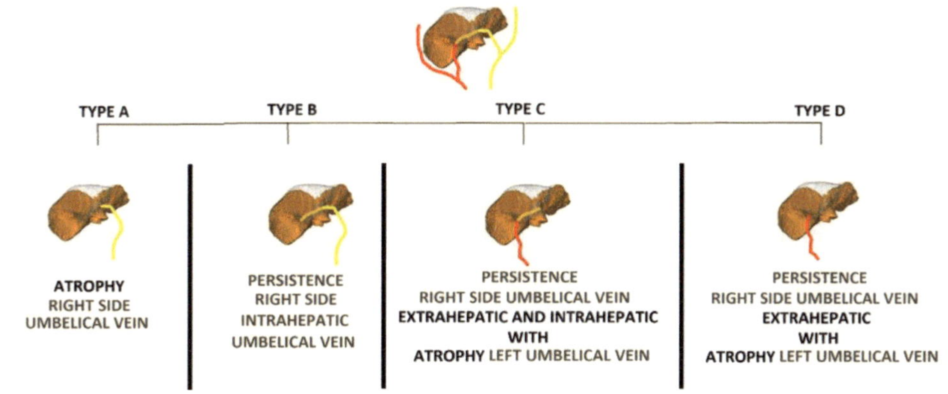

Figure 3.
Schematic evolution of right and left umbilical veins with different evolution processes. (Type A) Normal evolution with the persistence of the left umbilical vein. (Type B) Persistence of the left umbilical vein and intrahepatic umbilical vein. (Type C) Persistence of the right umbilical vein and persistence of the intrahepatic umbilical vein with atrophy of left umbilical vein. (Type D) Persistence of the right umbilical vein only (in red: right umbilical vein; in orange: intrahepatic umbilical vein; in yellow: left umbilical vein).

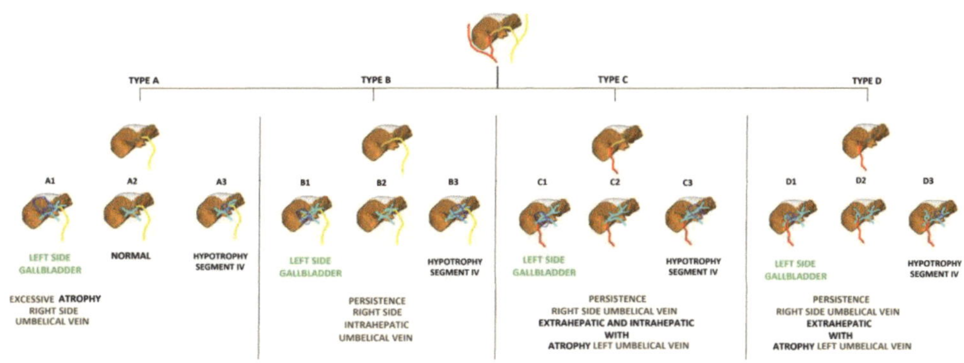

Figure 4.
Combination of the evolution process of right and left umbilical veins with atrophy mechanism of segment 5 and 4 (in red: right umbilical vein; in orange: intrahepatic umbilical vein; in yellow: left umbilical vein; in light blue: portal vein and its branches; and in blue: area of hypotrophy). A1-B1-C1-D1 corresponding to atrophy of segment 5 area; A2-B2-C2-D2 absence of liver atrophy; A3-B3-C3-D3 corresponding to atrophy of segment 4 area.

Types C and D represent the cases in which a persistence of the right umbilical vein occurs instead of the normal left umbilical vein, classifying this as "true right side round ligament."

Combining these variations with how lower liver atrophy can occur, the following classifications can be determined (**Figure 4**):

Type A:

A1: The right umbilical vein goes into complete atrophy and is accompanied by an excessive involution of segments 8-5-4b. In this case, the gallbladder will present to the left of the round ligament.

A2: The right umbilical vein goes into atrophy completely, and there is no parenchymal atrophy. This is the normal anatomy that is described.

A3: The right umbilical vein goes into atrophy completely and is accompanied by involution of segment 4b with hypotrophy of the latter.

Type B:

B1: The right external umbilical vein goes into atrophy, and the right intrahepatic umbilical vein persists. An involution in the segment 5 site is associated. In this case, there is the presence of left side gallbladder with the persistence of the right portal branch only for segments 6 and 7 and hypertrophy of the portal branch of segment 4.

B2: The right external umbilical vein goes into atrophy, and the right intrahepatic umbilical vein persists. There is no involution of the hepatic parenchyma with normal portal trifurcation.

B3: The right external umbilical vein goes into atrophy, and the right intrahepatic umbilical vein persists. It is associated with segment 4b hypotrophy. This determines the absence of the left portal branch and vascularization of segments 2 and 3 from the right portal branch through the persistent right umbilical vein portion.

Type C:

C1: The right extrahepatic and intrahepatic umbilical veins persist with atrophy of the left umbilical vein. An involution in the segment 5 site is associated. In this case, there is the presence of left side gallbladder with the persistence of the right portal branch only for segments 6 and 7 and the absence of segment 5 or 5 and 8. The vascularization of segments 2 and 3 and 4 occurs through the persistent right intrahepatic umbilical vein portion.

C2: The right extrahepatic and intrahepatic umbilical veins persist with atrophy of the left umbilical vein. No involution of the hepatic parenchyma occurs. The vascularization of the liver is arched from right to left giving, in sequence, the branch for segments 6 and 7, that of segments 5 and 8 and ending with the vascularization of segments 2 and 3 and 4 through the persistent intrahepatic right umbilical vein.

C3: The right extrahepatic and intrahepatic umbilical veins persist with atrophy of the left umbilical vein. An involution in the segment 4b site is associated. The vascularization of the liver is arched from right to left giving the branch for segments 6 and 7, the branch for segments 5 and 8 and ending with the vascularization of segments 2 and 3 through the persistent intrahepatic right umbilical vein.

Type D:

D1: The right extrahepatic umbilical vein persists with atrophy of the left umbilical vein. An involution in the segment 5 site is associated. In this case, there is the presence of left side gallbladder with the persistence of the right portal branch that vascularizes segments 6 and 7 and the absence of segment 5 or 5 and 8, and the left portal branch that vascularizes segments 2 and 3 and 4.

D2: The right extrahepatic umbilical vein persists with atrophy of the left umbilical vein. There is no involution of the hepatic parenchyma. In this case, the right portal branch that vascularizes segments 6–7 and 5–8 and the left portal branch that vascularizes segments 2 and 3 and 4 persist.

D3: The right extrahepatic umbilical vein persists with atrophy of the left umbilical vein. An involution is associated with segment 4b. In this case, the right portal branch that vascularizes segments 6–7 and 5–8 and the left portal branch that vascularizes segments 2 and 3 persist.

The principle of the fusion of the planes is necessary to be added at the classification performed by rotating or increasing the volume of one of the two hepatic lobes.

In this way, we can reposition the ligament tears in the position in which it is located once the complete fetal development has taken place. To clarify, we have modified the left liver portion by rotating it counterclockwise as shown in **Figure 5**.

We can see how this classification allows us to catalog the cases of literature described or represented with images, the portal modifications found: Kawai et al. [18] describe the absence of the left portal vein and a branch for the left liver originating from the right portal branch that we identify as an atrophy of left

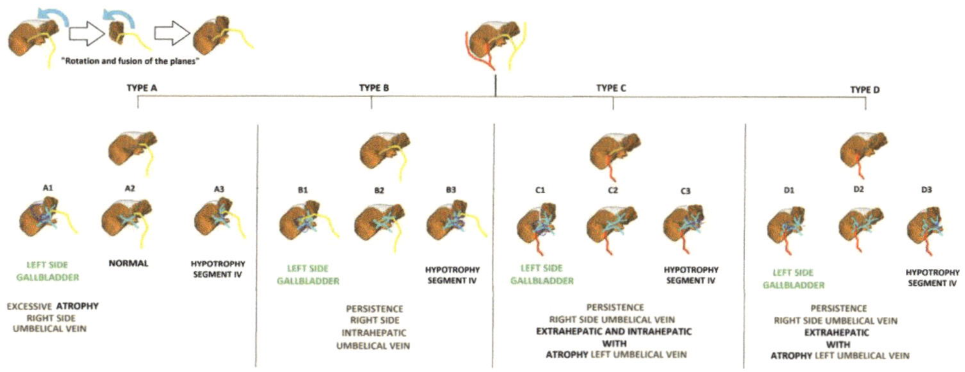

Figure 5.
Combination of the evolution process of right and left umbilical veins with atrophy mechanism of segments 5 and 4, associated rotation and fusion of the right and left liver.

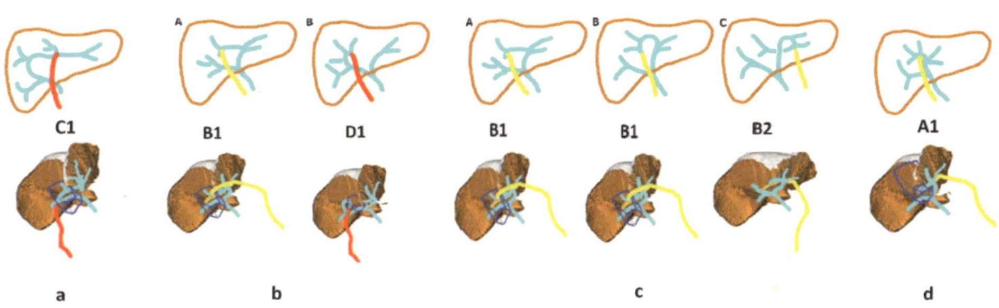

Figure 6.
Schematic representation published in the literature with comparison and reclassification with our nomenclature. (a) Kawai description (12) corresponding to Type C; (b) Nagai description (3) corresponding to Types B1 and D1; (c) Maetani description (20) corresponding to Type B1-B1-B2; and (d) Banchini description (9) corresponding to Type A1.

umbilical vein Type C1 (**Figure 6a**); Nagai et al. [90] describe a case with the absence of the right anterior portal branch, corresponding to Type B1, and the other absence of the left portal branch that we call Type D1 (**Figure 6b**); Lin [42] describes tree cases of the absence of the right anterior portal branch, corresponding to Type B; Maetani et al. [45] also describe two cases that we classify as Type B1 and one case with the absence of the right anterior portal branch and a vascularization of segments 5 and 8 from the left portal one that we consider Type B2 (**Figure 6c**); Banchini et al. [20] describe the agenesis of segments 5 and 8 with the absence of the right anterior portal branch, Type A1 (**Figure 6d**). On the contrary, the classification we propose differs from Shindon's classification [121] in defining the true right side ligamentum teres. Comparing the three types of portal bifurcation listed by Shindon, we consider the "independent right lateral" one as Type A1, the "bifurcation" one as Type D, and "trifurcation" one as an intermediate of Types A1–A3 (**Figure 7**), concluding that only the "bifurcation type" could be considered as "true right side ligamentum teres." It is evident that these three variables of fusion, atrophy, and umbilical vein evolution can be combined in a considerably higher number of ways and may result in intermediate presentations. Likewise, using this principle, we can also hypothesize how the biliary tract variations occur. Even if we will not deal in this chapter, we underline that, as evidenced by Nishitai et al. [122], the Biliary tree could differ a lot from the corresponding portal branches, making this a further challenge.

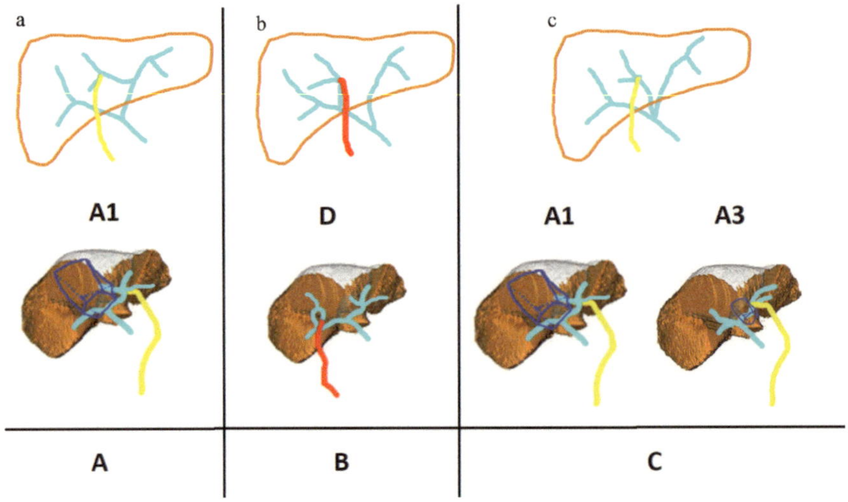

Figure 7.
Schematic representation of Shindon's classification (21) with comparison and reclassification with our nomenclature. (A) "Type A Shindon" corresponding to Type A1; (B) "Type B Shindon" corresponding to Type D; (C) "Type C Shindon" corresponding to intermediate Types A1–A3.

Considering the numerous possibilities with which a left gallbladder can present, we recommend an accurate study of the entire hepatic anatomy, with the need to recognize the portal, arterial, and biliary changes, in all patients presenting this diagnosis in the preoperative setting.

4. Clinical implication

As pointed out in the previous paragraph, the presence of LSG is associated with a high number of variations both internal and external to the liver, regardless of the type of classification we want to use.

However, the presence of this anomaly does not seem to be associated with either a particular clinical manifestation or cancer, thus representing a simple anatomical variation presents in the population. The absence of symptoms makes the diagnosis of LSG an occasional event, consequent to its finding during investigations performed for other factors. Likewise, as in the normal population, gallstones follow the physiological mechanism of formation. However, gallbladder malpositioning does not seem to change the afferent pain pathways, and, as reviewed by Iskandar et al. [6] on 32 articles, the related symptoms are those of biliary colic or classic acute cholecystitis, with pain in the right upper quadrant or epigastric pain.

The diagnosis of gallbladder gallstones is mostly performed with ultrasound, but it has a very low diagnostic capacity in case of unknown LSG. Therefore, patients presenting with symptoms of biliary colic or acute gallbladder cholecystitis have a high probability to find this anomaly only during surgery. This condition exposes the patient and the surgeon to considerable risk. In the literature, cases of biliary lesions during cholecystectomy in LSG range from 4.4 [115] to 7.3% [5].

Laparoscopic cholecystectomy does not seem to be contraindicated, but some precautions are necessary to avoid risks of complications. Many authors advocate different techniques in trocar placement or in the patient's position, but this strategy could be applicable only in the case of preoperative diagnosis.

Anyway, the main risk factor seems to be the passage of the gallbladder anterior to the liver pedicle. This rotation moves Calot's triangle from horizontal and lateral to a vertical and anterior position, bringing the gallbladder closer to the biliary tract (**Figure 8**).

In normal cholecystectomy, the opening of the Calot allows moving the gallbladder and cystic duct away from the biliary tract. This isolation is performed with a dissection directed from the superficial to the deep plane and is done by pulling the gallbladder laterally. The dissection finishes posterolaterally by finding an area free of tissue, corresponding to the posterior side on Calot's triangle. In the case of LSG, if we perform the dissection of the Calot using this method, we risk finding a posterior plane occupied by the biliary tract and liver peduncle instead of a free one (**Figure 9**).

Taking into account this condition, it is necessary to look for a dissection modality that allows maintaining the distance from the biliary tract and the hepatic peduncle. We advocate performing laparoscopic cholecystectomy with fundus first technique [24] to achieve a proper distance from the hepatic pedicle. Once the body of the gallbladder is detached from the liver surface and Calot's triangle is joined, we recommend to follow the dissection close to the gallbladder border. The border dissection allows minimizing the removal of peripedicle fat tissue, avoiding unintended biliary duct discovery. In order to augment the distance from the pedicle and the biliary way, once the peritoneum of the Calot has been opened, it is advisable to pull the gallbladder on the lateral side to horizontalize the triangle itself. This traction can move the gallbladder on the right side of the hepatic pedicle, repurposing the normal anatomy. After this mobilization, it could be useful to apply the Strasberg criteria for the visualization of all structures [123], so that the cystic duct and cystic artery can be dissected and clipped distant from the biliary tract, after their recognition. In case of doubt, it is useful to perform an intraoperative cholangiography or visualize the biliary tract with the indocyanine green or finally proceed with the conversion to have a direct view.

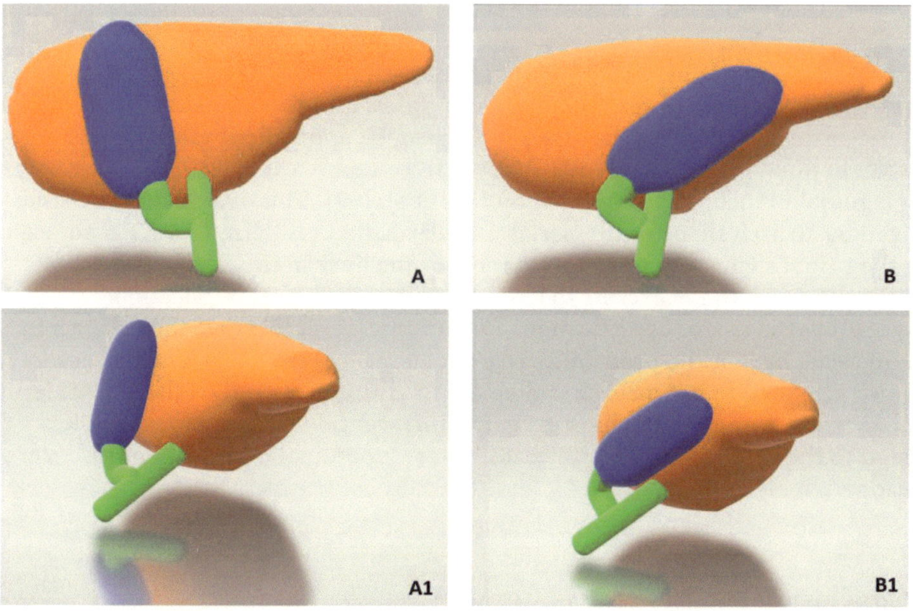

Figure 8.
Blue gallbladder; green cystic duct and biliary way; brown liver. (A) Normal gallbladder frontal view; (A1) normal gallbladder left lateral view; (B) left side gallbladder frontal view; and (B1) left side gallbladder left lateral view.

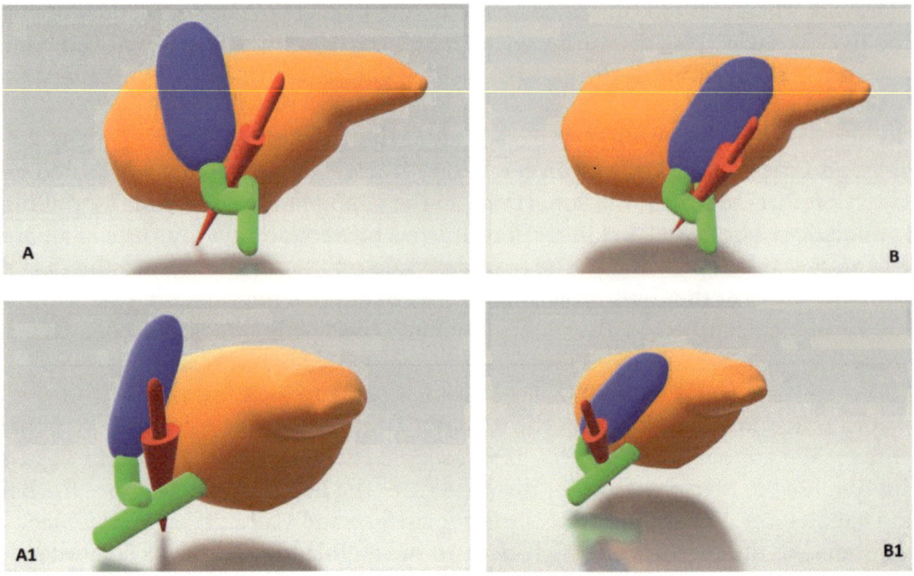

Figure 9.
(A) Normal gallbladder frontal visual; (A1) normal gallbladder left lateral visual; (B) left side gallbladder frontal vision; (B1) left side gallbladder left lateral. Visual red arrow: direction of dissection in Calot's triangle.

While accurate dissection and recognition of structures in cholecystectomy can prevent iatrogenic lesions, it is different in the case of liver resections. The anatomical variations that can occur are so high that a detailed study of portal, arterial, and biliary structures is mandatory. This necessity stems from the fact that the portal variations may not correspond to arterial or biliary anomalies, and therefore, all three of these structures must be considered separately. CT scan could be sufficient for portal and arterial study, and in particular, 3D CT could be particularly effective. On the opposite, the CT scan is not sufficient to demonstrate biliary variations, and for this reason, a magnetic resonance cholangiopancreatography is mandatory before elective major hepatectomy to ensure patient's safety [122].

Defining the types of resection is too complex, and therefore, each patient will require an on-demand treatment depending on the anomalies found. The main issue to keep in mind is that, in the case of LSG, liver supply can be sustained by only a single portal branch, as pointed out by Hsu et al. [97]. This eventuality is characterized by an arch shape of the portal vascularization visualized on CT scan, exposing the risk of extending resection to most of the liver itself.

The approach to LSG seems to have a significant clinical implication, augmenting the risk of complications in both liver resection and cholecystectomy. On one side, even if the probability to perform liver resection in LSG is very low, the risk is related to the major intrahepatic modification, on the other, considering cholecystectomy one of the most frequent interventions in surgery, the risk is related to the high probability to treat LSG as symptomatic gallbladder discovered intraoperatively.

5. Conclusion

Left side gallbladder is a rare and little known anomaly that is diagnosed, in most cases, during cholecystectomy for biliary colic or cholecystitis symptoms. The disposition of the gallbladder over the liver pedicle and the simultaneous presence of variations in the liver vascularization result in an increased risk during surgery. To prevent complications, we recommend performing a cholecystectomy with safety criteria, starting from the fundus and isolating Calot's triangle along the edge of the gallbladder. In the case of hepatic resection, an accurate study of the portal, arterial, and biliary branches should be done before surgery. This makes possible to plan an intervention tailored to the patient's anatomical condition.

Acknowledgements

A particular acknowledgment gives to "Associazione Carlo Malchiodi per le Ricerche in Chirurgia ONLUS" for funding publication.

Conflict of interest

The author declares no conflict of interest.

Author details

Filippo Banchini* and Patrizio Capelli
Department of General Surgery, Guglielmo da Saliceto Hospital, Piacenza, Italy

*Address all correspondence to: filippobanchini@virgilio.it

References

[1] Hochstetter F. Anomaliem der pfortader und der nabelvene in verbindung mit defect oder Linkscage der gall-en-blase. Archiv für Mikroskopische Anatomie und Entwicklungsmechanik. 1886;**3**:369-384

[2] Abe K, Kajiyama N, Harimoto T, Gion K, Shirabe T. Nagaie, resection ofmetastatic liver cancer in a patient with a left-sided gallbladder andintrahepatic portal vein and bile duct anomalies: A case report. International Journal of Surgery Case Reports. 2012;**3**(5):147-150. Available from: https://www.sciencedirect.com/science/article/pii/S2210261212000090?via%3Dihub

[3] Ishii H, Noguchi A, Onishi M, et al. True left-sided gallbladder withvariations of bile duct and cholecystic vein. World journal of gastroenterology. 2015;**21**(21): 6754-6758. DOI: 10.3748/wjg.v21.i21.6754

[4] Noritomi T, Watanabe K, Yamashita Y, Kitagawa S, Oshibuchi M, Shirakusa T. Left-sided gallbladder associated with congenital hypoplasia of the left lobe of the liver: A case report and review of literature. International Surgery. 2004;**89**:1-5

[5] Abongwa HK, De Simone B, Alberici L, Iaria M, Perrone G, Tarasconi A, et al. Implications of left-sided gallbladder in the emergency setting: Retrospective review and top tips for safe laparoscopiccholecystectomy. Surgical Laparoscopy, Endoscopy & Percutaneous Techniques. 2017;**27**(4): 220-227. DOI: 10.1097/SLE.0000000000000417

[6] Iskandar ME, Radzio A, Krikhely M, Leitman IM. Laparoscopic cholecystectomy for a left-sided gallbladder. World Journal of Gastroenterology. 2013;**19**(35): 5925-5928

[7] Ogawa T, Ohwada S, Ikeya S, Shiozaki H, Aiba S, Morishita Y. Left sided gallbladder with anomalies of the intrhepatic portal vein and anomalous junction of the pancreatico-biliary ductal system: A case report. Hepatogastroenterology. 1995;**42**: 645-649

[8] Alharthi S, Bernon M, Krige JE. Beware the left-sided gallbladder. South African Journal of Surgery. 2012;**50**: 88-89

[9] Jona G, Szaho L, Tasnadi L. A case of left sided gallbladder. Magyar Radiologia. 1961;**13**:115

[10] Ogino T, Ohwada S, Morishima I, Takahashi H, Ogawa T, Takei H, et al. Left-sided gallbladder resected by laparoscopic cholecystectomy (in Japanese with English abstract). Journal of Japan Surgical Association. 1996;**57**: 1203-1205

[11] Almodhaiberi H, Hwang S, Cho YJ, Kwon Y, Jung BH, Kim MH. Customized left-sided hepatectomy and bile duct resection for perihilar cholangiocarcinoma in a patient with left-sided gallbladder and multiple combined anomalies. Korean Journal of Hepato-Biliary-Pancreatic Surgery. 2015;**19**:30-34

[12] Jung HS, Huh K, Shin YH, et al. Left-sided gallbladder: A complicated percutaneous cholecystostomy and subsequent hepatic embolisation. The British Journal of Radiology. 2009;**82**: e141-e144

[13] Oshima I. A case of a left-sided gallbladder with right-sided round ligament which was performed partial

hepatectomy (in Japanese with English abstract). Geka. 2004;**66**:959-962

[14] Aoki H, Tagaya N, Kubota K. Laparoscopic cholecystectomy with miniaturized instruments for a left-sided gallbladder: A case report (in Japanese with English abstract). Japan Society for Endoscopic Surgery. 2001;**6**: 261-265

[15] Kanazumi N, Fujiwara M, Sugimoto H, Fujii T, Nomoto S, Inoue S, et al. Laparoscopic cholecystectomy for left-sided gallbladder: Report of two cases. Hepato-Gastroenterology. 2007; **54**:674-676

[16] Ozeki Y, Onitsuka A, Hayashi M, Sasaki E. Left-sided gallbladder: Report of a case and study of 26 cases in Japan. Nippon Geka Gakkai Zasshi. 1987;**88**: 1644-1650

[17] Asonuma K, Shapiro AM, Inomata Y, Uryuhara K, Uemoto S, Tanaka K. Living related liver transplantation from donors with the left-sided gallbladder/portal vein anomaly. Transplantation. 1999;**68**: 1610-1612. DOI: 10.1097/ 00007890-199911270-00031

[18] Kawai K, Miyata N, Yuasa E, Takeuchi Y, Goto H, Miyake H, et al. Kobayashi, true left-sidedgallbladder with a portal anomaly: Report of a case. Surgery Today. November 2012;**42**(11): 1130-1134. DOI: 10.1007/s00595-011-0093-5

[19] Pradeep VM, Ramachandran K, Sasidharan K. Anomalous position of the gallbladder: Ultrasonographic and scintigraphic demonstration in four cases. Journal of Clinical Ultrasound. 1992;**20**:593-597

[20] Banchini F, Ekpo EF, Conti L, Capelli P. Left side gallbladder with agenesis of right anterior sector and absence of right hepatic duct. A case report. International Journal of Surgery Case Reports. 2019;**60**: 249-252. DOI: 10.1016/j. ijscr.2019.06.034

[21] Kehr H. Hine seltene anomalie der gall en gange. Muench Med Weschr. 1902;**49**:229

[22] Quah GS, Ng IE, Punch G, Richardson AJ. True left-sided gallbladder: A rare anatomical anomaly and its associated surgical challenges. ANZ Journal of Surgery. 2019;**89**:E333-E334

[23] Banzo I, Carril JM, Arnal C. Left sided gallbladder. An incidental finding on hepatobiliary scintigraphy. Clinical Nuclear Medicine. 1990;**15**:358-359

[24] Kelly Michael D. Laparoscopic retrograde (fundus first) cholecystectomy. BMC Surgery. 2009;**9**: 19. DOI: 10.1186/1471-2482-9-19

[25] Qureshi Z. Awad, aberrant presentation of the gallbladder duringlaparoscopic cholecystectomy. JSLS. 2009;**13**(4):605-607. DOI: 10.4293/108680809X12589999538075

[26] Bender EA, Springhetti S, Shemisa K, Wittenauer J. Leftsided gallbladder (sinistroposition) with duplication of the common bile duct. JSLS. 2007;**11**:148-150

[27] Kim EJLJ, Song SY, Lee KG, Park HK, Lee KS. Left-sided gallbladder with intra-hepatic portal vein anomalies: A single centre experience. Korean Journal of Hepato-Biliary-Pancreatic Surgery. 2010;**14**:241-247

[28] Rafailidis S, Varelas N, Kotsidis D. Rafailidis, two congenital anomalies in one: An ectopic gallbladder with phrygian cap deformity. Case Reports in Radiology. 2014;**2014**:246476

[29] Bonomo BR, Veenstra TM, Komar HM. Richter,

single-incisioncholecystectomy for left-sided gallbladder. JSLS. 2014;**18**(2): 338-341. DOI: 10.4293/108680813X13693422518632

[30] Kinoshita H, Sahai K, Kubo S, Ohno K. Two cases of leftsided eallbladder associated with cholelithiasis: Review of the literature in Japan. Osaka City Medical Journal. 1964; **88**:494-497

[31] Reddy PK, Subramanian RV, Yuvaraja S. Laparoscopic cholecystectomy for left-sided gallbladder (sinistroposition). JSLS. 2005;**9**:356-357

[32] Chrungoo SL, Kachroo AK, Sharma AB, Khan AS. Nadim, left-sided gallbladder: Report of two cases. Journal of Minimal Access Surgery. 2007;**3**(3):108-110. DOI: 10.4103/0972-9941.37194

[33] Kubo S, Lee S, Yamamoto T, Edagawa A, Kinoshita H. Leftsided gallbladder associated with anomalous branching of the portal vein detected by sonography. Osaka City Medical Journal. 2000;**46**:95-98

[34] Rocca JP, Rodriguez-Davalos MI, Burke-Davis M, Marvin MR, Sheiner PA, Facciuto ME. Living-donor hepatectomy in right-sided round-ligament liver: Importance of mapping the anatomy to the left medial segment. Journal of Hepato-Biliary-Pancreatic Surgery. 2006;**13**:454-457

[35] Chuang VP. The aberrant gallbladder: Angiographic and radioisotopic considerations. American Journal of Roentgenology. 1976;**127**: 417-421

[36] Lee DK, Park YH, Kim JS. Clinical significance and characteristics of left-sided gallbladder: Case series study of 10 patients. Annals of Surgical Treatment and Research. 2019;**97**(6): 302-308

[37] Rozsos I, Ferenczy J, Vincze K, Rainer S. Left sided gallbladder [in Hungarian]. Magyar Sebészet. 2002; **55**(5):329-330

[38] Chung CC, Leung KL, Lau WY, Li AK. Ectopic gallbladder revisited, laparoscopically: A case report. Canadian Journal of Surgery. 1997;**40**: 464-466

[39] Leone V, Consolea BN. Management of incidental left-side gallbladder in laparoscopiccholecystectomy. Journal of Current Surgery. 2013;**3**(1):41-43

[40] Saafan T, Hu JY, Mahfouz AE, Abdelaal A. True left-sided gallbladder: A casereport and comparison with the literature for the different techniques oflaparoscopic cholecystectomy for such anomalies. International Journal of Surgery Case Reports. 2018;**42**:280-286. DOI: 10.1016/j.ijscr.2017.12.029

[41] Cirla A, De Vecchi A. Left sided ectopic gallbladder. Quaderni di Radiologia. 1965;**30**:749-758

[42] Lin HY. Is right-sided ligamentum teres hepatis always accompanied by left-sided gallbladder? Case reports and literature review. Insights into Imaging. 2018;**9**:955-960. DOI: 10.1007/s13244-018-0671-9

[43] Sadhu S, Jahangir TA, Roy MK. Left-sided gallbladder discovered during laparoscopic cholecystectomy in a patient with dextrocardia. Indian Journal of Surgery. 2012;**74**:186-188. DOI: 10.1007/s12262-011-0261-2

[44] Colovic R, Colovic N, Barisic G, Atkinson HD, Krivokapic Z. Left-sided gallbladder associated with congenital liver cyst. HPB (Oxford). 2006;**8**: 157-158. DOI: 10.1080/13651820410016642

[45] Maetani Y, Itoh K, Kojima N, et al. Portal vein anomaly associated with deviation of the ligamentum teres to the

right and malposition of the gallbladder. Radiology. 1998;**207**:723-728

[46] Sakihara H, Yokota R, Yamaga S, Nagabuchi E, Kuribayashi H. A case of laparoscopic cholecystectomy for a left-sided gallbladder, diagnosed intraoperatively (in Japanese with English abstract). Japan Society for Endoscopic Surgery. 2008;**13**:625-630

[47] Dhulkotia A, Kumar S, Kabra V, Shukla HS. Aberrant gallbladder situated beneath the left lobe of liver. HPB (Oxford). 2002;**4**:39-42. DOI: 10.1080/136518202753598726

[48] Makni A, Magherbi H, Ksantini R, Rebai W, Safta ZB. Left-sided gallbladder: An incidental finding on laparoscopic cholecystectomy. Asian Journal of Surgery. 2012;**35**:93-95. DOI: 10.1016/j.asjsur.2012.04.011

[49] Schiffino L, Mouro J, Levard H, Dubois F. A case of a left-sided gallbladder treated surgically via laparoscopy. Annali Italiani di Chirurgia. 1993;**64**:229-231

[50] Donthi R, Thomas DJ, Sanders D, Schmidt SP. Report of laparoscopic cholecystectomy in two patients with left-sided gallbladders. JSLS. 2001;**5**:53-56

[51] Masood R, Samiullah, Chaudhary IA, Taimur. Laparoscopic cholecystectomyfor left sided gall bladder: An unusual case. Journal of Ayub Medical College, Abbottabad. 2009;**21**(1):162-163

[52] Seiberman J et al. Left sided gallbladder. A rare anatomic variant. Chirnag. 1986;**57**:653-654

[53] Ergun R. Sinistrac position of the gallbladder. Turk Tip Cem Mec. 1960; **52**:344

[54] Matsumoto N, Hasegawa H, Shiroko T, Komatsu S, Kurumiya Y, et al. A case of laparoscopic cholecystectomy for acute cholecystitis associated with the left sided gallbladder and an aberrant hepatic duct. Japanese Journal of Gastroenterological Surgery. 2008;**41**:1704-1709

[55] Shen BY. Sinistroposition of the gallbladder and common bile duct. Hepatobiliary & Pancreatic Diseases International. 2005;**4**:313-315

[56] Etter LE. Left sided gallbladder: Necessity for film of the entire abdomen incholecystography. American Journal of Roentgenology. 1953;**70**:987

[57] Matsumura N, Tokumura H, Yasumoto A, Sasaki H, Yamasaki M, Musya H, et al. Laparoscopic cholecystectomy and common bile duct exploration for cholecystocholedocholithiasis with a left-sided gallbladder: Report of a case. Surgery Today. 2009;**39**:252-255. DOI: 10.1007/s00595-008-3837-0

[58] Shimizu T, Hayashi M, Inoue Y, Komeda K, Asakuma M, Hirokawa F, et al. Living-donor liver transplantation from donor with a left-sided gallbladder with portal vein anomaly. Transplantation. 2012;**94**:e60-e61

[59] Feldman L, Venta L. Percutaneous cholecystectomy of an ectopic gallbladder. Gastrointestinal Radiology. 1988;**13**:256-258

[60] Matsuoka N, Morimoto T, Yasui Y, Kita S, Yanai H, Matsuo K, et al. A case of a left-sided gallbladder (in Japanese with English abstract). J Kyoto City Hospital. 2007;**27**:22-25

[61] Shirono K, Kounosu H, Kubo H, et al. Case of left-sided gallbladder accompanying the anomalous intrahepatic portal and hepatic venous branching. Japanese Journal of Gastroenterological Surgery. 1990;**23**: 1477 [in Japanese]

[62] Fujita N, Shirai Y, Kawaguchi H, Tsukada K, Hatakeyama H. Left-sided gallbladder on the basis of a right-sided round ligament. Hepato-Gastroenterology. 1998;**45**:1482-1484

[63] Mazzamurro G, Di Lella V, Di Segni R. Comments on a case of left sided gallbladder. Radiologia Medica (Torino). 1981;**67**:476-480

[64] Siebermair J. Die linksseitige gallenblase eine selteneanatomische variante. Der Chirurg. 1986;**57**:653-654

[65] Fujita T, Ajiki T, Matsumoto T, Okazaki T, Matsumoto I, Kuroda Y, et al. Laparoscopic cholecystectomy for a left-sided gallbladder (in Japanese with English abstract). Japan Society for Endoscopic Surgery. 2007;**12**:403-407

[66] McGowan JM, Nussbaum CC, Burroughs EW. Cholecystitis due to giardia lambdia in a left sided gallbladder. Annals of Surgery. 1948; **128**:1032-1037

[67] Si-Youn R, Poong-Man J. Left-sided gallbladder with rightsided ligamentum teres hepatis: Rare associated anomaly of exomphalos. Journal of Pediatric Surgery. 2008;**43**:1390-1395. DOI: 10.1016/j.jpedsurg.2008.03.033

[68] Fukuda Y, Fujio N, Ihara T, Tsukazaki T, Koyama I, Tsukazaki Y, et al. A case of laparoscopic cholecystectomy for the left-sided gallbladder (in Japanese with English abstract). Geka. 2006;**68**:343-346

[69] Mendoza-Calderon JWS, Davila-Arriaga AR. Gallbladder to the left side of the falciform ligament in absence of Situs Inversus "Sinistroposition"—Case series of 2 patients with this anomaly who underwent mini-laparoscopic cholecystectomy. International Journal of Surgery Case Reports. 2018;**50**:36-41

[70] Strong RW, Fawcett J, Hatzifotis M, Hodgkinson P, Lynch S, O'Rourke T, et al. Surgical implications of a left-sided gallbladder. American Journal of Surgery. 2013;**206**:59-63. DOI: 10.1016/j.amjsurg.2012.10.035

[71] Funakoshi T, Kamiyama T, Nakagawa T, Sato N, Matsushita M, Todo S, et al. Resection of echinococcosis of the liver with the left-sided gallbladder and anomalous intrahepatic portal vein system: A case report (in Japanese with English abstract). Rinsyogeka. 2004;**59**: 743-746

[72] Mizray L. A case of left gallbladder. El Día Médico. 1960;**31**:2364

[73] Surjan RDT, Pinheiro JLS, Pinheiro PHS, da Silva IBM, do Prado Silveira S, Frugis MO. True left-sided gallbladder concomitant to direct insertion of the cystic duct into the duodenum: An extremely rare anatomic variation. Relatos Casos Cir. 2019;**5**(4): e2364. DOI: 10.30928/2527-2039e-20192364

[74] Futamura N, Matsumoto M, Yasumura M, Tateyama K, Tarao M, Sakamoto K, et al. A case of left-sided gallbladder (in Japanese). Gekachiryo. 2004;**90**:361-363

[75] Mohammed AA, Arif SH. Midline gallbladder makes a challenge for surgeons during laparoscopiccholecystectomy; case series of 6 patients. Annals of Medicine and Surgery. 2019;**40**:14-17

[76] Szanto I, Voros A, Altorjai A, Kiss J. Gallbladder in the left side of the lower abdomen. Endoscopy. 1996;**28**:49

[77] Gondra MD, Urien ID, Pturrioz T. Vesicula Biliar a la izquierda. Prensa Médica Argentina. 1954;**41**:124

[78] Moo-Young T, Picus DD, Teefey S, Strasberg SM. Common bile duct injury following laparoscopic cholecystectomy in the setting of sinistroposition of the gallbladder and bilairy confluence: A case report. Journal of Gastrointestinal Surgery. 2009;**14**:166-170

[79] Tachibana H, Tachibana R, Tachibana T. Two case reports of left sided gallbladder. Shindan to Chiryou. 1978;**66**:135-140 (in Japanese)

[80] Gui D, Magalini S, Prete F, Sermoneta D. What's right when the gallbladder's left? A case report. Surgical Endoscopy. 2002;**16**:1637

[81] Moravik J. Left sided gallbladder—Laparoscopic cholecystectomy. Surgical Endoscopy. 2015;**29**:S188

[82] Takemura S, Yamasaki O, KwanChoon L, Mori A, Ikeda K, Kinoshita H, et al. A case of left-sided gallbladder and anomalous branching of the intrahepatic portal vein in which a Biliary cystadenoma of the liver was resected (in Japanese with English abstract). Japanese Journal of Gastroenterological Surgery. 1994;**27**:2243-2247

[83] Hasbahceci M, Erol C, Seker M, Basak F, Alimoglu O. Standard laparoscopic cholecystectomy for malposition of the gallbladder caused by right-sided ligamentum teres. Journal of Minimal Access Surgery. 2013;**9**:177-179

[84] Moriyama S, Mori T, Umegae S. Two cases of left sided gallbladder with intrahepatic portal vein anomaly. Japanese Journal of Gastroenterological Surgery. 1990;**23**:2813-2817

[85] Takiguchi S, Sekimoto M, Matsui S, Yano H, Tateishi H, Kinuta M, et al. A case of left-sided gallbladder combined with an anomalous intrahepatic portal vein, confirmed by laparoscopic cholecystectomy (in Japanese with English abstract). Japanese Journal of Gastroenterological Surgery. 1996;**29**:2294-2298

[86] Herrington JL Jr. Gallbladder arising from the left hepatic lobe. American Journal of Surgery. 1966;**112**:106-109

[87] Naganuma S, Ishida H, Konno K, Hamashima Y, Hoshino T, Naganuma H, et al. Sonographic findings of anomalous position of the gallbladder. Abdominal Radiology. 1998;**23**:67-72

[88] Tomiyama M, Okamura K, Kondo S, Kato H. A case of a leftsided gallbladder treated with laparoscopic cholecystectomy (in Japanese with English abstract). Japan Society for Endoscopic Surgery. 2002;7:65-69

[89] Hirohata et al. Hirohata laparoscopic cholecystectomy for acute cholecystitis in a patient with left-sided gallbladder: A case report. Surgical Case Reports. 2019;**5**:54. DOI: 10.1186/s40792-019-0614-9

[90] Nagai M, Keiichi K, Seiji K, et al. Are left-sided gallbladders really located on the left side? Annals of Surgery. 1997;**225**(3):274-280

[91] Uesaka K, Yasui K, Morimoto T, et al. Left-sided gallbladder with intrahepatic portal venous anomalies. Journal of Hepato-Biliary-Pancreatic Surgery. 1995;**2**:425-430

[92] Nagendram S, Lynes K, Hamade A. A case report on a left sided gallbladder: A rare finding during cholecystectomy. International Journal of Surgery Case Reports. 2017;**14**(41):398-400. DOI: 10.1016/j.ijscr.2017.11.004

[93] Velimezis G, Vassos N, Kapogiannatos G, et al. Left-sided gallbladder in the era of laparoscopic cholecystectomy: A single-center experience. The American Surgeon. 2015;**81**:1249-1252

[94] Hopper N, Ryder JM, Swarnkar K, Stephenson BM. Laparoscopic left hepatic lobe cholecystectomy. Journal of Laparoendoscopic & Advanced Surgical Techniques. Part A. 2003;**13**:405e406

[95] Nakakubo Y, Tanaka K, Tamoto E, Okushiba S, Kawamura K, Kondo S. A case of a left-sided gallbladder treated

using a laparoscopic cholecystectomy (in Japanese with English abstract). Rinsyogeka. 2006;**61**:995-997

[96] Watanabe O, Tsuchiya Y, Makino H, Tsutsui M, Nashimoto A, Sano M, et al. A case of left-sided gallbladder confirmed by laparoscopic cholecystectomy (in Japanese). Shujutsu. 1994;**48**:2241-2243

[97] Hsu T-YC, Huang T-L, Sun C-K, Mconcejero A, Tsang LL-C, Cheng Y-F. Left-sided gallbladder: Its clinical significance and imaging presentations. World Journal of Gastroenterology. 2007;**13**(December):6404-6409

[98] Namikawa T, Tamura K, Morita M, et al. Laparoscopic cholecystectomy for a patient with left-sided gallbladder. Surgical Technology International. 2015; **26**:120-123

[99] Wong J, Rusby T. Ismail, left-sided gall bladder: A diagnostic and surgicalchallenge. ANZ Journal of Surgery. 2001;**71**:557-558. DOI: 10.1046/j.1440-1622.2001.02195.x

[100] Huang T, Yamasaki Y, Yamasaki H, Fukui Y, Hatanaka N, Okuno S, et al. Six cases of laparoscopic cholecystectomy to leftsided gallbladder (in Japanese with English abstract). Journal of Japan Surgical Association. 2000;**61**:458-461

[101] Nastos C, Vezakis A, Papaconstantinou I, Theodosopoulos T, Koutoulidis V, Polymeneas G. Methods of safe laparoscopic cholecystectomy for left-sided (sinistroposition) gallbladder: A report of two cases and a review of safe techniques. International Journal of Surgery Case Reports. 2014;**5**:769-773

[102] Wu TC, Lee RC, Chiang JH, Chang CY. Reappraisal of left-sided gallbladderand its accompanying anomalies: A report of two cases and literature review. Acta Radiologica. 2005;**46**:233-236. DOI: 10.1080/02841850510012706

[103] Hwang S, Lee SG, Park KM, et al. Hepatectomy of living donors with a left-sided gallbladder and multiple combined anomalies for adult-toadult living donor liver transplantation. Liver Transplantation. 2004;**10**:141-146

[104] Nemours, Auguste, Barrag. Sur un cas de vesicule biliare flottante a gauche. Arch Mal Appar Dig. 1951;**40**:453

[105] Yamazaki M, Takahashi K. Left sided gallbladder. Rinsho Hoshasen. 1970;**15**:341-345

[106] Iaccarino AI, Done A. Su di un caso di cholecisti a sinistra G. Tal Chir. 1955; **11**:1073

[107] Newcombe JF, Henley FA. Left-sided gallbladder. A review of the literature and a report of a case associated with hepatic duct carcinoma. Archives of Surgery. 1964;**88**:494-497

[108] Yu T, Wu SD, Min L. Incidental left-sided gallbladder during laparoscopic cholecystectomy for cholelithiasis. The American Surgeon. 2012;**78**:492-493

[109] Idu M, Jakimowicz J, Iuppa A, Cuschieri A. Hepatobiliary anatomy in patients with transposition of the gallbladder: Implications for safe laparoscopic cholecystectomy. British Journal of Surgery. 1996;**83**:1442-1443

[110] Nguyen TH, Nguyen TS, Van Nguyen PD, Dang TN, Talarico EF Jr. Sinistroposition: A case report of true left-sided gallbladder in a Vietnamese patient. International Journal of Surgery Case Reports. 2018;**51**:82-85

[111] Zografos GC, Lagoudianakis EE, Grosomanidis D, Koronakis N, Tsekouras D, Chrysikos J, et al. Management of incidental left-sided

gallbladder. JSLS. 2009;**13**(April–June): 273-275

[112] Ikoma A, Tamaka K, Hamada N. Left sided gallbladder with accessory liver accompanied by intra-hepatic cholangiocarcinoma. Journal of the Japanese Surgical Society. 1992;**93**: 434-436 [in Japanese]

[113] Nishio H, Hasegawa H, Ogiso S. A case of the left-sided gallbladder with gallstones treated with laparoscopic cholecystectomy. Tan to Sui. 1995;**16**: 697-701

[114] Zoulamoglou M, Flessas I, Zarokosta M, et al. Left-sided gallbladder(Sinistroposition) encountered during laparoscopic cholecystectomy: A rarecase report and review of the literature. International Journal of Surgery. 2017;**31**:65-67. DOI: 10.1016/j.ijscr.2017.01.011

[115] Ryan P, Talbir S, John A, Sam B, Eslick Guy D, Cox Michael R. Left-sided gallbladder: A systematic review of a rare biliary anomaly. ANZ Journal of Surgery. 2019;**89**:1392-1397. DOI: 10.1111/ans.15041

[116] Gross RE. Congenital anomalies of the gallbladder. A review of 148 cases, with report of a double gallbladder. Archives of Surgery. 1936;**32**:131-162

[117] Radha S, Shyam S, Gupta SK, Sameer R. Anatomical variations of cystic ducts in magnetic resonance cholangiopancreatography and clinical implications. Radiology Research and Practice. 2016. p. 6. Article ID 3021484. DOI: 10.1155/2016/3021484

[118] Arey LB. Developmental Anatomy; A Text Book and Laboratory Manual of Embryology. 7th ed. Philadelphia: WB Saunders Co; 1965

[119] Matsumoto H. A newer concept of the segments of the liver. Japanese Journal of Medical Ultrasonics. 1986;**13**:551-552

[120] Olivier L, Jacques T, Eric S, Mehdi C, Laurent H, Grenier Philippe A. Fusion of the midplane with the left intersectional plane: A liver anatomical variation revisited with multidetector-row CT. European Radiology. 2006;**16**: 1699-1708. DOI: 10.1007/s00330-006-0245-y

[121] Shindoh J, Akahane M, Satou S, Aoki T, Beck Y, Hasegawa K, et al. Vascular architecture in anomalous right-sided ligamentum teres: Three-dimensional analyses in 35 patients. HPB. 2012;**14**:32-41

[122] Nishitai R, Shindoh J, Yamaoka T, Akahane M, Kokudo N, Manaka D. Biliary architecture of livers exhibiting right-sided ligamentum teres: An indication for preoperative cholangiography prior to major hepatectomy. HPB. 2016;**18**:929-935. DOI: 10.1016/j.hpb.2016.08.002

[123] Strasberg SM, Brunt LM. Rationale and use of the critical view of safety in laparoscopic cholecystectomy. Journal of the American College of Surgeons. 2010;**211**(July). DOI: 10.1016/j.jamcollsurg.2010.02.053

Chapter 8

Stereotactic Image-Guidance for Ablation of Malignant Liver Tumors

Iwan Paolucci, Raluca-Maria Sandu, Pascale Tinguely, Corina Kim-Fuchs, Martin Maurer, Daniel Candinas, Stefan Weber and Anja Lachenmayer

Abstract

Stereotactic percutaneous ablation is a rapidly advancing modality for treatment of tumors in soft solid organs such as the liver. Each year, there are about 850,000 cases of primary liver cancer worldwide. Although surgical resection still is the gold standard for most cases, only 20–30% of patients are candidates for it, due to the advanced stage of the disease. Surgery can also be a huge burden to the patient and his/her quality of life might be temporarily severely reduced due to long hospital stays, complications, and slow recovery. To overcome these disadvantages, thermo-ablation of tumors of up to 3 cm has become a more viable alternative especially in the last decade, offering a potentially equally effective but minimally invasive and tissue sparing treatment alternative. In conjunction with improved CT imaging, stereotactic image-guidance techniques and image fusion technology were introduced to increase safety, efficacy, and accuracy of this treatment. Stereotactic image-guidance leads to a simple, fast, and accurate placement of the ablation probe into the liver tumor, which is a prerequisite for a complete destruction of the tumor by ablation. More and more physicians, including surgeons, consider ablation a viable alternative to resection whenever feasible. Patients undergoing such a minimally invasive treatment benefit from a shorter hospital stays, reduced complication rates, and faster recovery.

Keywords: image-guidance, ablation, microwave/radiofrequency ablation, irreversible electroporation, liver tumors

1. Introduction

Thermal ablation of liver tumors is a minimally invasive locally destructive treatment alternative to surgical resection, which is the current gold standard for curative care. Not only is ablation considered for patients not amenable for surgical resection (<20%) but also increasingly for resectable tumors even with a curative intent [1–3]. Percutaneous ablation is generally performed under image-guidance based on CT, MRI, or ultrasound. Stereotactic image-guidance leads to a simple, fast, and accurate placement of the ablation needle into the liver tumor. Patients undergoing a percutaneous ablation benefit from an improved quality of life due to the shorter hospital stay compared to patients undergoing surgery [1].

IntechOpen

The key challenges in percutaneous ablations are complete coverage of the tumor with ablation necrosis including a 5- to 10-mm margin. Insufficient coverage of the ablation necrosis is related to local tumor progression, which is also associated with poor survival prognosis. While there are many unknown factors influencing the ablation process, one of the prerequisites is the accurate placement of the ablation needle in the tumor to ablate the tumor from the inside out. Stereotactic image-guidance aims to provide technical means to plan and accurately place an ablation needle into the tumor and verify its complete destruction.

1.1 Indications

For primary liver tumors (hepatocellular carcinoma, HCC), ablation is considered in cases of very early to early stage disease (BCLC 0/A) with less than three lesions that are smaller than 3 cm in diameter, according to the Barcelona Clinic Liver Cancer (BCLC) staging system guidelines [4]. For liver metastases from colorectal cancer (CRLM), ablation is still mostly performed for lesions not amenable to resection; however, first comparative studies suggest equal oncological outcomes (local recurrence, survival) after ablation versus resection of potentially resectable lesions [5]. The application as alternative to resection for HCC > 1 cm and CRLM is currently studied in various clinical trials; however, the oncologic non-inferiority of ablation has still to be confirmed in prospective trials. While the guidelines do not specify the access (open surgical vs. laparoscopic vs. percutaneous), it has been shown that the percutaneous access has lower complication rates and hospital stay with similar oncologic outcomes. Therefore, percutaneous ablations are generally preferred over surgical ablations. However, surgical ablations are performed in lesions that are difficult to target percutaneously or when ablation is combined with surgical resection. Stereotactic image-guidance offers a procedure to accurately target a lesion percutaneously, even in very difficult cases, in a predictable time.

In recent years, studies have been conducted to show that stereotactic image-guidance also allows to treat larger lesions by combining multiple ablation zones to fully cover the lesion [6], and also as an option for downstaging or bridging candidates for liver transplantation [7]. Larger lesions can also be treated with transcatheter arterial chemoembolization (TACE), but complete necrosis is barely achieved due to incomplete embolization and tumor angiogenesis. Therefore, approaches have been studied where TACE is combined with thermal ablation for HCCs >3 cm and found a synergetic effect [8]. For this combined treatment approach, an image-guidance approach has also been proposed, and preliminary animal experiments conducted [9].

1.2 Available image-guidance systems

There are currently three stereotactic image-guidance systems available on the market. The CAS-One IR (CAScination AG, Switzerland) and IMACTIS (IMACTIS, France) systems are pure image-guidance systems, whereas the MAXIO (Perfint, India) is a system with an integrated robotic arm for needle alignment. There are also several research devices in use in specialized clinics and it is expected that more devices will be available in the future.

1.3 Ablation modalities

Tumor ablation is defined as the local delivery of thermal, chemical, or electrical energy to a specific tumor in order to achieve its complete destruction. The most commonly used ablation techniques in conjunction with stereotactic image-guidance are thermal, chemical, and electrical ablation, which are described in the following sections.

1.3.1 Thermal ablation

Radiofrequency ablation (RFA) refers to energy sources that generate energy within the RF spectrum between 300 and 500 KHz. The RF electrode destroys all the cells at the target zone by heating up the tissue as a result of a high alternating electrical field that oscillates in the high-frequency range [10]. In Microwave ablations (MWA), a high-frequency electromagnetic field in the range of 900 MHz–2.45 Ghz forces water molecules to continuously realign, which results in high kinetic energy that is converted to heat in the tissue. Both RFA and MWA techniques destroy the tumor cells by coagulation necrosis using heat above 60°C. Compared to RFA, MWA heats the tissue faster due to the different heat distribution and therefore is also less affected by adjacent vessels (heat sink effect) [11, 12].

To date, most evidence supporting local ablation for small HCC lesions is based on works reporting RFA treatment and the comparison of RFA versus surgical resection. However, more recently, the theoretical and clinical advantages of MWA have often been highlighted. These include shorter application times, and the generation of higher temperatures resulting in larger ablation zones. Currently, several works comparing RFA versus MWA have reported partially contradicting results, especially regarding local tumor control after bot treatments [13, 14]. Overall, it can be assumed that no significant difference between RFA and MWA regarding overall and recurrent-free survival in patients with HCC exists [15]. However, there seems to be a tendency toward superiority of MWA regarding local recurrence rates in larger tumors as well as regarding operating times.

Cryoablation destroys tissue with freezing temperatures, alternating freezing and thawing or slight heating. The rapid freezing of tissue disrupts the cellular membranes by direct intracellular ice crystal formation. The most commonly used cooling agents are argon gas or liquid nitrogen [16].

1.3.2 Chemical ablation

Percutaneous ethanol injection (PEI) is the most commonly employed chemical ablation technique, but was demonstrated to have inferior results to thermal ablation [17]. PEI denaturizes the cellular proteins through cytoplasmic dehydration, which eventually also causes local coagulation necrosis. However, when compared to the other techniques, PEI shows significant disadvantages such as high local tumor progression rate, unpredictable ablation volumes, and lower overall survival rates.

1.3.3 Irreversible electroporation

Irreversible electroporation (IRE) is non-thermal ablation technique that delivers short pulses of high-voltage electrical energy directly to a tumor. This technique disrupts the cell membrane irreversibly and induces cell death by apoptosis (also known as natural cell death). The advantage of IRE is that it preserves blood vessels and therefore there is a high incentive to use IRE especially where vital structures and blood vessels can be easily damaged by thermal ablation methods [18]. IRE requires placing multiple needles in parallel and at a specific configuration and distance and therefore stereotactic image-guidance provides a precise placement of the needles. As IRE is a relatively new treatment, there are also less data available about its outcomes.

2. Components of a stereotactic image-guidance system

In this chapter, the general components of stereotactic image-guidance devices are described. In general, such a system consists of (**Figure 1**):

a. a tracking system that measures the position and orientation of the patient and the instruments in 3D space

b. software packages for

- trajectory and ablation planning
- trajectory and ablation validation
- visualization aids for needle placement

c. an alignment device that allows an accurate placement of the ablation needle into the tumor

2.1 Tracking systems

The tracking system measures the position and orientation of the needle guidance device and the patient in space. There are currently two different tracking modalities used for these procedures, namely optical and electromagnetic tracking. Optical tracking systems use a stereo infrared camera and locate retroreflecting spheres mounted on a rigid body— the so-called marker shields. Based on the geometry of these marker shields, the camera is able to identify them (e.g., needle guidance device). The second tracking modality is electromagnetic tracking, which generates an electromagnetic field and measures the current induced into small coils, which are attached to the device [19]. The position and orientation of the instrument are calculated from the current and a chip attached to the sensor provides information for identification.

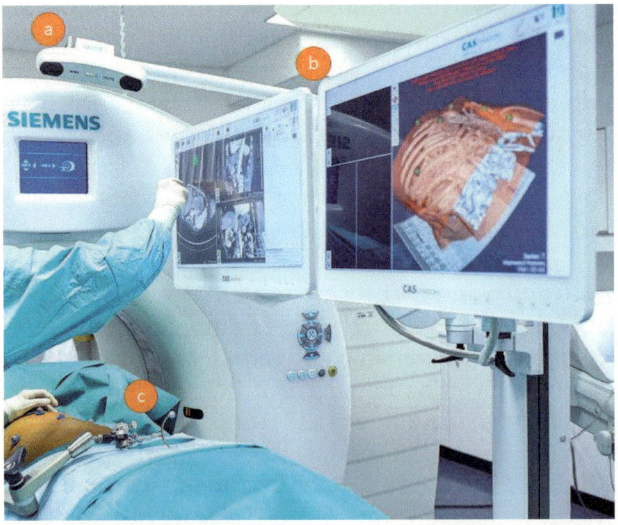

Figure 1.
Components and setup of a stereotactic image-guidance system.

Optical tracking systems tend to be more accurate but have the problem of a line-of-sight. Therefore, if the line-of-sight is occluded (e.g., by blood, radiologists' hand), the tracking device will lose track of the marker. Electromagnetic tracking relies on a known magnetic field and therefore is heavily affected by ferromagnetic and electrically conducting materials. Therefore, which system to use heavily depends on the target environment where the system will be used.

2.1.1 Patient tracking

A stereotactic image-guidance system needs to know where the patient is located relative to the tracking device in order to calculate the position of the needle guidance device relative to the planned needle trajectory (**Figure 2**). One option is to place retroreflective spheres on the patient that are detectable by the optical tracking system [20]. These spheres are also detectable on the CT scan and can therefore be used to register the CT to the patient [21]. Another approach, typically used with EM-based systems, is to place a position sensor on the patient's abdomen, which can be detected by the EM-tracking system. Both methods allow to track the patient in space. However, organ deformations due to breathing or repositioning of the patient cannot be calculated by these tracking methods. Nevertheless, when using multiple spheres or sensors, large deformations can be recognized, which allows to display a warning to the user.

2.2 Navigation software

The navigation software consists of planning tools, validation tools, and visualization aids for the radiologist to accurately align the needle guide and place the ablation needle.

2.2.1 Trajectory and ablation planning software

With the trajectory planning component, the radiologist plans trajectories to the tumor and also estimates the amount of energy needed to successfully ablate the tumor. In the most basic form, the software allows to plan a single straight-line trajectory to the tumor. In a more advanced setting, the software compensates for the offset between the needle tip and the active zone (which depends on the type of ablation device) and also supports multi-needle ablations with overlapping ablation

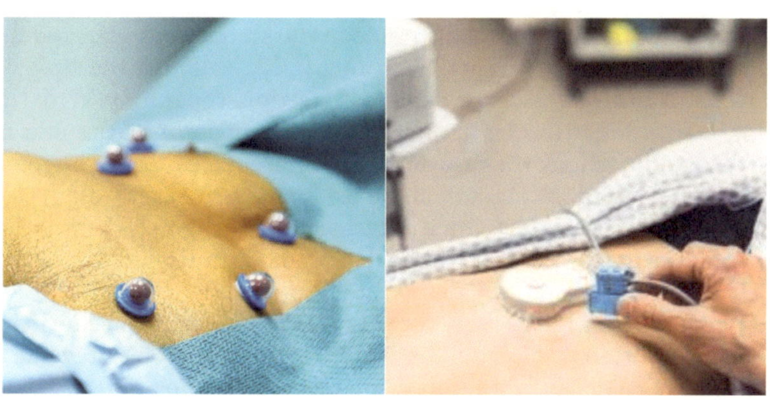

Figure 2.
(left) Patient tracking method using multiple retroreflective spheres (right) or using a single EM position sensor (© IMACTIS).

zones [6]. A trajectory for an ablation consists of a target point (tumor center) and an entry point on the skin. Depending on the location of the tumor, this trajectory passes nearby critical structures (e.g., *major* blood vessels, ribs) where specialized views along the needle trajectory are used to keep sufficient distance from these structures.

In cases where the tumor is not visible on the CT scan or the contrast agent cannot be administered to the patient, a pre-operative MRI scan can be fused with the intra-operative CT. The image-guidance system then allows to plan the trajectory on the MRI scan and then calculates the location on the CT scan.

2.2.2 Navigation visualization

The visualization component for navigation typically consists of a crosshair viewer and/or CT slice with a real-time overlay of the needle trajectory. This allows the radiologist to align the needle guidance device with the planned trajectory and then to place the needle at the correct depth. An indication of the deformation or motion of the patient is also visualized for monitoring and estimation of the accuracy.

2.2.3 Ablation validation

The ablation validation component fuses the pre- and post-ablation CT scans and visualizes them using alpha blending. The radiologist can switch between the pre- and post-ablation scan by choosing the blending level. More advanced systems allow to segment the tumor and the ablation zone and present a coverage.

2.3 Needle guidance devices

2.3.1 Freehand stereotactic navigation

With freehand navigation, a position sensor is attached to the ablation needle and the position and orientation of the needle are measured by the tracking device. The radiologist can freely move the needle and the navigation screen helps to place the needle according to the defined plan.

2.3.2 Stereotactic arms

When using a stereotactic arm (**Figure 3**), the tracking device measures the position and orientation of the needle guide in the stereotactic arm and uses this information to guide the radiologist. Such an arm typically has multiple handles, which allow to adjust and lock each degree of freedom separately. With this, the radiologist first aligns the arm roughly to the entry point on the skin and then pulls the handle to lock the position of the stereotactic arm. The remaining handles can then be used to fine-adjust the orientation to exactly align the device to follow the planned trajectory. Once the trajectory is aligned, the needle can be placed through the needle guide with the depth that is indicated on the navigation screen [22].

Another advantage of the stereotactic arm is that it holds the needle in place during a control CT scan and during the ablation procedure. This prevents movement of the needle, which would result in an uncontrolled ablation and potential tissue damage. Because the stereotactic arm holds the ablation needle during the control CT scan, the radiologist does not need to be in the CT room and thus is also not exposed to radiation [23].

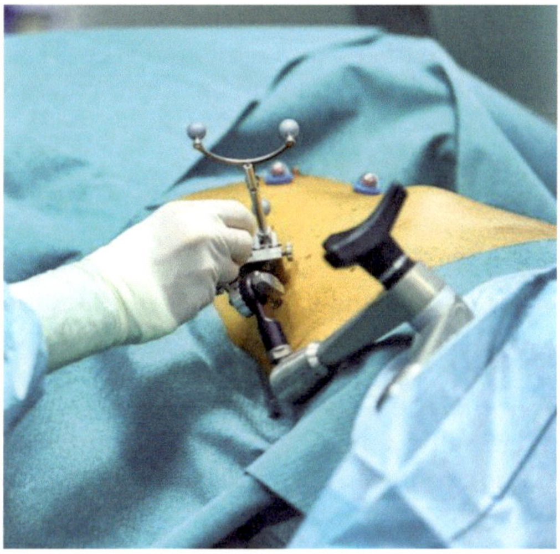

Figure 3.
Stereotactic arm during the adjustment of the needle trajectory.

2.3.3 Robotic devices

These devices are motorized articulated arms for alignment of ablation needles, providing a 6-dimensional alignment of a trajectory with respect to the target. The radiologist delivers the needle by hand and the robots passively guide it. There is a commercial provider, which has shown superior results in terms of accuracy and precision when compared to freehand targeting [24]. The findings from pre-clinical models and also from available clinical data show that passive needle guidance robots do not significantly increase available accuracy compared to stereotactic arms. Therefore, it is rather a matter of choice which kind of system to use.

3. Procedure

In the following chapter, a typical workflow (**Figure 4**) for a stereotactic image-guided percutaneous ablation of a liver tumor is presented.

3.1 Patient preparation

An important part when applying stereotactic guidance is that the organ of interest is properly fixated. In the case of the liver, that not only means to fixate the patient but also reduce the motion of the liver due to breathing. The fixation of the patient is generally done using a vacuum mattress. Once the patient is under

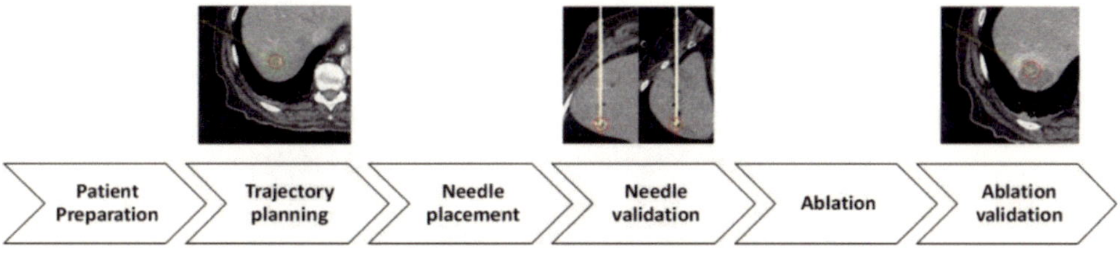

Figure 4.
Workflow of a percutaneous ablation of a liver tumor using stereotactic image-guidance.

anesthesia, the vacuum mattress is pressed toward the patient and the vacuum applied. This will prevent the patient from moving on the CT table.

To minimize the motion of the liver due to breathing, there are a number of alternatives:

- *Apnea*: where the ventilation is stopped on the ventilation device to hold a predefined air pressure inside the lung.

- *Tube disconnection*: where the endotracheal tube is disconnected from the ventilation device and all air is exhaled from the lungs.

- *High-frequency jet ventilation (HFJV)*: where short pulses of small volumes of pressurized air are delivered with high respiratory rates. This technique of mechanical ventilation results in minimal movement of lung and abdominal organs and is feasible for long durations [25].

Apnea and tube disconnection are applied during the CT scans and during the needle placement, while during the rest of the procedure, normal ventilation is applied. Jet ventilation can be applied during the whole procedure or also only during the CT scans and the needle placement.

3.1.1 Marker for patient tracking

Before starting the procedure, the patient tracker has to be placed on the patient's abdomen. Depending on the system, there are also specific requirements on how and where to place these markers for optimal accuracy of the system.

3.2 Trajectory planning

A trajectory for an ablation consists of a target point (the center of the tumor) and an entry point (entry on the skin) (**Figure 5**). Most ablation systems do not have their active center (the center of the ablation) at the tip. Therefore, the ablation system and the needle type can be selected, and the navigation system then computes a modified trajectory, such that the center of the ablation is in the center of the tumor. Additional to the trajectory, software guidance can also support the decision of the time and energy level to apply during the ablation. To avoid the puncture of

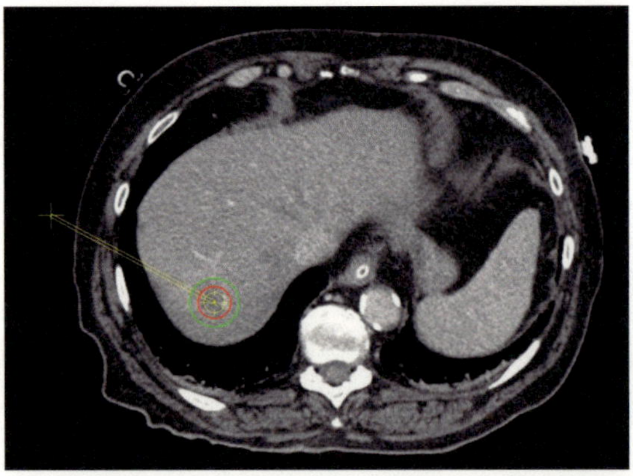

Figure 5.
Planning of a trajectory and the optimal ablation energy through an inter-costal trajectory.

blood vessels or other organs at risk, the navigation system presents a slice of the CT scan along the planned trajectory. This is especially useful in ablations in the superior segments where usually a sub- or inter-costal trajectory is required.

In case the tumor is not visible on the CECT scan, a pre-operative MRI scan can be fused with the intra-operative CT scan. The trajectory can then be planned on the MRI scan and the navigation system calculates the position of the trajectory on the intra-operative CT scan. One thing to consider is that the liver might have deformed with respect to the MRI scan depending on the positioning of the patient. Therefore, it is crucial to visually assess the accuracy of the fusion before planning a trajectory.

3.3 Navigated needle placement

During the navigated needle placement, the radiologist aligns the stereotactic arm with the planned trajectory according to the crosshair viewer. Additionally, the system presents a real-time overlay of the needle trajectory on the CT scan (**Figure 6**). Once the stereotactic arm is aligned, the needle can be placed into the tumor according to the depth information on the display.

Depending on the patient tracking method, the system presents a real-time estimation of the deformation of the organ and stops the navigation display if the estimated deformation is too large.

3.4 Needle validation

To ensure correct needle position before applying the energy of the ablation needle, a non-enhanced CT scan is acquired and fused with the planning scan by the navigation system. The image-guidance system then either detects the needle automatically or the radiologist selects it manually. Based on this selection and the planned trajectory, the needle placement accuracy is measured and displayed on the screen (**Figure 7**). If the placement accuracy is insufficient (>3 mm), the radiologist would repeat the needle placement step.

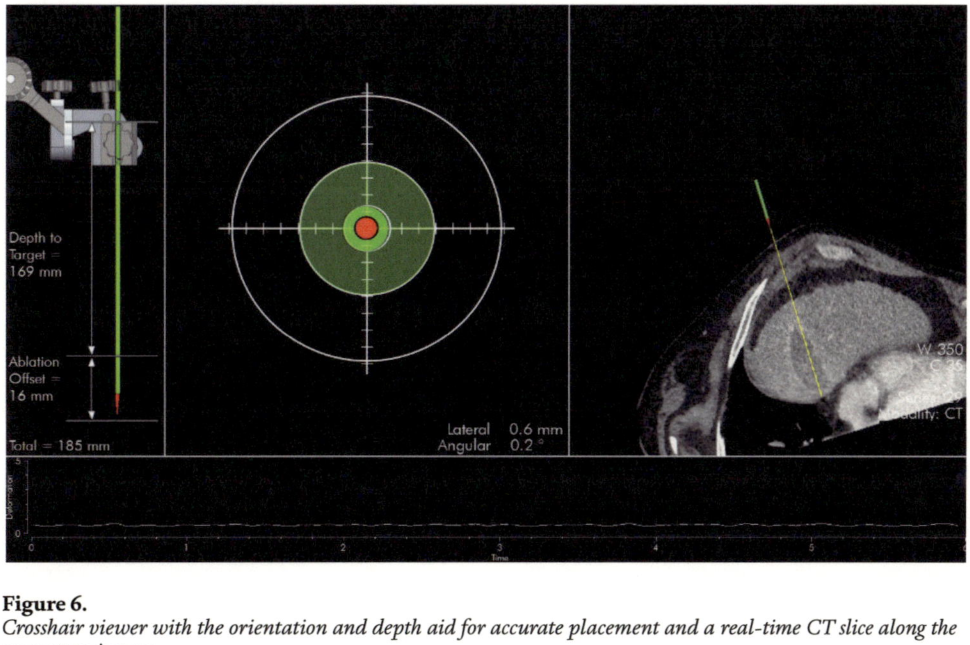

Figure 6.
Crosshair viewer with the orientation and depth aid for accurate placement and a real-time CT slice along the current trajectory.

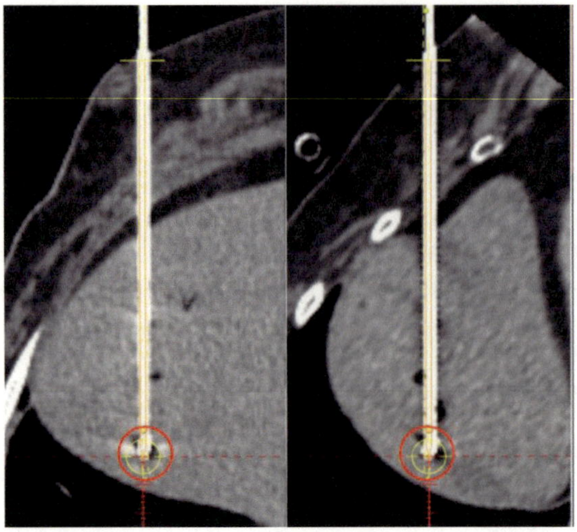

Figure 7.
Needle validation on a CT slice along the actual needle trajectory.

In lesions that are close to critical structures (vena cava, heart, etc.), the needle can be placed at three-fourths of the final depth and correct orientation can be measured on the needle validation scan before the needle is inserted into the final target.

3.5 Ablation

Once correct needle placement is confirmed, the energy is applied by the ablation device. The amount of energy needed can also be planned with the planning software. However, recent studies have shown that the resulting ablation zones differ from the prediction based on the ex-vivo results that are provided by the ablation device manufacturers [26] and also depend on the tumor type [27].

3.6 Ablation validation

In this step, the radiologist evaluates the coverage of the tumor by the ablation necrosis, which has been shown to be an independent predictor in determining local

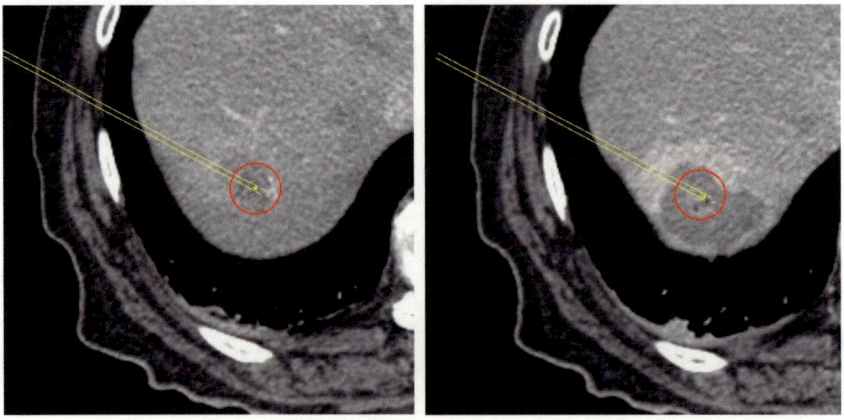

Figure 8.
Ablation zone validation with the tumor on the pre-ablation scan (left) and the ablation necrosis on the post-ablation scan (right).

tumor recurrence with a larger ablation margin resulting in a lower risk of local tumor recurrence [28]. The ablation coverage and margin are evaluated by visual assessment where the radiologist compares the pre- and post-ablation scans, which can be displayed side-by-side on a radiological screen or overlaid with transparency (**Figure 8**). An image-guidance system or external software can display the segmented tumor and the planned ablation margin, which makes the visual ablation validation more accurate, reproducible, and less subjective by providing visual markers and boundaries. If the radiologist identifies residual tumor or insufficient margin on the fused pre- and post-ablation scan, then another ablation is performed in the same procedure. Therefore, a new trajectory is planned based on the post-ablation scan to also cover the remaining tumor.

4. Current evidence and future perspectives

Using stereotactic ablation reduces the exposure to radiation and procedure time while improving the needle placement accuracy at the same time [29]. The interventional radiologist can leave the CT room during the acquisition, and therefore is not exposed to ionizing radiation at all. There are also large retrospective studies showing the potential benefits and applications of stereotactic image-guided ablations. While these studies do not show better oncological outcomes when using stereotactic ablation over conventional ablation, they state that the number of patients treated with a curative intent largely increased with the introduction of stereotactic guidance [1, 30, 31]. Furthermore, it has been shown in case-reports that stereotaxy was especially useful in very difficult cases when the tumor would not be reachable with conventional CT guidance [32].

Despite the current evidence showing that stereotactic image-guidance improves ablation needle accuracy and reduces procedure time and radiation dose, the ablation treatment itself has limitations, which are part of the current research—both clinical and engineering research.

4.1 Ablation of larger tumors

One of the short-term improvements of thermal ablations is the reproducible ablation of tumors larger than 3 cm. Current evidence shows that the LTP rate is higher in tumors larger than 3 cm and therefore such tumors are not recommended to treat with ablation [30, 33]. There are studies reporting larger ablation zones when using multiple needles in parallel, which could cover tumors larger than 3 cm [34]. With stereotactic image-guidance, such treatments can be delivered more reproducibly [6]. However, using multiple needles heavily increases the cost for the procedure at some institutions, which can be a major limitation.

4.2 Ablation zone prediction

The planning of the ablation employs the information from the ablation device manufactures' brochures, which presents the expected ablation necrosis that can be obtained for a specific energy delivered. The ablation model presented in the brochures is described as an ellipsoidal or spherical volume, which was obtained from measuring the ablation necrosis in ex-vivo, non-perfused, healthy animal livers. Recent studies have shown that the in-vivo ablation volumes differ significantly from the ex-vivo data, with the in-vivo ablation volumes being much smaller than the ex-vivo data predicts [26, 35]. Future models will be based on retrospective in-vivo data and also take any clinical parameters into account, such as the pathology of the tissue, the patient's clinical background, other treatments being administered (e.g., chemotherapy), and the influence of adjacent blood vessels on the expansion of the ablation volume.

4.3 Quantitative ablation assessment

Recently, there has been a high interest in quantitative ablation assessment to decrease the local tumor progression rates by ensuring complete ablation coverage and sufficient (<5mm) ablation margin using 3D image analysis software [36]. There are several studies that have attempted to describe the ablation success or coverage using numerical metrics derived from 3D tumor and ablation segmentations based on a follow-up scan at 4–8 weeks after ablation [37]. However, a fast intra-operative tool for assessing the ablation outcome would enable an immediate re-ablation and achievement of complete tumor destruction in the same treatment session. The Ablation fit (Ablation-fit, Italy) software is currently the only software available on the market for intra-operative quantitative 3D ablation assessment. However, evidence of the predictive value of intra-operative assessment is still limited as it has been evaluated only at a single center so far and due to the unknown tissue shrinkage after thermal ablation treatment [38].

4.4 Robotics

As in other disciplines in medicine, robotics will also be introduced in interventional oncology on a larger scale. While there are robotic devices available for stereotactic ablations, these are merely motorized arms for alignment. The radiologist still has to be sterile at the CT table and place the needle by hand. However, the future most likely will go toward autonomous robots that plan the trajectory, place the needle, and choose the right amount of energy for ablation. The radiologist might then be able to control the procedure in the control CT room monitoring and approving the robots' decisions [39–41].

5. Conclusion

In conclusion, stereotactic image-guidance provides technical support for accurately planning and placing ablation needles at the desired location and verifying the complete destruction of the tumor. These highly complex systems not only decrease radiation dose, contrast, and needle punctures, but also give a predictable procedure time even in technical challenging cases, which allows to optimally allocate the resources in an interventional radiology suite and most importantly offers the patient a safe and efficient minimally invasive procedure.

Conflict of interest

No conflict of interest.

Author details

Iwan Paolucci[1*], Raluca-Maria Sandu[1], Pascale Tinguely[2], Corina Kim-Fuchs[2], Martin Maurer[3], Daniel Candinas[2], Stefan Weber[1] and Anja Lachenmayer[2]

1 ARTORG Center for Biomedical Engineering, University of Bern, Bern, Switzerland

2 Department of Visceral Surgery and Medicine, University Hospital of Bern, Bern, Switzerland

3 Department of Diagnostic and Interventional Radiology, University Hospital of Bern, Bern, Switzerland

*Address all correspondence to: iwan.paolucci@artorg.unibe.ch

References

[1] Beermann M, Lindeberg J, Engstrand J, Galmén K, Karlgren S, Stillström D, et al. 1000 consecutive ablation sessions in the era of computer assisted image guidance—Lessons learned. European Journal of Radiology Open. 2019;**6**:1-8. Available from: https://www.sciencedirect.com/science/article/pii/S2352047718301072?via%3Dihub [cited March 12, 2019]

[2] Dupré A, Jones RP, Diaz-Nieto R, Fenwick SW, Poston GJ, Malik HZ. Curative-intent treatment of recurrent colorectal liver metastases: A comparison between ablation and resection. European Journal of Surgical Oncology. 2017;**43**(10):1901-1907. Available from: https://linkinghub.elsevier.com/retrieve/pii/S0748798317306467 [cited August 13, 2019]

[3] Leoni S, Piscaglia F, Serio I, Terzi E, Pettinari I, Croci L, et al. Adherence to AASLD guidelines for the treatment of hepatocellular carcinoma in clinical practice: Experience of the Bologna liver oncology group. Digestive and Liver Disease. 2014;**46**(6):549-555. Available from: https://www.sciencedirect.com/science/article/pii/S1590865814002448?via%3Dihub [cited August 13, 2019]

[4] Sastre J, Díaz-Beveridge R, García-Foncillas J, Guardeño R, López C, Pazo R, et al. Clinical guideline SEOM: Hepatocellular carcinoma. Clinical and Translational Oncology. 2015;**17**(12):988-995

[5] Meijerink MR, Puijk RS, van Tilborg AAJM, Henningsen KH, Fernandez LG, Neyt M, et al. Radiofrequency and microwave ablation compared to systemic chemotherapy and to partial hepatectomy in the treatment of colorectal liver metastases: A systematic review and meta-analysis. Cardiovascular and Interventional Radiology. 2018;**41**(8):1189-1204. DOI: 10.1007/s00270-018-1959-3

[6] Bale R, Widmann G, Stoffner DIIR. Stereotaxy: Breaking the limits of current radiofrequency ablation techniques. European Journal of Radiology. 2010;**75**(1):32-36. Available from: https://www.sciencedirect.com/science/article/pii/S0720048X10001774?via%3Dihub [cited July 10, 2019]

[7] Bale R, Schullian P, Eberle G, Putzer D, Zoller H, Schneeberger S, et al. Stereotactic radiofrequency ablation of hepatocellular carcinoma - A histopathological study in explanted livers. Hepatology. 2018:hep.30406. Available from: https://onlinelibrary.wiley.com/doi/abs/10.1002/hep.30406 [cited July 10, 2019]

[8] Wang X, Hu Y, Ren M, Lu X, Lu G, He S. Efficacy and safety of radiofrequency ablation combined with transcatheter arterial chemoembolization for hepatocellular carcinomas compared with radiofrequency ablation alone: A time-to-event meta-analysis. Korean Journal of Radiology;**17**(1):93-102

[9] Tinguely P, Schwalbe M, Fuss T, Guensch DP, Kohler A, Baumgartner I, et al. Multi-operational selective computer-assisted targeting of hepatocellular carcinoma-evaluation of a novel approach for navigated tumor ablation. PLoS One. 2018;**13**(5):e0197914. Available from: http://www.ncbi.nlm.nih.gov/pubmed/29791518 [cited September 04, 2019]

[10] Lencioni R, Crocetti L. Local-regional treatment of hepatocellular carcinoma. Radiology. 2012;**262**(1):43-58. Available from: http://www.ncbi.nlm.nih.gov/pubmed/22190656

[11] Tombesi P, Di Vece F, Bianchi L, Sartori S. Thermal ablation of liver tumours: How the scenario has changed in the last decade. The European Medical Journal. 2018;**6**:88-94

[12] Vogl TJ, Nour-Eldin NEA, Hammerstingl RM, Panahi B, Naguib NNN. Microwave Ablation (MWA): Basics, Technique and Results in Primary and Metastatic Liver Neoplasms - Review Article [Internet]. Vol. 189, RoFo Fortschritte auf dem Gebiet der Rontgenstrahlen und der Bildgebenden Verfahren. 2017. p. 1055-66. Available from: http://www.ncbi.nlm.nih.gov/pubmed/28834968 [cited August 22, 2019]

[13] Potretzke TA, Ziemlewicz TJ, Hinshaw JL, Lubner MG, Wells SA, Brace CL, et al. Microwave versus radiofrequency ablation treatment for hepatocellular carcinoma: A comparison of efficacy at a single center. Journal of Vascular and Interventional Radiology. 2016;**27**(5):631-638. DOI: 10.1016/j.jvir.2016.01.136

[14] Kamal A, Elmoety AAA, Rostom YAM, Shater MS, Lashen SA. Percutaneous radiofrequency versus microwave ablation for management of hepatocellular carcinoma: A randomized controlled trial. The Journal of Gastrointestinal Oncology. 2019;**10**(3):562-571

[15] Facciorusso A, Di Maso M, Muscatiello N. Microwave ablation versus radiofrequency ablation for the treatment of hepatocellular carcinoma: A systematic review and meta-analysis. International Journal of Hyperthermia. 2016;**32**(3):339-344

[16] Ryan MJ, Willatt J, Majdalany BS, Kielar AZ, Chong S, Ruma JA, et al. Ablation techniques for primary and metastatic liver tumors. World Journal of Hepatology. 2016;**8**(3):191-199

[17] Zhu GQ, Sun M, Liao WT, Yu WH, Zhou SL, Zhou ZJ, et al. Comparative efficacy and safety between ablative therapies or surgery for small hepatocellular carcinoma: A network meta-analysis. Expert Review of Gastroenterology and Hepatology. 2018;**12**(9):935-945. Available from: https://www.tandfonline.com/doi/full/10.1080/17474124.2018.1503531 [cited August 22, 2019]

[18] Yu H, Burke CT. Comparison of percutaneous ablation technologies in the treatment of malignant liver tumors. Seminars in Interventional Radiology. 2014;**31**(2):129-137. Available from: http://www.ncbi.nlm.nih.gov/pubmed/25071303 [cited August 19, 2019]

[19] Franz AM, Haidegger T, Birkfellner W, Cleary K, Peters TM, Maier-Hein L. Electromagnetic tracking in medicine—A review of technology, validation, and applications. IEEE Transactions on Medical Imaging. 2014;**33**(8):1702-1725. Available from: http://www.ieee.org/publications_standards/publications/rights/index.html [cited Sepetember 7, 2016]

[20] Oliveira-Santos T, Peterhans M, Hofmann S, Weber S. Passive single marker tracking for organ motion and deformation detection in open liver surgery. Lecture Notes in Computer Science (including Subser Lect Notes Artif Intell Lect Notes Bioinformatics). 2011;6689 LNCS:156-167

[21] Oliveira-Santos T, Klaeser B, Weitzel T, Krause T, Nolte L-P, Peterhans M, et al. A navigation system for percutaneous needle interventions based on PET/CT images: Design, workflow and error analysis of soft tissue and bone punctures. Computer Aided Surgery. 2011;**16**(5):203-219

[22] Toporek G, Wallach D, Weber S, Bale R, Widmann G. Cone-beam computed tomography-guided stereotactic liver punctures: A

phantom study. Cardiovascular and Interventional Radiology. 2013;**36**(6):1629-1637. Available from: http://link.springer.com/10.1007/s00270-013-0635-x [cited July 7, 2016]

[23] Wallach D, Toporek G, Weber S, Bale R, Widmann G. Comparison of freehand-navigated and aiming device-navigated targeting of liver lesions. International Journal of Medical Robotics and Computer Assisted Surgery. 2014;**10**(1):35-43. Available from: http://doi.wiley.com/10.1002/rcs.1505 [cited August 13, 2019]

[24] Beyer LP, Pregler B, Niessen C, Dollinger M, Graf BM, Müller M, et al. Robot-assisted microwave thermoablation of liver tumors: A single-center experience. International Journal of Computer Assisted Radiology and Surgery. 2016;**11**(2):253-259

[25] Engstrand J, Toporek G, Harbut P, Jonas E, Nilsson H, Freedman J. Stereotactic CT-guided percutaneous microwave ablation of liver tumors with the use of high-frequency jet ventilation: An accuracy and procedural safety study. The American Journal of Roentgenology. Jan 2017;**208**(1):193-200. [Internet] Available from: http://www.ajronline.org/doi/10.2214/AJR.15.15803

[26] Ruiter SJS, Heerink WJ, de Jong KP. Liver microwave ablation: A systematic review of various FDA-approved systems. European Radiology. Springer. 2019;**29**:4026-4035. Available from: http://www.ncbi.nlm.nih.gov/pubmed/30506218 [cited August 15, 2019]

[27] Heerink WJ, Solouki AM, Vliegenthart R, Ruiter SJS, Sieders E, Oudkerk M, et al. The relationship between applied energy and ablation zone volume in patients with hepatocellular carcinoma and colorectal liver metastasis. European Radiology. 2018;**28**(8):3228-3236. Available from: http://www.ncbi.nlm.nih.gov/pubmed/29536242 [cited June 6, 2019]

[28] Wang X, Sofocleous CT, Erinjeri JP, Petre EN, Gonen M, Do KG, et al. Margin size is an independent predictor of local tumor progression after ablation of colon cancer liver metastases. Cardiovascular and Interventional Radiology. 2013;**36**(1):166-175. Available from: http://link.springer.com/10.1007/s00270-012-0377-1 [cited August 10, 2019]

[29] Beyer LP, Pregler B, Nießen C, Schicho A, Haimerl M, Jung EM, et al. Stereotactically-navigated percutaneous irreversible electroporation (IRE) compared to conventional IRE: A prospective trial. Peer Journal. 2016;**4**:e2277. Available from: http://www.ncbi.nlm.nih.gov/pubmed/27602266 [cited June 9, 2017]

[30] Tinguely P, Frehner L, Lachenmayer A, Banz V, Weber S, Candinas D, et al. Stereotactic image-guided microwave ablation for malignant liver tumors—A multivariable accuracy and efficacy analysis (In review)

[31] Lachenmayer A, Tinguely P, Maurer M, Frehner L, Knöpfli M, Peterhans M, et al. Stereotactic Image-Guided Microwave Ablation of Hepatocellular Carcinoma using a computer-assisted navigation system. Liver International. 2019:liv.14187. Available from: https://onlinelibrary.wiley.com/doi/abs/10.1111/liv.14187

[32] Fischer T, Lachenmayer A, Maurer MH. CT-guided navigated microwave ablation (MWA) of an unfavorable located breast cancer metastasis in liver segment I. Radiol Case Reports. 2019;**14**(2):146-150. Available from: https://www.sciencedirect.com/science/article/pii/S1930043318301109?via%3Dihub [cited August 13, 2019]

[33] Leung U, Kuk D, D'Angelica MI, Kingham TP, Allen PJ, Dematteo RP, et al. Long-term outcomes following microwave ablation for liver malignancies. The British Journal of Surgery. 2015;**102**(1):85-91. Available from: http://www.ncbi.nlm.nih.gov/pubmed/25296639 [cited August 19, 2019]

[34] Mulier S, Jiang Y, Jamart J, Wang C, Feng Y, Marchal G, et al. Bipolar radiofrequency ablation with 2 × 2 electrodes as a building block for matrix radiofrequency ablation: Ex vivo liver experiments and finite element method modelling. International Journal of Hyperthermia. 2015;**31**(6):649-665

[35] Amabile C, Ahmed M, Solbiati L, Meloni MF, Solbiati M, Cassarino S, et al. Microwave ablation of primary and secondary liver tumours: Ex vivo, in vivo, and clinical characterisation. International Journal of Hyperthermia. 2017;**33**(1):34-42. Available from: https://www.tandfonline.com/doi/full/10.1080/02656736.2016.1196830 [cited August 19, 2019]

[36] Hocquelet A, Trillaud H, Frulio N, Papadopoulos P, Balageas P, Salut C, et al. Three-dimensional measurement of hepatocellular carcinoma ablation zones and margins for predicting local tumor progression. Journal of Vascular and Interventional Radiology. 2016;**27**(7):1038-1045.e2. Available from: https://www.sciencedirect.com/science/article/pii/S1051044316003821?via%3Dihub [cited August 19, 2019]

[37] Kaye EA, Cornelis FH, Petre EN, Tyagi N, Shady W, Shi W, et al. Volumetric 3D assessment of ablation zones after thermal ablation of colorectal liver metastases to improve prediction of local tumor progression. European Radiology. 2019;**29**(5):2698-2705. Available from: http://link.springer.com/10.1007/s00330-018-5809-0 [cited August 19, 2019]

[38] Solbiati M, Muglia R, Goldberg SN, Ierace T, Rotilio A, Passera KM, et al. A novel software platform for volumetric assessment of ablation completeness. International Journal of Hyperthermia. 2019;**36**(1):337-343. Available from: https://www.tandfonline.com/doi/full/10.1080/02656736.2019.1569267 [cited August 19, 2019]

[39] Ben-David E, Shochat M, Roth I, Nissenbaum I, Sosna J, Goldberg SN. Evaluation of a CT-guided robotic system for precise percutaneous needle insertion. Journal of Vascular and Interventional Radiology. 2018;**29**(10):1440-1446

[40] Hiraki T, Matsuno T, Kamegawa T, Komaki T, Sakurai J, Matsuura R, et al. Robotic insertion of various ablation needles under computed tomography guidance: Accuracy in animal experiments. European Journal of Radiology. 2018;**105**:162-167

[41] Hiraki T, Kamegawa T, Matsuno T, Komaki T, Sakurai J, Kanazawa S. Zerobot®: A remote-controlled robot for needle insertion in CT-guided interventional radiology developed at Okayama University. Acta Medica Okayama. 2018;**72**(6):539-546. Available from: http://www.ncbi.nlm.nih.gov/pubmed/30573907 [cited August 19, 2019]

Chapter 9

Hepatitis E: Disease in Humans

Adriana Turculeanu

Abstract

Hepatitis E virus (HEV) is one of the 7 viruses with mainly hepatic tropism. HEV determines 20 million new infections worldwide every year, 3.4 million acute hepatitis E and 44,000 deaths in 2015 (3.3% of the mortality due to viral hepatitis). Transmitted by the digestive tract mainly (fecal- orally, particularly by water infected with feces), the virus reaches the liver where it does not have a direct cytolytic effect, but immunological phenomena, especially cellular, activated by the replication of the virus in the hepatocytes. Clinically, over 95% of cases of HEV infection are asymptomatic and sel- limiting; in immunocompetent patients in tropics HEV can cause acute hepatitis with clinical features. On rare situations the infection can result in a severe, fulminant hepatitis with acute liver failure. In immunocompromised patients (organ transplant recipients, hematologic malignancies, HIV-infected) HEV may determine chronic hepatitis. In pregnant women or the elderly people or people with underlying liver disease HEV can cause fulminant forms which can become fatal (E.g.: 30% deaths among pregnant women in some parts of the world). Acute and chronic E hepatitis may be accompanied by extrahepatic manifestations: neurological, kidney, pancreatic, hematological diseases, autoimmune diseases with a pathogenesis not fully elucidated.

Keywords: hepatitis E virus (HEV), acute hepatitis, acute liver failure (ALF), acute-on-chronic liver failure (ACLF), cellular immunity, pregnant women, extrahepatic manifestations

1. Introduction

Hepatitis E virus (HEV) infection is a global public health problem. The World Health Organization (WHO) estimates that there are about 20 million HEV infections worldwide per year with a 3.3 million symptomatic cases E and approximately 44,000 deaths in 2015 [1].

HEV infection is a disease transmitted by enterically mainly in worldwide, special in the tropical countries. The source for infection is represented by zoonotic HEV - pigs, wild boar, deer camels (Genotype 7- GT 7) [2]. Transmission can be done through: direct contact with HEV infected animals, through heat processed meat incorrectly or through water of lagoons, streams and rivers polluted with the feces of sick animals. As such, other marine filter animals can become infected and transmit the disease (E.g. mollusks and seafood) or fruits and vegetables irrigated with infected fecaloid water. Organ transplantation in industrialized countries and blood products represent other ways of contamination for humans [2]. The virus can also be vertically transmitted from infected mother to fetus [3].

Hepatitis E occurs most commonly in adult men and with a lower prevalence in children [4].

In terms of clinical manifestations most infections caused by HEV in immunocompetent persons are asymptomatic (over 95%) and self-limiting; acute liver failure is rare [5]. In immunocompromised patients (solid organ transplant recipients, the patients with pre-existent chronic liver diseases, HIV infected patients, hematologycal diseases) HEV can cause chronic hepatitis, which may have an unfavorable evolution to acute fulminant hepatitis with to acute liver failure (ALF) or to cirrhosis [6]. In pregnant women, acute hepatitis can be benign or sever [7]; sever forms may occur during the third trimester with severe damage to the mother and fetus and their death (around 30% in India) [7, 8].

Extra-hepatic manifestations can also occur in patients with acute or chronic HEV infection such as neurological abnormalities (Guillain–Barre syndrome- GBS, neuralgic amyotrophy- NA, encephalitis and myelitis), acute pancreatitis, hematological disorders, kidney failure [9].

The pathogenesis of HEV infection is very complex and still unexplained. It involves the intervention of two categories of factors: the host organism and HEV. The host organism tries to stop the infection caused by HEV, and HEV tries to overcome the opposite barriers by the human body. This fight results in various clinical pictures of HEV infection.

There is a genetic predisposition of the human body to HEV infection, an increased susceptibility to this virus, to which is added the innate immunity and the adaptive response of the human body [7]. However, HEV uses different means to escape the defense of the human body, especially the genetic variation that leads to the appearance of genotypes, subgenotypes and quasi-species of HEV or a recombinant variants HEV-host cell with a different pathogenicity [2, 7], in general severe pathogenicity. HEV is not cytopathic in the liver, but it activates immune means, especially cellular immunity in determining liver damage.

One particular aspect is related to the pathogenicity of HEV in pregnancy when HEV infection can become fatal. In this situation there is a constellation of factors (immune, hormonal, viral, fetal) that can lead to severe clinical forms of hepatitis E with the death of the mother and fetus [10].

2. Clinical features- the main clinical manifestations of HEV infection

2.1 *A*cute hepatitis E in immunocompetent people

In developing countries most infections caused by HEV in immunocompetent persons are asymptomatic (over 95%) [6] and lead to spontaneous clearance of the virus [11] and acute liver failure is rare [5].

Clinically, manifest forms are found in only 5% of cases, especially in men aged 15–30 years as E acute hepatitis. These forms have an incubation period of 2–8 weeks (median 30 days) [12].

Clinical onset is characterized by non-specific symptoms: fever, nausea, vomiting, abdominal pain, anorexia, malaise and hepatomegaly; jaundice occurs only in 60% of cases accompanied by itching and light-colored stool and darkened urine [12].

The laboratory shows: increase in ALT (alanine aminotransferase), AST (aspartate aminotransferase) values (ALT is greater than AST), frequently accompanied by altered bilirubin, alkaline phosphatase and gamma-glutamyl transferase (GGT) [10].

E Acute Hepatitis is self-limiting illness, with full resolution of symptoms within weeks (usually) to months (less commonly) of onset. Viremia usually peaks during the early symptomatic phase and becomes undetectable about two weeks thereafter; excretion of the virus in the feces remains 2–3 weeks longer [10]. Progression of acute HEV infection to fulminant liver failure (FLF) remains rare and in the literature there are only 2 examples of HEV induced acute fulminant failure requiring emergency transplantation [13].

This clinical manifestations are especially present in the Tropics where HEV-infections are endemic or epidemic (e.g. Asia and Africa-Western Africa, Latin America- as Mexico) and contaminated water and reduced hygienic conditions represents the source for fecal- orally transmission.

In developed countries, patients infected with HEV are usually middle-aged or elderly men (>55 years). In developed countries, in immunocompetent persons HEV infections is less severe. Severe HEV infections were not described in pregnant women. Severe forms can be found in these countries, in rare situations, in immunocompromised patients such as the elderly people or patients with chronic liver disease of other etiology, in whom HEV can cause acute liver failure [11].

2.2 Acute hepatitis E in chronic liver diseases patients

Acute hepatitis E is a concern in patients with underlying chronic liver disease. This is a particular problem in elderly patients where acute hepatitis may take a more severe course [2]. In patients with chronic liver disease, acute HEV infection causes a rapid deterioration of liver function (acute-on-chronic liver failure-ACLF) with the appearance of complications such as: ascites, hepatic encephalopathy and/or hepatic coagulopathy, which can lead to death (up to 70% of cases) [13].

2.3 Acute hepatitis E in pregnancy

In pregnant women, acute hepatitis with HEV etiology may have various clinical aspects. The clinical features of E acute hepatitis depend on several factors.

One of these factors is the geographical area in which the pregnant woman lives. So, HEV infection in pregnant women may be present with a higher or lower incidence and may be benign or severe, accompanied by an increased mortality rate or not. Example: in Northern India where HEV infection is endemic, HEV infection in pregnant women has a high incidence (representing 60% of viral hepatitis) and clinically is severe, evolving in 55% of cases with fulminant liver failure (FLF) that can leads to a maternal mortality of 41% [14]; in Egypt, another country where HEV infection is endemic, the incidence of HEV infection in pregnant women is lower and severe forms are rarely, although Egypt is part of the category of HEV endemic countries, compared to Northern India [14].

Another factor that influences the incidence and clinical appearance of HEV infection in pregnant women is the level of sanitation in that area, so there is a difference in the incidence and clinical feature of the disease in developed countries compared to the tropical region where the level of hygiene it is reduced and favors the fecal-oral transmission (especially water contaminated with feces) of HEV to pregnant women [14].

Other factors that may influence the clinical manifestation in pregnant women are:

- exposure to HEV infection, especially in early childhood, which leads to a protective immune fund, producing long-lasting immunity and/or modify subsequent responses to exposure to the virus; so the incidence of HEV infection may be lower and the severity of the disease rare [3, 15];

- different virulence of infectious HEV strains. E.g. HEV genotype(s) in Egypt could be less virulent than those in Asia [14];

- the pregnancy status, that means hormonal factors specially [8]

Conclusion: the clinical features of HEV infection of pregnant women can be benign or severe, with fulminant hepatic insufficiency that can lead to death, depend on a constellation of factors related to: the host (hormonal factors, immune status, nutritional, genetic status, infectious history), the infectious viral strain and external factors (e.g.: the hygienic-sanitary level, the prevalence of HEV infection in the respective area/country).

The mortality rate in pregnant women can be as high as 30% and usually occurs in the 3rd trimester [3] by obstetric complications such as hemorrhage or eclampsia, fulminant liver failure, premature delivery, low-birth-weight neonates and still-births, as well as the vertical transmission to infants, which leads to increased neonatal morbidity and mortality [10, 16]. HEV infection during pregnancy is also associated with more frequent miscarriages, preterm deliveries and perinatal mortality [7].

2.4 Acute and chronic HEV infectious in immunocompromised hosts

In immunocompromised patients, including solid organ transplant (SOT) [17] and those coinfected with the human immunodeficiency virus (HIV) with a T CD4+ count <200/mm^3 [7], patients with hematological disease receiving chemotherapy, those given stem cell transplants or patients with rheumatic disorders with heavy immunosuppression secondary the immunotherapy [7], HEV can determines acute or chronic hepatitis.

Acute HEV in immunocompromised patients generally presents asymptomatically [17]; in the case of clinical manifestation the symptoms are non-specific as well: jaundice, fatigue, diarrhea and myalgia [11].

Chronic hepatitis HEV infection in immunocompromised patients defined as HEV replication that persists for more than 3 months [18], can progress rapidly to cirrhosis in 10% of the chronically infected patients [7, 19]. Some of these patients may die from decompensated cirrhosis 2–3 years after 1the diagnosis [7]. HEV-infected transplant recipients did not develop fulminant forms [20].

The incubation period for the virus in the context of immunosuppression is longer than seen in immunocompetent hosts at 60 days, with chronicity itself being defined by viral persistence after the acute phase for either 3 or 6 months [21]. Chronic HEV infection in immunocompromised patients is almost exclusively secondary to HEV G3 infection; one case of chronic HEV G4 infection has been noted but none due to HEV G1 or G2 [21].

2.5 Extra-hepatic manifestations

Extra-hepatic manifestations can also occur in patients with acute or chronic HEV infection such as neurological (Guillain–Barré syndrome; GBS), neuralgic amyotrophy and meningoencephalitis, myositis, Bell's palsy, vestibular neuritis and peripheral neuropathy), acute pancreatitis, hematological disorders (aplastic anemia, hemolytic anemia, cryoglobulinemia, thrombocytopenia, monoclonal immunoglobulin), kidney failure and others (myocarditis, autoimmune thyroiditis, arthritis) [2].

3. Pathogenesis

The pathogenesis of hepatitis E is complex and still to be studied. Infection in humans with HEV is the result of 2 categories of factors: viral factors and factors related to the host organism.

3.1 Viral factors

HEV enters the human body through the digestive tract, especially fecal-oral. The intestine is the first site where HEV suffers the replication [22] or lymph nodes or colon [6] via the blood as a quasi-enveloped particle and reaches the liver for which it manifests a high tropism where it replicates, especially in the hepatocytes, without being directly cytotoxic, but with the initiation of immune phenomena, especially on the cell line by activating cytotoxic T lymphocytes and natural killer (NK) cells, that causes necro-inflammatory liver damages [23]. After replication in the hepatocyte cytoplasm, the virus is eliminated in the bile (at the apical membrane) [23, 24] and blood; most HEV particles are released at the apical membrane, then bile salts strip the lipids from the virus shed in the stool.

In the liver, the virus must enter the hepatocyte into which it will be replicated. In this process, the first stage of attaching the virus to the surface of the hepatocytes is extremely important in the viral development cycle replication, so as to HEV infection can be initiated or not. The attachment of the virus to the surface of the hepatocytes is achieved by fixing it at certain receptors from the surface of the hepatocytes resulting in viral inoculum.

3.1.1 The attachment of viral particles to the surface of the hepatocytes is different, depending on the morphology of the viral particles

HEV was discovered in 1983 by Dr. Mikhail Balayan who described the HEV particle as non-enveloped in the feces, with icosahedral symmetry, 27–30 nm, with spikes on the surface [6]. But in infected people, viral particles were also found in the blood. Under the electron microscope these particles appear enveloped, the capsid encased in limiting host-derived membranes; these particles have been called „quasienveloped" forms or „eHEV" [6, 7]. So, there are 2 categories of viral particles: enveloped and non-enveloped (naked). Each of them uses a specific means of attachment to the host cell. This is a very important step for HEV pathogenesis because the rate of attachment and penetration of the virus into hepatocytes influences the value of the viral inoculum, one of the viral pathogenic factors.

3.1.1.1 Attachment of non-enveloped particles

The receptor for HEV is unknown. However, the host cell provides a number of factors that can be used as receptors for the non-enveloped (naked) viral particles, so:

Heparan Sulfate Proteoglycans (HSGPs) - are glycans present on the cell surface that are involved in cell attachment of many nonenveloped and enveloped viruses. HSGPs, particularly syndecans, play a role in the binding of HEV VLPs to human hepatoma cells [25].

Glucose-Regulated Protein 78 (GRP78)- is a molecular chaperone in the ER, implicated in the attachment and entry of both enveloped and nonenveloped viruses [26].

Asialoglycoprotein Receptor (ASGPR)- is a protein receptor present on the basolateral membrane of hepatocytes that binds glycoproteins that lack sialic acid modifications. Experimentally, through different techniques, a direct interaction between the ectodomain of both ASGR1 and ASGR2 and HEV ORF2 was highlighted [27].

ATP Synthase Subunit 5β (ATP5B)- is largely a mitochondrial protein, but a small fraction is expressed on the cell surface and is implicated in other viral infections [28]. Experimentally, the link between ATP5B and viral proteins p239 VLP has been demonstrated [28].

Integrin Alpha 3 (ITGA3)- a new HEV entry factor into the cell: overexpression of α3 integrin in nonpermissive cells made the cells permissive to HEV, while removal of α3 integrin in permitted cells abrogated permissiveness [29].

Conclusion: for non-enveloped (naked) viral particles, the range of receptors offered by the host cell is large, as such there is the possibility of making a high value viral inoculum that can cause even severe clinical manifestations.

3.1.1.2 Attachment of „quasienveloped" particles or "eHEV"

Quasi-coated HEV particles do not have viral proteins on the surface of their envelope, so, they must use different attachment factors and/or cellular receptors to initiate entry into the host cell. Thus, these qvasiparticles use for attachment to the host cell, as in the case of exosomes, the phosphatidylserine present at their outer membrane to bind at the TIM-1 receptor. However, this attachment to the surface of the host cell is less efficient than in the case of non-enveloped particles, which led to the theory that other unidentified substances present on the surface of non-enveloped particles participate in attaching of these particles to the host cell surface and make it inefficient [29]. On the other hand, this less efficient connection of this type of particles to the surface of the hepatocytes would explain their presence in the blood and could facilitate its penetration of immunologically privileged sites such as the central nervous system and other tissues and causes extrahepatic manifestations [30].

Similar to naked particles, eHEV enters hepatocytes mainly through the clathrin- and dynamin-dependent pathway [30, 31] or use a particular pathway that involves in degradation of the lipid membrane in the lysosome [30].

Conclusion: non-enveloped viral particles bind much more efficiently to the surface of hepatocytes, compared with eHEV; this aspect influences the clinical manifestations of the disease: the non-enveloped particles are located mainly in the liver and usually cause liver damages, while the eHEV cause especially extrahepatic manifestations.

3.1.2 Viral genetic variability- another pathogenic factor

So far, 8 HEV genotypes are known [8] with different hosts, including humans, and a certain geographical spread. Genotypes 1–4 and 7 are present in humans; genotype 1 (HEV-1) is predominant in Asia and Africa, HEV-2 in Mexico and parts of Africa, HEV-3 circulates among human, swine, rabbit and deer and has a world-wide distribution, HEV-4, mostly present in Southeast Asia, circulates between human and swine; HEV-5 and HEV-6, phylogenetically close to HEV-4, were identified in Japanese wild boars [31]; HEV-7 and the last, HEV-8 were identified as camel genotypes in the Middle East [32]; HEV-7 was implicated in chronic HEV infection in a liver transplant recipient consuming camel milk and meat [31], which suggests the possible transmission of this genotype to human and the possibility to affecting human health [23].

3.1.2.1 The correlation clinical features - viral genotypes

There is a close correlation between the clinical features caused by HEV and the viral genotypes, which demonstrates a different pathogenicity of HEV. So:

In case of acute hepatitis in immunocompetent hosts - genotypes G1 and G2 from tropical countries and endemic areas determine more aggressive forms of acute hepatitis [12] with clinical manifestations and changes in biochemical parameters [2], compared to genotypes G3 and G4 [12]. The evolution of acute HEV infection to fulminant liver failure remains rare and there are only two examples in the literature of HEV acute fulminant liver failure that required emergency transplantation [11, 33].

In case of acute hepatitis in pregnancy: in pregnant women, particularly in the third trimester, HEV infection is associated with devastating maternal and fetal outcomes [21]. In this context, acute hepatitis with HEV is associated with the G1 genotype [11].

In case of immunocompromised hosts (SOT patients, HIV-infected patients or patients with chronic granulomatous diseases or connective tissue disorders like SLE or patients with hematological diseases receiving chemotherapy, those given stem cell transplants or patients with rheumatic disorders on heavy immunosuppression immunotherapy [7, 20, 34]: the incubation period for the virus in the context of immunosuppression is longer than seen in immunocompetent hosts at 60 days, with chronicity itself being defined by viral persistence after the acute phase for either 3 or 6 months [21]; they are not able to spontaneously clear the virus and as early as 12 months after HEV infection can involve significant hepatic fibrosis [35]. The genotype associated with these pathological conditions is HEV G3 [21].

In patients with pre-existing chronic liver diseases: HEV infection may exacerbate chronic liver failure (ACFL). The HEV genotype involved is G3 in Europe and G1 and G2 in China and India where the mortality rate can reach 67%, with an average of 34% [13].

In case of extrahepatic manifestations: acute pancreatitis is associated with HEV G1; kidney injury (membranous glomerulonephritis, membranoproliferative glomerulonephritis and even relapses of IgA nephropathy) is associated with HEV G3 [36]. A possible mechanism for these renal dysfunction in HEV infected patients is through the development of cryoglobulinaemia [36].

3.1.2.2 HEV quasispecies and pathogenicity

HEV may also present numerous quasispecies with different pathogenicity, in general more aggressive. These quasi-HEV species can be the consequence of:

- a high heterogeneity ORF1 and ORF 2 during the acute phase of the infection; these HEV quasi-species are associated with HEV persistence [6], so with a predisposition to chronicity;
- a high heterogeneity of the M domain at the viral capsid, a domain that contains epitopes for T cells, expressed by a low value of the Ka/Ks ratio (an indirect indicator of the selection pressure on a quasispecies) in patients with chronic HEV infection who are not able to achieve spontaneous HEV clearance [6] which means viral persistence and a tendency to chronicity;
- the heterogeneity of the P domain at the viral capsid that determines the progression to liver fibrosis in patients with chronic hepatitis E. Nearly 10% of SOT patients with HEV develop cirrhosis within 3–5 years following the primary infection [6].

3.1.2.3 The recombinant HEV-host variants

The recombinant HEV-host variants with replicative advantage in vitro [6, 37] in chronically infected patients. These HEV variants presented fragments of human genes (ribosomal genes S17 or S19, inter alpha trypsin inhibitor) in the PPR regions and duplications and insertions of the HEV genome [6].

3.2 The host organism

The human host can influence the pathogenicity of HEV and secondarily the clinical manifestations [6] by:

3.2.1 The presence of Apolipoprotein E (ApoE)

The presence of Apolipoprotein E (ApoE) considered a protective factor of the human body against HEV pathogenicity. ApoE is a plasma lipid transporter, but can also be found associated with lipids in the structure of cell membranes. In HEV infection, its intense activity was highlighted, suggesting its intervention in the pathogenesis of HEV infection [6]. An argument in this regard: the protection against HEV by ApoE highlighted in American non-Hispanic blacks by certain isoforms of ApoE (ApoE ε3 and ε4) [38]. The protection by ApoE against HEV action would be achieved by: blocking the attachment of HEV to the surface of the host cell by competition with the heparan-sulfate receptor, modulation of the entry of HEV particles in the host cell, given its presence in the membrane associated with eHEV particles in the blood, modulation of the anti-HEV immune response by regulating T lymphocytes activation and proliferation [6].

3.2.2 Genetic polymorphism in the promoter regions

Genetic polymorphism in the promoter regions for tumor necrosis factor alpha (TNF-α) and interferon gamma (IFN-γ) in HEV infection *that stimulates their synthesis,* leading to severe clinical manifestations [39]. E.g.: a (G/A) polymorphism in 308 position of the promotor region of TNF-α will increase TNF production 7 times; a single nucleotide polymorphisms in the promotor IFN-γ (IFN-γ +874 T/A) will associate with a higher IFN-γ production and with symptomatic cases [39].

3.2.3 Innate immune response of the host

The synthesis of different types of IFN (interferon alpha, IFN beta) can influence the pathogenicity of HEV. HEV is more susceptible to IFN action, but has developed means of resistance to its action. There are experimental studies in animals (chimpanzees) that have demonstrated the role of interferon alpha (IFN-α) in the pathogenesis of hepatitis E, HEV being more susceptible than HCV to the innate immunity induced by IFN-α [40]. Studies in human cell cultures (human lung epithelial cells A549 [40] and Huh7 hepatocellular carcinoma cells [41]) have shown that HEV through the ORF3 region can inhibit IFN-induced phosphorylation of signal transducer and activator of transcription STAT1; the result is decreased synthesis of 2 key antiviral proteins: dsRNA-activated protein kinase and 2′,5′-oligoadenylate synthetase. Other authors [41] using other cell lines have shown that HEV by ORF3 protein enhanced type I IFN production by interacting directly with the pattern recognition receptor (PRR) retinoic acid-inducible gene I (RIG-I) [41]. In the same cell line was demonstrated the intervention of another HEV protein, namely ORF1 with inhibitory effect on the signaling and secretory pathway for IFN beta (IFN-β) by de-ubiquitination of RIG-I and tank binding kinase (TBK) [42]. So, gene suppression of key component of the Janus kinase (JAK)-STAT cascade of the IFN signaling, including JAK1, STAT1, and interferon regulatory factor (IRF) 9 stimulates replication of HEV [41].

An increased production of proinflammatory cytokines such as IL-6, IL-8, TNF-α and RANTES (regulated on activation, normal T cell expressed and secreted), as well as the activation of both nuclear factor kappa-light-chain-enhancer of B cells (NF-κB) and IFN regulatory factor 3 (IRF3), two transcription factors activated in innate immune signaling pathways [42] *in vitro*, using HEV-infected A549 cell line.

NK and natural killer T (NKT) cells could also play a major role in the innate immune response to HEV [6]. Natural killer (NK) and natural killer T (NKT) cells constitute a major fractions of the lymphocytes in the liver, where they are important for the pathogenesis of viral hepatitis. In the peripheral blood of acute infected patients is present a higher proportion of $CD4^+$ cells than in uninfected controls [43]. This increase in CD4+ cells is not associated with an expansion of HEV ORF2-specific CD4+ CD69+ cells producing helper T cell type 1 (IFN-γ and TNF-α) T cytokines or helper T cell type 2 (IL-4) cytokines [43]. The expansion of $CD4^+$ cells could reflect an increase in NKT cells, which can be either $CD3^+$ $CD4^+$ or $CD3^+$ $CD4^-$ $CD8^-$ [43]. In acute hepatitis E the proportion and activation status of NK and NKT cells among PBMCs varies reversibly; there is generally a low proportion of NK ($CD3^-$/$CD56^+$) and NKT cells ($CD3^+$/$CD56^+$) in the periphery, but an excessive accumulation of them in the liver [43]. This aspect was supported by immunohistochemical liver biopsies obtained from patients infected with HEV with acute hepatic failure [44].

3.2.4 Adaptive response of the host

Humoral Immune Response

HEV elicits the appearance of IgM and IgG antibodies,. IgM anti- HEV appear in the early stages of the disease and may persist for several months (usually no longer than three to four months). IgG anti- HEV appear shortly after the appearance of IgM and may persist for several years with increasing antibody avidity over time [2]. Anti-HEV IgG antibodies are of the neutralizing type, directed against the neutralizing epitopes of the HEV capsid protein and are protective [45]. These antibodies can also occur after vaccination and confers protection against hepatitis E infection for up to 4.5 years [45] special in the China, although the minimum protective concentration of antibodies has not been determined. WHO suggests that an antibody concentration of 2.5 units of the WHO/ml postvacciunation is protective [45]. But in solid organ transplant recipients, HEV reinfection has been described at an IgG concentration below 7 WHO units/mL [46].

Cellular Immune Response

In acute HEV infection effector T cells are activated with CD8+ increased especially in the liver [44] and high proportions of PBMCs producing IFN-γ (after stimulation with recombinant ORF2 or ORF3 HEV proteins) [44].

An increased expression of CD11a integrin in naïve CD45RA+ T cells, as well as overexpression of CCR5 and CCR9, two chemokine receptors that play important roles in cell trafficking and homing, was also reported in peripheral blood of acutely infected patients. The expanded CD45RA+ CD11a high subpopulations present during the early phase of acute infection suggests the recruitment of these cells from the periphery to the liver, thus contributing to the pathogenesis of the infection [7]. This suggests that the immunosuppressive immune response is involved in the acute phase of the infection, but its exact role remains to be clarified.

General conclusion: the human body can modulate HEV infection using different resources (**Table 1**).

3.3 Specific/particular aspects of pathogenicity in HEV infection

3.3.1 Pathogenesis of fulminant hepatitis E

Fulminant hepatitis with HEV etiology may be present in patients with hepatic chronic diseases and in pregnant women.

	Pathogenic	Mechanisms	Changes present in HEV infection
HEV	Attachment of viral particles to the surface of the host cell	Naked- HEV particles Quasienveloped HEV particles („eHEV")	Inoculum value: the increased inoculum correlates with the severity of the infection
	Viral genetic variability:		
	• Genotypes	GT1–8 (HEV1–8)	• In immunocompetent hosts - genotypes G1 and G2 • In pregnancy: G1 genotype • In immunocompromised hosts: G3 genotype • In patients with pre-existing chronic liver diseases: G3 in Europe and G1 and G2 in China and India • Acute pancreatitis is associated with HEV G1 kidney injury: G3 genotype
	• Subtypes	—	—
	• Quasispecies	—	• A high heterogeneity ORF1 and ORF 2 • A high heterogeneity of the M domain at the viral capsid, • The weaker heterogeneity of the P domain at the viral capsid
	The recombinant HEV-host variants	—	The replicative advantage
	The rhythm of viral replication	—	Increased viral replication
HOST	Genetic susceptibility factors	Apolipoprotein E	Intense activity
		Genetic polymorphism in the promoter regions for tumor necrosis factor alpha (TNF-α) and interferon gamma (IFN-γ)	• G/A polymorphism in 308 position of the promotor region of TNF-α • the polymorphism in the promotor IFN-γ (IFN-γ +874 T/A)
		Surface receivers provided for attachment of HEV	HSGPs, GRP78, ASGPR, ATP5B, ITGA3 for naked- HEV
	Innate Immune Response of the Host	The synthesis of different types of IFN(IFN alpha, IFN beta)	HEV through ORF3 region can inhibit IFN-induced phosphorylation of signal transducer and activator of transcription STAT1
		The proinflammatory cytokines: IL-6, IL-8, TNF-α and RANTES	• An increased production of proinflammatory cytokines: IL-6, IL-8, TNF-α and RANTES • activation of both nuclear factor kappa-light-chain-enhancer of B cells (NF-κB) and IFN regulatory factor 3 (IRF3)
		NK and natural killer T (NKT) cells	Low proportion of NK ($CD3^-$/$CD56^+$) and NKT cells ($CD3^+$/$CD56^+$) in the periphery, but an excessive accumulation of them in the liver

Pathogenic	Mechanisms	Changes present in HEV infection
Adaptive Response of the Host.	Humoral Immune Response (IgM and IgG antibodies anti- HEV)	I- gM anti- HEV appear in the early stages of the disease and may persist for several months (usually no longer than three to four months). • IgG anti- HEV appear shortly after the appearance of IgM and may persist for several years
	Cellular Immune Response: CD4+, CD8+, CD11a integrin in naïve CD45RA+ T cells, CCR5, CCR9	• CD8+ increased especially in the liver • High proportions of PBMCs producing IFN-γ • An increased expression of CD11a integrin in naïve CD45RA+ T cells, • Overexpression of CCR5 and CCR9

Table 1.
Pathogenesis of HEV infection.

3.3.1.1 Fulminant hepatitis E in the general population

The pathogenesis of the fulminant liver failure (FHF) with HEV is unclear, but there are a number of issues related to HEV and the host organism that can be correlated with FLF.

It is discussed about associating FLF with the presence of IgM and IgG anti-HEV antibodies and some researchers believe that the humoral immune response is dominant in this fulminant forms [47], associated with increased amounts of IFN-γ, TNF-α, IL-2, and IL-10 produced by PBMCs stimulated by ORF2 HEV. FLF is also associated with changes in the cellular immune response anti-HEV, lower cellular immune response, but with the very important humoral immune response anti-HEV [47]. There is a difference between the peripheral blood and liver in FHF in terms of cellular immunity, so, in the periphery, the cellular immunity was lower, but in the liver the proportion of CD4 + and CD8 + T lymphocytes was increased [48]. CD8 + cytotoxic lymphocytes may play an essential role in the pathogenesis of liver injury in FHF caused by HEV [20].

On the other hand, FHF could be linked to the *viral genotype and/or the subgenotype*, perhaps due to specific mutations in the polyprotein of HEV such as F179S, A317T, T735I, L1110F, V1120I and FG1439Y in the ORF1 E polyprotein [49] or H105R, D29N, V27A mutations in the methyltransferase region of the HEV genome [50] or the association of FLF with HEV-4 [51]. These mutations could correlate with increased pathogenicity of HEV strains and progression to FLF [7].

3.3.1.2 Pathogenesis of HEV infection in pregnancy

Hepatitis E has both a high incidence and severe course in pregnant women in some geographic regions of HEV endemic countries, such as Northern India, [8] while in other HEV endemic countries, such as Egypt, it has been shown to have a benign course with little or no morbidity [7].

During pregnancy, especially in the third trimester, the course of acute hepatitis caused by HEV can be towards acute fulminant hepatitis which can lead to acute liver failure (ALF) and death. The pathogenic aspects of this evolution in pregnant women are related to: immunity, hormonal factors and the peculiarities of the virus [7]. In the initial period of pregnancy up to 20 weeks gestational age, all immune, hormonal factors are oriented to the protection of the fetus during the implantation period [7].

Immune status in pregnancy is characterized by a constellation of factors that lead to decreased cellular immunity that can no longer act on the fetus seen as an allograft. The decrease of cellular immunity is achieved by changing the immune status of the pregnant woman from the Th1 dominant state to that of "Th2 bias", a change initiated by the increased progesterone during pregnancy. The progesterone stimulate the synthesis of progesterone-induced binding factor (PIBF) by lymphocytes [52]. High concentrations of PIBF promote differentiation of $CD4^+$ T cells into helper T cell type 2 (Th2) cells that secrete high concentrations of anti-inflammatory cytokines, including IL-4, IL-5, and IL-10 which causes a decrease in the inflammatory effect of Th1 (e.g., production of IFN-γ), both at the maternal-fetal interface and systemically in humans [53]. These cytokines influence the functionality of monocytes/macrophages. As such, the decrease in cellular immunity protects the fetus, but it also alters the immune response mounted against infections [54]. Th2 status has been demonstrated in pregnant women infected with HEV and this status is likely to favor HEV replication, but its implication for the severity of a hepatitis E infection is unknown [54].

Decreased cellular immunity can also be caused by the placenta through the structural outer layer - the trophoblast. The trophoblast can cause a decrease in cellular immunity through various mechanisms:

- the cells of trophoblast does not express on their surface the major histocompatibility complex (MHC) which mediate antigen presentation; as a result T lymphocytes cannot be activated and cannot act on the fetus [16]. But, the NK cells, another immune cell effector, do not require MHC proteins for their activation. As such, the trophoblast also acts on them by expressing on its surface a special Human Leukocyte Antigen (HLA) molecule called *HLA-G*, which binds to NK receptors CD 16, and CD 56 and inactivates them [54].

- the trophoblast secretes an enzyme indoldeamin 2,3-dioxigenase, the enzyme that breaks down tryptophan, an amino acid essential for the function of T lymphocytes; as such, cellular immunity at the placental interface is suppressed [55].

- the placenta and trophoblast secrete cytokines, especially TGF-β, IL-4, IL-10 which inhibits cell-mediated immunity with protective effect on the fetus. Experimental laboratory animal studies have shown low levels of IL-1β, IL-2, IL-6, IL-10, IL-12 (p40), IL-12 (p90), IL-17, TNF-α in early pregnancy and significantly increased in the latter part of pregnancy and postpartum [56].

Another mechanism that leads to a decrease in cellular immunity in pregnant women is a decrease of the total T lymphocytes and TCD4 + lymphocytes, namely in the first part of pregnancy and then an increase or normalization towards the end of pregnancy or postpartum. This decrease in T lymphocytes and cellular immunity in pregnancy in general, protects the fetus, but would favor viral infections generally, including HEV infection [16, 57].

To summarize, the immunological changes during pregnancy promote the maintenance of the antigenic fetus in the maternal environment by suppression of T cell mediated immunity. Whether this suppressed immune system translates into increased risk of infections during pregnancy is still not clear [16].

Hormonal factors in pregnancy

Pregnancy is characterized by a hormonal storm, namely by the increase of progesterone, estrogens and human chorionic gonadotropin (HCG) [16, 57]. Hormones contribute significantly to the outcome of immune-related diseases during pregnancy by altering the functioning of immune cells. Hormones can have additional effects on the outcome of infection during pregnancy. Experimentally in animals it has been shown that estrogens and progesterone acts on the thymus. So, progesterone determines the involution of the thymus with disorders in the development of T cells with lyTh1 inhibition and promoting lyTh2 status; this involution of the thymus is related to the expression of progesterone receptors at the thymic level; it can also cause the inadequate, early transition of pro-T to pre-T ly in the process of differentiating these cells [58]. The result will be: decreased cellular immunity of the pregnant woman.

The suppression of cellular immunity by progesterone may be correlated with another phenomenon: the mutations in the progesterone gene (the PROGINS haplotype) that will cause decreased progesterone receptor expression and progesterone-induced blocking factor (PINF) with NK cell inhibition and suppression of cellular immunity with anti-abortive effect [58].

Estrogens causes thymus contraction with the depletion of CD4+ and CD8+ ly T, thus the suppression of cellular immunity [59, 60]. This aspect can be correlated with other studies that show an increased predisposition to viral infections in certain states with high estrogens [61], especially in the third trimester of pregnancy, with an intensification of viral HEV replication (elevated levels of HEV RNA) by inhibiting estrogen receptors and type I IFNs synthesis [61].

Increased progesterone and estrogens in pregnancy can affect also the B lymphocyte population in the bone marrow and decrease mainly pre-B and immature (fractions B–D) bone marrow B cells of pregnant mice [16].

HCG is a chemoattractant protein secreted by the blastocyst after fertilization [62] which mediates migration of regulatory T cells to the pregnant uterus. Regulatory T cells are hypothesized to orchestrate immune tolerance of the fetus during pregnancy in mammals [62].

Steroid hormones are other hormonal markers that can influence viral replication through a mechanism similar to Cytomegalovirus that causes increased replication in pregnancy [16].

To summarize: Progesterone, estrogen, steroid hormones, HCG cause decreased immunity, especially on the cell line, favoring the acquisition of viral infections, including HEV.

HEV genotype

Previous studies have shown the correlation of HEV3 - pregnancy as dominant in the case of poorer outcome of HEV infection [63]. Histopathological HEV3 determines increased apoptosis and necrosis at the maternal- fetal interface with alterations in the architecture of the placental barrier and changes in the cytokine microenvironment - triggers the production of pro-inflammatory cytokines like IL-6 and chemokines [63]. HEV3 also correlates with elevated levels of pro-inflammatory cytokines (TNF-α, IL-6, IFN-γ and TGF-β1) in peripheral blood with „poor outcome" of HEV infection [64]. Subsequent studies have shown that the dominant genotype is not HEV3, but HEV1. The genotype HEV1 replicates more efficiently than HEV3 *in vivo* in tissue explants of decidua basalis and fetal placenta, and also in stromal cells [63].

Other factors that may influence the evolution of hepatitis E in pregnancy to acute liver failure are: the nutritional status of the pregnant woman including micronutrient or folate deficiencies [65] and the differences in the expression of MHC, molecule that can influence the immune response in pregnant women [16].

In certain regions of the world, the pregnancy is associated with acute fulminant E hepatitis and ALF can have an unfavorable evolution, accompanied by a very high maternal mortality (30% - 41% in Northern India) [8, 15].

Pathogenic mechanisms involved in this **high maternal mortality** remains unclear, but the factors involved in this situation are the same as in a common form pregnancy, but in much higher quantities and with a strong effect and much more deeply cellular immunity which favors HEV replication at a very high rate. Thus:

- Th2 "bias status", considered a major cause of death in pregnant women with fulminant HEV hepatitis (e.g., in Asia) [6, 16];
- higher CD8+ count and lower CD4+ count (Ly CD8 + seems to play an important role in the pathogenesis of fulminant hepatitis in pregnancy, being highlighted in large numbers in the liver of patients with fulminant hepatitis E) [59];
- MHC variations of the host pregnancy that mediate antigen presentation may explain the geographical variations in mortality in pregnant women infected with HEV [16];
- high concentrations of cytokines (TNF-α, IL-6, IFN-γ and TGF-β1) may also be associated with an adverse pregnancy outcome [64];
- elevated levels of estrogens, progesterone and beta -HCG can also contribute to a poor outcome in HEV-positive pregnant women who develop FHF [57];
- a reduced expression of toll-like receptor (TLR) 3/TLR7/TLR9 of the host body of the pregnant woman with acute liver failure, the key pattern recognition receptor in innate immunity. The consequence will be: an inadequate innate immune response with decreased phagocytosis capacity of macrophages/monocytes and the possibility of appearance the severe acute liver failure in pregnancy [66];
- genetic factors in the host- an aspect more discussed in the case of pregnant women of Asian origin. The human genetic factor is not considered relevant in this case. The opposite argument: if the priority intervention of this factor is accepted in the evolution of HEV infection in pregnant women, the mortality rate should be very high in pregnant women with HEV infection in the endemic regions, an aspect that is not found in medical practice [67].

To these factors is added:

- **steroid hormones** present in increased amounts in pregnancy with unfavorable evolution in the presence of HEV infection. These steroid hormones may promote viral replication [16] and also has a direct inhibition on hepatic cells, which may predispose to hepatic dysfunction/failure when exposed to infectious pathogens [16]. Steroid hormones promote viral replication through the immunosuppressive effect [16] and mediate lymphocyte apoptosis by NF-kB factor [16]. NF-κB is a eukaryotic dimeric transcription factor which has a multiple cellular effects, including liver development and regeneration and its implications on the immune response [16]. NF-κB, physiologically down regulated during pregnancy, also plays an important role in sustaining the fetus during pregnancy [68]. An important role in the development and regeneration of the liver is the p65 protein, a component of the NF-kB factor. Experimentally, proteins p65 and p50 - another component of NF-kB - were studied in pregnant women with severe hepatitis E infection. The absence of p65 protein was associated with a minimal or even absence of HEV in mononuclear cells in peripheral blood and in liver biopsy samples obtained post-mortem from pregnant women with fatal evolution of HEV infection. So, the absence of p65 in the NF-kB complex produced fulminant liver damage [68].

Conclusion: the NF-kB factor is a very important protective factor in the pregnant woman influencing her immune status; the modification of its structure determines the severe immune deficiency and favors high replication of HEV.

- **viral genotype.** Numerous studies have highlighted the role of HEV genotype or its subtypes in producing the severity of HEV infection in pregnant women, leading to a high percentage of deaths in some geographical areas [16, 67]. HEV1 in developing countries is associated as the cause of elevated maternal mortality (30%, with most deaths occurring in the third trimester) of pregnant women [16, 67]. Genotype 1 has been further classified into 4 subtypes and most of them have been grouped to genotype 1A. Sub-genotype shift, may have been responsible for the different geographic morbidity in pregnant women in Southern India and Egypt [16].

- **fetal infection with HEV**- may be responsible for the increased severity of the disease in the mother [69].

- In certain geographical areas **the use of herbal medicines by pregnant women** may influence the severity of HEV infection. This would explain the difference in mortality in certain geographical regions and could be used as a prognostic factor in the evolution of a fulminant liver failure due to other etiologies [70].

Conclusion: Severe pregnancy lesions due to HEV infection are caused by viral factors, host-related factors, immunological factors and hormonal factors and environmental factors.

3.3.1.3 Pathogenesis of chronic infection in immunocompromised patients

In immunocompromised patients HEV infection is present as chronic liver disease. HEV infection is present in a proportion of 0.9–3.5% in patients with **SOT** and the rates of chronicity ranging from 21% - 50% [7]. Chronic infection with HEV is characterizes by persistence of HEV in the organisms that are not able to realize the clearance of the virus. HEV persistence may be related to **the immunosuppressive condition of the patient** characterized by:

- a significantly lower of CD2+, CD3+ and CD4+ T cells comparative with the patients who spontaneously eliminate the virus [7].

- a lower concentration of IL-Ra and IL-2R, to which are added to higher concentrations of chemokines in the acute phase [37]

- refractory response of infected HEV cells to the action of interferon due to increased expression of interferon stimulated gene (ISG) [7]; these cells are not able to realize the clearance of the virus; in patients with kidney transplantation has been described this aspect and also *in vitro* in human hepatoma cell cultures and primary human hepatocytes despite the continuous production of type III IFNs [71] and the persistent activation of the JAK/STAT signaling that confers to infected cells refractory to exogenous IFN [26].

- secondary immunosuppression due to HIV infection: in HIV-infected patients with low CD4+ T cell count $<200/mm^3$, HEV infection may become chronic [2].

- secondary immunosuppression due to the use of immunosuppressive drugs in the treatment of various diseases. In humans, HEV is more likely to be persistent in SOT patients treated with tacrolimus and cyclosporin or treatment used in rheumatoid arthritis. Cyclosporin and tacrolimus are both immunosuppressive drugs by inhibition the calcineurin phosphatase in lymphocytes (inhibition of cyclolines A and B); this immunosuppression promote viral replication [72].

Thrombocytopenia by HEV is another change associated with HEV infection in this category of patients: the decrease in platelet count is associated with the persistence of HEV infection and the reduction in the number of antiviral cytotoxic ly T in the liver. HEV-infected patients had low platelet counts [73], but, how HEV induces thrombocytopenia is unknown. It could be immune-mediated as in other virus infections or be linked to the development of fibrosis with splenomegaly [73].

Viral factors meaning the different types, subtypes, quasispecies belonging to HEV can be involved in the chronic evolution of the infection. Arguments:

- chronic infection HEV was found to be rare in a large cohort of Japanese liver transplant recipients, suggesting that there are differences in HEV subtype, strains, or host genetic factors that influence HEV persistence [74].

- greater heterogeneity of quasispecies in ORF1 and ORF 2 during the acute phase of infection is associated with HEV persistence [6, 7].

- the value of Ka/Ks ratio, an indirect indicator of selection pressure on quasispecies in the M domain of HEV capsid protein; M domain of HEV capsid contains epitopes for Ly T. This ratio is lower in patients with chronic HEV infection hence the importance of the cellular immune response in HEV clearance [7].

- the weak diversity of the P capsid domain of HEV, another component of the viral capsid, that can undergo to the evolution to liver fibrosis by the selection of aggressive variants of virus. Nearly 10% of SOT patients with HEV develop cirrhosis within 3 to 5 years after the primary infection [7].

- chronic HEV infection is associated with recombinant host-HEV variants, These recombinant variants have *in vitro* a replicative advantage. The PPR regions of these HEV variants contain fragments of different genes of human origin (e.g. ribosomal genes S17, S19, inter alpha trypsin inhibitor) [7].

Conclusion: HEV infection in immunocompromised patients is characterized by chronic hepatitis due to viral persistence. Viral persistence can be caused by multiple factors related to the immunosuppression of the host organism, but also to HEV.

3.3.1.4 Pathogenesis of extrahepatic manifestations in HEV infection

Neurological disorders have been reported in patients with acute or chronic HEV infections, namely: Guillain–Barré syndrome (GBS), neuralgic amyotrophy

(NA), encephalitis/meningoencephalitis, myositis, Bell's palsy, and polyradiculopathy [16].

Clinically, the evolution of these diseases is more severe in the presence of HEV infection. E.g.: cases of NA that clinically showed bilateral damage, with clamping of the brachial plexus, the phrenic nerve [22].

The pathophysiology of HEV-associated neurological injury remains uncertain. Some of these neurological conditions such as GBS and NA are immune-mediated, due to molecular mimicry [22], secondary to the immune response triggered by the virus. This immune response that cross-reacts with axolemmal or Schwann cell antigens damages peripheral nerves [22]. In case of NA direct infection of the brachial plexus cannot be excluded because HEV RNA was demonstrated in all HEV-associated patients at the start of their illness [19]. Another arguments for direct virus neurotropism:

- HEV variants found in the cerebrospinal fluid were different from those found in the serum of the same patient, which would lead to the theory that HEV may have variants with neurological tropism and replication in the central nervous system. [75]. Neurological disorders can be associated with special genotypes as HEV-1 in infected Asians and HEV-3 in infected Europeans [75, 76].

- the presence of HEV ORF 2 in the cytoplasm or nucleus of cells in brain and spinal cord tissues of the HEV RNA positive rabbits, such as glial cells, microglial cells, choroid epithelium cells, and neural cells, especially in cells located in perivascular areas. These aspects suggest that perivascular cells and neural cells are targets for HEV present in cerebrospinal fluid (CNS) [77] described in HEV infected gerbils the thickening of the basement membrane of blood vessels even reduplicated in brain and spinal cord tissues as a compensatory response to blood–brain barrier (BBB) disruption permeability. In conclusion: HEV can cross the BBB directly into the central nervous tissue. [77]

In summary, HEV entry to the brain. The BBB of brain is a potential target of HEV invasion into the CNS in experimentally infected rabbits. Components of the BBB include tight junction (TJ) and adhesion junction (AJ) between endothelial cells (EC), pericytes (PC), astrocytes endfoot (EF), as well as basement membrane (BM) surrounded ECs and PCs; HEV causes a decrease in TJ proteins, including ZO-1, Occludin, and Claudin5 and an increase in AJ protein VE-cadherin expression; the result will be in breaking the junctional complexes integrity between capillary ECs, facilitating HEV invasion into the brain tissue. This is the key factor in HEV pathogenicity at the CNS level [78].

Kidney injuries and impaired renal function

Both acute and chronic HEV infections can lead to kidney injuries and impaired renal function [79]. Both HEV antigen and RNA have been detected in the urine of patients with acute or chronic HEV4 [80] or HEV3 infections [41]. Experimentally, immunohistochemistry also detected ORF3 protein in the kidneys of infected rabbits [81]. This suggests that the kidneys or the urinary tract could be an HEV reservoir. Kidney biopsies from patients with glomerular disease and HEV infection revealed histological features of membranoproliferative glomerulonephritis (MPGN), with or without cryoglobulinemia, membranous glomerulonephritis [79, 82] and a relapse of immunoglobulin A nephropathy [79].

The pathophysiology of HEV infection at these patients is linked to the deposition of immune complexes formed from the HEV antigen, anti-HEV IgG antibodies, and a rheumatoid factor in the glomerulus [33]. It is also possible that the HEV antigen with lower molecular weight by-products of ORF2s could be secreted into the urine by cross the glomerular filtration barrier [83] Both HEV antigen and RNA were detected in the urine of patients chronically infected with HEV [80] Kidney biopsies showed interstitial inflammatory cell infiltrates at tubule-interstitial. [36, 80]. But, there is still no evidence neither about viral replication of HEV in human renal cells nor of the direct nephrotoxic effect [7].

Hematological manifestations in HEV infection

Anemia and severe thrombocytopenia may be associated with HEV infection. Anemia related to HEV infection can be: hemolytic anemia due to deficiency of glucose 6-phosphate dehydrogenase (G6PD) [84, 85] or aplastic anemia secondary to severe forms of HEV infection [85].

Thrombocytopenia may be associated with HEV infection [29]. 11% HEV-infected patients had thrombocytopenia [86]. The pathogenic mechanisms involved by HEV could be: immune-mediated or be linked to the development of fibrosis with splenomegaly [86].

Cryoglobulenemia: there were only a few cases of Hepatitis E-associated cryoglobulenemia reported in the medical literature,; all of these patients are chronic hepatitis patients, immunocompromised, all from western Europe, with genotype 3 confirmed in eight cases, with all MC type 2 or 3 [22].

HEV-induced acute pancreatitis have been reported.

2.1% of patients with acute pancreatitis in a study conducted in India had serological arguments about a recent HEV infection. Acute pancreatitis associated with hepatitis E usually has a good prognosis. The mechanism of pancreatitis in patients with acute viral hepatitis (nonfulminant) is unknown, and it may be multifactorial. One proposed pathogenesis of pancreatitis associated with hepatitis is the development of edema of the ampulla of Vater with obstruction to the outflow of pancreatic fluid. A more plausible mechanism for virus-associated acute pancreatitis is the direct inflammation and destruction of pancreatic acinar cells by the virus [22].

4. Laboratory diagnosis

The laboratory is essential for establishing the etiological diagnosis.

4.1.Serology is the main way to diagnose HEV infection. It consists of highlighting IgG and IgM antibodies anti- HEV [8]. IgM rises rapidly within a month of acquiring the infection, the peak corresponds to the onset of clinical symptoms and increased liver enzymes (ALT, AST) and disappear up to 32 weeks to 5months after the initial disease onset; IgG occurs after the disappearance of IgM and they persist for a long time after infection (not yet defined), occasionally disappearing before the one year mark [8]. In endemic regions in acute infections, IgM antibodies may coexist with IgG antibodies for a certain period of time.

Clinical significance of the 2 types of anti-HEV antibodies: the presence of IgM antibodies means a recent acute HEV infection; presence of anti-HEV IgG antibodies means past HEV infection or post-vaccination status (protective value over 2.5 U/mL according to WHO) [87].

4.2. HEV RNA detection in blood or in the stool by Real-Time Polymerase Chain Reaction (RT-PCR).

HEV RNA detection is a method used to diagnose the infection in early stage. HEV viremia disappears after 3 weeks, and from feces HEV disappears after another 2 weeks [2].

NOTE: HEV RNA measurement is required in immunocompromised patients in whom antibodies tests may be negative, 3 months after an HEV infection to determine whether it becomes chronic, for monitoring antiviral therapy, or in blood donors as a screening test [8].

4.3. HEV antigen (HEV Ag) detection is another method for early acute HEV infection, comparable to RT-PCR. Antigen detection can be a good cost-effective alternative to real-time PCR [88].

4.4. HEV isolation *in vitro*, from serum or feces, using certain cell cultures, such as PLC/PRF/5 (human hepatocarcinoma) and A549 cells (human lung adenocarcinoma) or in hepatocytes derived from pluripotent stem cells. In these cell lines HEV replicates, the replication being dependent on the value of the inoculum [89, 90].

4.5. HEV genotyping to identify types, subtypes, variants, quasispecies HEV that has been shown to be correlated with the severity of the disease, with certain epidemiological aspects, with the area of spread of HEV infection [8].

5. Conclusions

Hepatitis E is a liver infection not yet sufficiently investigated, with an unclear pathophysiology, in which the confluence of several viral factors, the host or environmental factors can lead to different clinical features. Although most infections are subclinical, there are cases with severe forms of the disease that can progress unfavorably either to fulminant forms with acute liver failure, cirrhosis and death, or to chronicity, and during pregnancy can take benign or extremely severe forms that can lead to death. Mother and fetus. As such, hepatitis E is a topic that should be investigated in future studies.

Acknowledgements

Thanks to Mateo Pullok for the collaboration initiative.

Conflict of interest

No conflict of interest.

Funding

This work received no external funding.

Author details

Adriana Turculeanu[1,2]

1 Prof. University of Medicine and Pharmacy, Craiova, Romania

2 Dir. Regional Blood Bank, Craiova, Romania

*Address all correspondence to: adriana_turculeanu@yahoo.com

References

[1] WHO Hepatitis E. Available from: http://www.who.int/mediacentre/factsheets/fs280/en/. [Last accessed on 8 July 2019].

[2] Dalton HR, Kamar N, Baylis SA, et al. EASL Clinical Practice Guidelines on hepatitis E virus infection. J Hepatol, 2018; 68: 1256–1271ş DOI: https://doi.org/10.1016/j.jhep.2018.03.005

[3] Perez-Gracia M.T., Suay-Garcia B., Mateos-Lindemann M.L: Hepatitis E and pregnancy: Curren https://doi.org/10.1016/j.jhep.2018.03.005t state. Rev. Med. Virol. 2017;27(3):e1929. DOI: 10.1002/rmv.1929

[4] Arankalle VA, Chadha MS, Chitambar SD, Walimbe AM, Chobe LP, Gandhe SS.: Changing epidemiology of hepatitis A and hepatitis E in urban and rural India (1982–98). J. Viral Hepat. 2001; 8:293–303. DOI: 10.1046/j.1365-2893.2001.00279.x.

[5] Aggarwal, R.; Goel, A. Natural History, Clinical Manifestations, and Pathogenesis of Hepatitis E Virus Genotype 1 and 2 Infections. Cold Spring Harb. Perspect. Med. 2018, *9*, a032136.

[6] Sébastien Lhomme, Olivier Marion, Florence Abravanel, Sabine Chapuy-Regaud, Nassim Kamar, and Jacques Izopet, Hepatitis E Pathogenesis, Viruses. 2016 Aug; 8(8): 212. DOI: 10.3390/v8080212

[7] Sébastien Lhomme, Olivier Marion, Florence Abravanel, Jacques Izopet and Nassim Kamar, Clinical Manifestations, Pathogenesis and Treatment of Hepatitis E Virus Infections, *J. Clin. Med.* 2020, *9*(2), 331; DOI: 10.3390/jcm9020331

[8] Ekta Gupta, Pragya Agarwala. Hepatitis E virus infection: An old virus with a new story!, Indian Journal of Microbilogy, 2018, Volume : 36, Issue : 3, Page : 317–23. DOI: 10.4103/ijmm.IJMM_18_149

[9] Dalton H. R., van Eijk J. J. J., Cintas P., Madden R. G., Jones C., Webb G. W., et al. Hepatitis E virus infection and acute non-traumatic neurological injury: a prospective multicentre study. J. Hepatol. 2017, 67, 925–932. DOI: 10.1016/j.jhep.2017.07.010.

[10] Thomas Horvatits, Julian Schulze zur Wiesch, Marc Lütgehetmann, Ansgar W. Lohse, and Sven Pischke, The Clinical Perspective on Hepatitis E Viruses. 2019 Jul; 11(7): 617. Published online 2019 Jul 5. DOI: 10.3390/v11070617

[11] Abhishek Chauhan, Gwilym Webbb, James Ferguson, Clinical presentations of Hepatitis E: A clinical review with representative case histories, Clin Res Hepatol Gastroenterol. 2019 Nov; 43(6): 649–657., DOI: 10.1016/j.clinre.2019.01.005

[12] Johannes Hartl, Malte H. Wehmeyer and Sven Pischke , Acute Hepatitis E: Two Sides of the Same Coin, *Viruses* 2016, *8*(11), 299; DOI: 10.3390/v8110299

[13] A Kumar, VA Saraswat, E HepatitisAcute-on-chronic liver failure, J Clin Exp Hepatol, 2013, 3, pp. 225–230, DOI: 10.1016/j.jceh.2013.08.013

[14] Udayakumar Navaneethan, Mayar Al Mohajer and Mohamed T Shata, Hepatitis E and Pregnancy-Understanding the pathogenesis, Liver Int. 2008 Nov; 28(9): 1190–1199. DOI: 10.1111/j.1478-3231.2008.01840.x

[15] Stoszek SK, Engle RE, Abdel-Hamid M, et al. Hepatitis E antibody seroconversion without disease in highly endemic rural Egyptian

communities. Trans R Soc Trop Med Hyg. 2006;100:89–94. DOI: 10.1016/j.trstmh.2005.05.019

[16] Khuroo M.S., Kamili S., Khuroo M.S. Clinical course and duration of viremia in vertically transmitted hepatitis E virus (HEV) infection in babies born to HEV-infected mothers. J. Viral Hepat. 2009;16:519–523. DOI: 10.1111/j.1365-2893.2009.01101.x.

[17] S Mc Pherson, et al. Summary of the British transplantation society UK guidelines for hepatitis E and solid organ transplantation, Transplantation, 2018 Jan;102(1):15–20. DOI: 10.1097/TP.0000000000001908

[18] Kamar, N.; Rostaing, L.; Legrand-Abravanel, F.; Izopet, J. How should hepatitis E virus infection be defined in organ-transplant recipients? *Am. J. Transplant.* 2013 Jul;13(7):1935–6, DOI: 10.1111/ajt.12253

[19] Joachim Denner, Hepatitis E virus (HEV)—The Future, Viruses. 2019 Mar; 11(3): 251. Published online 2019 Mar 13. DOI: 10.3390/v11030251

[20] EASL Clinical Practice Guidelines on hepatitis E virus infection, J Hepatol, 2018;68(6):1256–1271, DOI: 10.1016/j.jhep.2018.03.005.

[21] Veeraraghavan Meyyur Aravamudan, Shahab R. Khan, Sushanth Dosala, Ikram Hussain, Beyond the Liver, Hepatitis E Can Affect the Nerves, Pancreas, and Blood Vessels. Extrahepatic Manifestations of Hepatitis E: A Comprehensive Literature Review, 2019 Aug 27;11(8):e5499. DOI: 10.7759/cureus.5499.

[22] Marion O., Lhomme S., Nayrac M., Dubois M., Pucelle M., Requena M., Migueres M., Abravanel F., Peron J.M., Carrere N., et al. Hepatitis E virus replication in human intestinal cells. 2020 May;69(5):901–910. DOI: 10.1136/gutjnl-2019-319004.

[23] Capelli N., Marion O., Dubois M., Allart S., Bertrand-Michel J., Lhomme S., Abravanel F., Izopet J., Chapuy-Regaud S. Vectorial Release of Hepatitis E Virus in Polarized Human Hepatocytes. J. Virol. 2019;93 DOI: 10.1128/JVI.01207-18.

[24] Xin Yin and Zongdi Feng, Hepatitis E Virus Entry, Viruses. 2019 Sep 20;11(10):883. DOI: 10.3390/v11100883.

[25] Nain M., Mukherjee S., Karmakar S. P., Paton A.W., Paton J.C., Abdin M.Z., Basu A., Kalia M., Vrati S. GRP78 Is an Important Host Factor for Japanese Encephalitis Virus Entry and Replication in Mammalian Cells. J. Virol. 2017;91:e02274–16. DOI: 10.1128/JVI.02274-16.

[26] Zhang L., Tian Y., Wen Z., Zhang F., Qi Y., Huang W., Zhang H., Wang Y. Asialoglycoprotein receptor facilitates infection of PLC/PRF/5 cells by HEV through interaction with ORF2. J. Med. Virol. 2016;88:2186–2195. DOI: 10.1002/jmv.24570.

[27] Fongsaran C., Jirakanwisal K., Kuadkitkan A., Wikan N., Wintachai P., Thepparit C., Ubol S., Phaonakrop N., Roytrakul S., Smith D.R. Involvement of ATP synthase beta subunit in chikungunya virus entry into insect cells.Arch. Virol. 2014;159:3353–3364. DOI: 10.1007/s00705-014-2210-4.

[28] Shiota T., Li T.C., Nishimura Y., Yoshizaki S., Sugiyama R., Shimojima M., Saijo M., Shimizu H., Suzuki R., Wakita T., et al. Integrin alpha3 is involved in non-enveloped hepatitis E virus infection. Virology. 2019;536:119–124. DOI: 10.1016/j.virol.2019.07.025.

[29] Yin X., Ambardekar C., Lu Y., Feng Z. Distinct Entry Mechanisms for Nonenveloped and Quasi-Enveloped Hepatitis E Viruses. J. Virol. 2016;90: 4232–4242. DOI: 10.1128/JVI.02804-15.

[30] Kapur N., Thakral D., Durgapal H., Panda S.K. Hepatitis E virus enters liver cells through receptor-dependent clathrin-mediated endocytosis. J. Viral Hepat. 2012;19:436–448. DOI: 10.1111/j.1365-2893.2011.01559.x.

[31] Lee G.H., Tan B.H., Teo E.C., Lim S. G., Dan Y.Y., Wee A., Aw P.P., Zhu Y., Hibberd M.L., Tan C.K., et al. Chronic Infection with Camelid Hepatitis E Virus in a Liver Transplant Recipient Who Regularly Consumes Camel Meat and Milk. Gastroenterology. 2016;150: 55–57. DOI: 10.1053/j.gastro.2015.10.048.

[32] Sridhar S, Teng JL, Chiu TH, Lau SK, Woo PC. Hepatitis E virus genotypes and evolution: Emergence of camel hepatitis E variants. Int J Mol Sci 2017;18(4):869. DOI: 10.3390/ijms18040869.

[33] M Carre, et al.Fatal autochthonous fulminant hepatitis E early after allogeneic stem cell transplantation, Bone Marrow Transplant, 2017;52(4): 643–645. DOI: 10.1038/bmt.2016.337.

[34] Pischke, S.; Peron, J.M.; von Wulffen, M.; von Felden, J.; Honer Zu Siederdissen, C.; Fournier, S.; Lutgehetmann, M.; Iking-Konert, C.; Bettinger, D.; Par, G.; et al. Chronic Hepatitis E in Rheumatology and Internal Medicine Patients: A Retrospective Multicenter European Cohort Study. *Viruses* 2019, 11(2):186. DOI: 10.3390/v11020186.

[35] Kamar N, Garrouste C, Haagsma EB, et al. Factors associated with chronic hepatitis in patients with hepatitis E virus infection who have received solid organ transplants. Gastroenterology 2011; 140: 1481–1489. DOI: 10.3390/v11070617

[36] S Pischke, et al.Hepatitis E virus: Infection beyond the liver?, J Hepatol, 2017, 66(5):1082–1095. DOI: 10.1016/j.jhep.2016.11.016

[37] Shukla P., Nguyen H.T., Torian U., Engle R.E., Faulk K., Dalton H.R., Bendall R.P., Keane F.E., Purcell R.H., Emerson S.U. Cross-species infections of cultured cells by hepatitis E virus and discovery of an infectious virus-host recombinant. Proc. Natl. Acad. Sci. USA.2011;108:2438–2443. DOI: 10.1073/pnas.1018878108.

[38] Romy Weller , Daniel Todt , Michael Engelmann , Martina Friesland, Heiner Wedemeyer, Thomas Pietschmann, , Apolipoprotein E polymorphisms and their protective effect on hepatitis E virus replication, Hepatology. 2016;64(6):2274–2276

[39] Mishra N., Arankalle V.A. Association of polymorphisms in the promoter regions of TNF-alpha (−308) with susceptibility to hepatitis E virus and TNF-alpha (−1031) and IFN-gamma (+874) genes with clinical outcome of hepatitis E infection in India. J. Hepatol. 2011;55:1227–1234. DOI: 10.1016/j.jhep.2011.03.023.

[40] Dong C., Zafrullah M., Mixson-Hayden T., Dai X., Liang J., Meng J., Kamili S. Suppression of interferon-alpha signaling by hepatitis E virus. Hepatology. 2012;55:1324–1332. DOI: 10.1002/hep.25530

[41] Zhou X., Xu L., Wang W., Watashi K., Wang Y., Sprengers D., de Ruiter P.E., van der Laan L.J., Metselaar H.J., Kamar N., et al. Disparity of basal and therapeutically activated interferon signalling in constraining hepatitis E virus infection. J. Viral Hepat. 2016;23:294–304. DOI: 10.1111/jvh.12491.

[42] Nan Y., Yu Y., Ma Z., Khattar S.K., Fredericksen B., Zhang Y.J. Hepatitis E virus inhibits type I interferon induction by ORF1 products. J. Virol. 2014;88: 11924–11932. DOI: 10.1128/JVI.01935-14.

[43] Srivastava R., Aggarwal R., Bhagat M.R., Chowdhury A., Naik S.

Alterations in natural killer cells and natural killer T cells during acute viral hepatitis E. J. Viral Hepat. 2008;15:910–916. DOI: 10.1111/j.1365-2893.2008.01036.x

[44] Prabhu S.B., Gupta P., Durgapal H., Rath S., Gupta S.D., Acharya S.K., Panda S.K. Study of cellular immune response against Hepatitis E virus (HEV) J. Viral Hepat. 2011;18:587–594. DOI: 10.1111/j.1365-2893.2010.01338.x.

[45] Zhang J., Zhang X.F., Huang S.J., Wu T., Hu Y.M., Wang Z.Z., Wang H., Jiang H.M., Wang Y.J., Yan Q., et al. Long-term efficacy of a hepatitis E vaccine. N. Engl. J. Med.2015;372:914–922. DOI: 10.1056/NEJMoa1406011

[46] Abravanel F., Lhomme S., Chapuy-Regaud S., Mansuy J.M., Muscari F., Sallusto F., Rostaing L., Kamar N., Izopet J. Hepatitis E virus reinfections in solid-organ-transplant recipients can evolve into chronic infections. J. Infect. Dis. 2014;209:1900–1906. DOI: 10.1093/infdis/jiu032.

[47] Saravanabalaji S., Tripathy A.S., Dhoot R.R., Chadha M.S., Kakrani A.L., Arankalle V.A. Viral load, antibody titers and recombinant open reading frame 2 protein-induced TH1/TH2 cytokines and cellular immune responses in self-limiting and fulminant hepatitis e. Intervirology.2009;52:78–85. DOI: 10.1159/000214862

[48] Agrawal V., Goel A., Rawat A., Naik S., Aggarwal R. Histological and immunohistochemical features in fatal acute fulminant hepatitis E. Indian J. Pathol. Microbiol.2012;55:22–27. DOI: 10.4103/0377-4929.94849

[49] Mishra N., Walimbe A.M., Arankalle V.A. Hepatitis E virus from India exhibits significant amino acid mutations in fulminant hepatic failure patients. Virus Genes. 2013;46:47–53. DOI: 10.1007/s11262-012-0833-7

[50] Borkakoti J., Ahmed G., Rai A., Kar P. Report of novel H105R, D29N, V27A mutations in the methyltransferase region of the HEV genome in patients with acute liver failure. J. Clin. Virol. 2017;91:1–4. DOI: 10.1016/j.jcv.2017.03.017

[51] Jeblaoui A., Haim-Boukobza S., Marchadier E., Mokhtari C., Roque-Afonso A.M. Genotype 4 hepatitis e virus in France: An autochthonous infection with a more severe presentation. Clin. Infect. Dis. 2013;57:e122–e126. DOI: 10.1093/cid/cit291

[52] Julia Szekeres-Bartho, The Role of Progesterone in FetoMaternal Immunological Cross Talk, Med Princ Pract 2018;27:301–307, DOI: 10.1159/000491576

[53] Angélique L Veenstra van Nieuwenhoven, Annechien Bouman, Henk Moes, Maas-Jan Heineman, Cytokine production in natural killer cells and lymphocytes in pregnant women compared with women in the follicular phase of the ovarian cycle, Fertility and Sterility 77(5):1032–7 · June 2002, DOI: 10.1016/S0015-0282(02)02976-X ·

[54] Pal R., Aggarwal R., Naik S.R., Das V., Das S., Naik S. Immunological alterations in pregnant women with acute hepatitis E. J. Gastroenterol. Hepatol. 2005;20:1094–1101. DOI: 10.1111/j.1440-1746.2005.03875.x

[55] R Mellor AL, Sivakumar J, Chandler P, et al. Prevention of T cell–driven complement activation and inflammation by tryptophan catabolism during pregnancy. Nat Immunol. 2001; 2001 Jan;2(1):64–8. doi: 10.1038/83183.

[56] Orsi NM, Gopichandran N, Ekbote UV, Walker JJ. Murine serum cytokines throughout the estrous cycle, pregnancy and post partum period. Anim Reprod Sci. 2006;96(1–2):54–65. DOI: 10.1016/j.anireprosci.2005.11.010.

[57] Jilani N, Das BC, Husain SA, Baweja UK, Chattopadhya D, Gupta RK, Sardana S, Kar P. Hepatitis E virus infection and fulminant hepatic failure during pregnancy. J Gastroenterol Hepatol. 2007; 22(5):676–82. DOI: 10.1111/j.1440-1746.2007.04913.x.

[58] Bose P.D., Das B.C., Kumar A., Gondal R., Kumar D., Kar P. High viral load and deregulation of the progesterone receptor signaling pathway: Association with hepatitis E-related poor pregnancy outcome. J. Hepatol. 2011; 54(6):1107–1113. DOI: 10.1016/j.jhep.2010.08.037

[59] Rijhisinghami AG, Thompson K, Bhatia SK, Waldscmidt TJ. Estrogen blocks early T cell development in the thymus. Am. J. Reprod. Immunol. 1996; 36(5):269–77. DOI: 10.1111/j.1600-0897.1996.tb00176.x.

[60] Boll G, Reimann J. Estrogen treatment depletes extrathymic T cells from intestinal lymphoid tissues. Scand. J. Immunol. 1996;43(3):345–50. https://doi.org/10.1046/j.1365-3083.1996.d01-41.x

[61] Bi Y., Yang C., Yu W., Zhao X., Zhao C., He Z., Jing S., Wang H., Huang F. Pregnancy serum facilitates hepatitis E virus replication in vitro. J. Gen. Virol. 2015;96(5):1055–1061. DOI: 10.1099/vir.0.000054

[62] Dionne P. Robinson and Sabra L. Klein, Pregnancy and pregnancy-associated hormones alter immune responses and disease pathogenesis, Horm Behav. 2012 Aug; 62(3): 263–271. DOI: 10.1016/j.yhbeh.2012.02.023

[63] Gouilly J., Chen Q., Siewiera J., Cartron G., Levy C., Dubois M., Al-Daccak R., Izopet J., Jabrane-Ferrat N., El Costa H. Genotype specific pathogenicity of hepatitis E virus at the human maternal-fetal interface. Nat. Commun. 2018; 9(1):4748. DOI: 10.1038/s41467-018-07200-2.

[64] Kumar A., Devi S.G., Kar P., Agarwal S., Husain S.A., Gupta R.K., Sharma S. Association of cytokines in hepatitis E with pregnancy outcome. Cytokine. 2014;65(1):95–104. DOI: 10.1016/j.cyto.2013.09.022.

[65] Zanzoni Kmush B.L., Labrique A., Li W., Klein S.L., Schulze K., Shaikh S., Ali H., Engle R.E., Wu L., Purcell R.H., et al. The Association of Cytokines and Micronutrients with Hepatitis E Virus Infection During Pregnancy and the Postpartum Period in Rural Bangladesh. Am. J. Trop. Med. Hyg. 2016; 94(1):203–11. DOI: 10.4269/ajtmh.15-0238.

[66] Sehgal R., Patra S., David P., Vyas A., Khanam A., Hissar S., Gupta E., Kumar G., Kottilil S., Maiwall R., et al. Impaired monocyte-macrophage functions and defective Toll-like receptor signaling in hepatitis E virus-infected pregnant women with acute liver, Hepatology, 2015;62(6): 1683–96. DOI: 10.1002/hep.28143

[67] Rasheeda CA, Navaneethan U, Jayanthi V. Liver Disease in pregnancy and its influence on maternal and fetal mortality- A prospective study from Chennai, Southern India. Eur J Gastroenterol Hepatol. 2008;20(4): 362–4. DOI: 10.1097/MEG.0b013e3282f246d6

[68] Prusty BK, Hedau S, Singh A, Kar P, Das BC. Selective Suppression of NF-kBp65 in Hepatitis Virus-Infected Pregnant Women Manifesting Severe Liver Damage and High Mortality. Mol Med. 2007; 13(9–10):518–26. DOI: 10.2119/2007-00055.Prusty.

[69] Sunil Yadav, Sneha Shirodker, Swapnali Kshirsagar, Maternal and fetal outcome in pregnancy with hepatitis E virus infection, Int J Reprod Contracept Obstet Gynecol. 2016;5(10):3482–3490, DOI: http://dx.doi.org/10.18203/2320-1770.ijrcog20163428

[70] Bernuau JR, Durand F. Herbal medicines in acute viral hepatitis: a ticket for more trouble. Eur J Gastroenterol Hepatol. 2008; 20(3): 161–3. DOI: 10.1097/MEG. 0b013e3282f2bbf7.

[71] Yin X., Li X., Ambardekar C., Hu Z., Lhomme S., Feng Z. Hepatitis E virus persists in the presence of a type III interferon response. PLoS Pathog. 2017; 13(5):e1006417. doi: 10.1371/journal. ppat.1006417.

[72] McAlister V.C., Haddad E., Renouf E., Malthaner R.A., Kjaer M.S., Gluud L.L. Cyclosporin versus tacrolimus as primary immunosuppressant after liver transplantation: A meta-analysis. Am. J. Transplant. 2006 Jul;6(7):1578–85. DOI: 10.1111/j.1600-6143.2006.01360.x.

[73] Fateh Bazerbachi, Samir Haffar, Sushil K Garg, and John R Lake, Extra-hepatic manifestations associated with hepatitis E virus infection: a comprehensive review of the literature, Gastroenterol Rep (Oxf). 2016 Feb; 4 (1): 1–15. DOI: 10.1093/gastro/gov042

[74] Inagaki Y., Oshiro Y., Tanaka T., Yoshizumi T., Okajima H., Ishiyama K., Nakanishi C., Hidaka M., Wada H., Hibi T., et al. A Nation wide Survey of Hepatitis E Virus Infection and Chronic Hepatitis E in Liver Transplant Recipients in Japan. E BioMedicine 2020;104(2):437–444. DOI: 10.1097/ TP.0000000000002801.

[75] Abravanel F., Pique J., Couturier E., Nicot F., Dimeglio C., Lhomme S., Chiabrando J., Saune K., Peron J.M., Kamar N., et al. Acute hepatitis E in French patients and neurological manifestations. J. Infect. 2018;77(3): 220–226. doi: 10.1016/j.jinf.2018.06.007

[76] Dalton H.R., Kamar N., van Eijk J.J., McLean B.N., Cintas P., Bendall R.P., Jacobs B.C. Hepatitis E virus and neurological injury. Nat. Rev. Neurol. 2016;12(2):77–85. doi: 10.1038/ nrneurol.2015.234.

[77] Shi R., Soomro M. H., She R., Yang Y., Wang T., Wu Q., et al. Evidence of Hepatitis E virus breaking through the blood-brain barrier and replicating in the central nervous system. J. Viral. Hepat. 2016, 23(11), 930–939. DOI: 10.1111/jvh.12557

[78] Jijing Tian, Ruihan Shi, Tianlong Liu, Ruiping She, Qiaoxing Wu, Junqing An, Wenzhuo Hao, and Majid Hussain Soomro, Brain Infection by Hepatitis E Virus Probably via Damage of the Blood-Brain Barrier Due to Alterations of Tight Junction Proteins, Front Cell Infect Microbiol. 2019; 9: 52. DOI: 10.3389/fcimb.2019.00052

[79] Taton B., Moreau K., Lepreux S., Bachelet T., Trimoulet P., De Ledinghen V., Pommereau A., Ronco P., Kamar N., Merville P., et al. Hepatitis E virus infection as a new probable cause of de novo membranous nephropathy after kidney transplantation. Transpl. Infect. Dis. 2013;15(6):E211–E215. DOI: 10.1111/tid.12143.

[80] Geng Y., Zhao C., Huang W., Harrison T.J., Zhang H., Geng K., Wang Y. Detection and assessment of infectivity of hepatitis E virus in urine. J. Hepatol. 2016;64(1):37–43. DOI: 10.1016/j.jhep.2015.08.034.

[81] Wang L., Xia J., Wang L., Wang Y. Experimental infection of rabbits with genotype 3 hepatitis E virus produced both chronicity and kidney injury. Gut. 2017;66:561–562. DOI: 10.1136/gutjnl-2016-312023.

[82] Guinault D., Ribes D., Delas A., Milongo D., Abravanel F., Puissant-Lubrano B., Izopet J., Kamar N. Hepatitis E Virus-Induced Cryoglobulinemic Glomerulonephritis in a Nonimmunocompromised Person. Am. J. Kidney Dis. 2016;67(4):660–663. DOI: 10.1053/j.ajkd.2015.10.022

[83] Montpellier, C.; Wychowski, C.; Sayed, I.M.; Meunier, J.C.; Saliou, J.M.; Ankavay, M.; Bull, A.; Pillez, A.; Abravanel, F.; Helle, F.; et al. Hepatitis E Virus Lifecycle and Identification of 3 Forms of the ORF2 Capsid Protein. Gastroenterology 2018, 154(1), 211–223. DOI: 10.1053/j.gastro.2017.09.020

[84] Thapa R., Pramanik S., Biswas B., Mallick D. Hepatitis E virus infection in a 7-year-old boy with glucose 6-phosphate dehydrogenase deficiency. J. Pediatr. Hematol. Oncol. 2009;31(3): 223–224. DOI: 10.1097/MPH.0b013e3181984dab

[85] Fotios S. Fousekis, Ioannis V. Mitselos, Dimitrios K. Christodoulou, Extrahepatic manifestations of hepatitis E virus: An overview, *Clin Mol Hepatol.* 2020;26(1):16–23. DOI: https://doi.org/10.3350/cmh.2019.0082

[86] Woolson K.L., Forbes A., Vine L., Beynon L., McElhinney L., Panayi V., Hunter J.G., Madden R.G., Glasgow T., Kotecha A., et al. Extra-hepatic manifestations of autochthonous hepatitis E infection. Aliment. Pharmacol. Ther. 2014; 40(11–12):1282–91. DOI: 10.1111/apt.129862014

[87] Shrestha MP, Scott RM, Joshi DM, Mammen MP Jr., Thapa GB, Thapa N, *et al.* Safety and efficacy of a recombinant hepatitis E vaccine. N Engl J Med 2007;356(9):895–903. DOI: 10.1056/NEJMoa061847.

[88] Majumdar M, Singh MP, Pujhari SK, Bhatia D, Chawla Y, Ratho RK, *et al.* Hepatitis E virus antigen detection as an early diagnostic marker: Report from India. J Med Virol 2013;85(3):823–7. https://doi.org/10.1002/jmv.23529

[89] Tanaka T, Takahashi M, Kusano E, Okamoto H. Development and evaluation of an efficient cell-culture system for hepatitis E virus. J Gen Virol 2007; 88(Pt 3):903–11. DOI: 10.1099/vir.0.82535-0.

[90] Helsen N, Debing Y, Paeshuyse J, Dallmeier K, Boon R, Coll M, *et al.* Stem cell-derived hepatocytes: A novel model for hepatitis E virus replication. J Hepatol 2016;64(3):565–73. DOI: 10.1016/j.jhep.2015.11.013.

Chapter 10

Microbiota, Inflammation, and Gut Barrier Dysfunction in HCC

Amit Kumar Ram, Gavin Wright and Balasubramaniyan Vairappan

Abstract

Hepatocellular carcinoma (HCC), which represents 90% of all primary liver cancers, is the fifth most common cancer and the third cause of cancer mortality rate. It is a complex disease with a poor prognosis. Incidence and mortality rates are increasing in many geographical regions, indicating a need for better management strategies. Chronic inflammation is the major driving factors for HCC development, which typically develops on the background of chronic liver disease (CLD). Currently, a large body of literature has focused on the key role of the gut-liver axis as the major pathophysiological mechanism of hepatic disease severity and HCC development. This chapter will describe the role of gut microbiota, inflammation, and intestinal barrier dysfunction-associated mechanism in the progression of HCC. In particular, enteric dysbiosis, tight junction, and inflammatory mediators in the pathogenesis of liver cancer will be discussed. Furthermore, this chapter will identify the possible potential therapeutic approach for the control of gut bacterial overgrowth, inflammation and restoration of eubiosis, and tight junction integrity in HCC.

Keywords: gut-liver axis, HCC, inflammation, microbiota, zonula occludens-1

1. Introduction

Highlights

- Gut dysbiosis, inflammation, and increased intestinal permeability are synergistically contributed to the pathogenesis of hepatocellular carcinoma.
- Previous studies in animal models suggest that targeting the gut-liver axis can inhibit HCC development.
- Targeting the gut-liver axis with probiotics, antibiotics, FMT, TLR4 antagonists, FXR agonists, and natural compounds could be the promising strategies for HCC prevention.

Hepatocellular carcinoma (HCC) is a heterogeneous type of tumor that is likely to develop on the background of an inflammatory milieu in patients with advanced liver disease. It is the third leading cause of cancer death globally and is more prevalent in men than in women [1]. Over the past two decades, there is increasing evidence from studies suggesting a causal link between gut microbiota in the progression of HCC. Normal commensal gut microbiota acts as an important source of energy and is pivotal to host metabolism and innate immunity [2]. Not unsurprisingly therefore, alteration to gut microbial composition has been linked to the promotion of chronic inflammatory bowel disease (IBD) via local effects. However, activation of such inflammatory effects can have a broader response across all organ beds such as the liver, kidney, brain, heart, and the hematopoietic system and have been strongly associated with carcinogenesis [3]. Anatomical considerations provide us with a logical understanding on why gut microbiosis may have such an impact on disease development, especially in the liver. Since the liver is anatomically connected to the intestine via the portal vein, it is the first organ to receive nutrient-rich blood and also the first target of gut microbiota. Furthermore, the liver can elicit an inflammatory response through microbe-associated molecular patterns (MAMPs) and pattern recognition receptors (PRRs). Though translocation of gut microbiota from the intestinal lumen to the systemic circulation is counterchecked by multilayer intestinal epithelium, any change in its integrity can initiate inflammation and contribute to fibrosis and thus chronic liver disease (CLD) progression and thus a precursor to HCC development, which is itself usually only seen in the context of cirrhosis, the most advanced form of CLD [4]. In this chapter, we summarize the available literature on the key role of gut microbiome in HCC pathogenesis and novel therapeutic approaches developed to target these processes.

2. Gut microbiota

The gut microbiota resides in the gastrointestinal (GI) tract. The human gut harbors complex and diverse microbial community of 100 trillion microorganisms with more than 2000 distinct species of bacteria, in addition to fungi protozoans and viruses. These microorganisms are collectively called gut microbiota, which comprises of commensals, beneficial microbiota, and opportunistic pathogens residing in what is a complex and dense microenvironment. Immediately after birth commensal bacteria colonize the intestine and predominantly comprise *Proteobacteria*, *Lactobacillus*, and *Actinobacteria*, but as we mature into adults *Bacteroidetes* and *Firmicutes species* predominate [5]. The composition of microbiota also varies from the small intestine to the distal colon, due largely to the effects of nutrient availability, intestinal pH, and motility. Moreover the overall composition of the microbial community in the gut is further individualized by any alteration in our diet, age, lifestyle, disease, and also medication exposure [6]. A symbiotic relationship exists between gut microbiota and the human host, which are critical to our maintenance of health. For example, gut microbiota are involved in the metabolism of bile acids, synthesis of vitamins, digestion of complex polysaccharides, and production of short-chain fatty acids (SCFAs) [2]. SCFAs are a vital source of energy for enterocytes, which are integral in maintaining gut barrier integrity. In addition, gut microbiota are also involved in the development of local and innate immunity providing defense against not only the pathogenic invasion but also systemic infection [7]. Experimental studies from rodents and humans have demonstrated that the gut microbiota is involved in the progression of HCC by increasing LPS-mediated pro-inflammatory microenvironment in the liver.

3. Gut-liver axis

Gut microbiota are known to influence multiple extraintestinal organs; however the importance of the gut-liver axis has understandably received greater attention in recent years. The gut and liver share anatomy from the embryonic phase, with bidirectional interaction through the portal vein. The symbiotic relationship between the gut microbiota and the liver is modulated by the nutrition, immune, metabolic, and neuroendocrine crosstalk between them and thus shapes human health and disease [8]. Functionally, gut and liver coordination influences our physiology. The liver receives 70% of the blood supply from the gut via the portal circulation. The nutrient-rich blood from the gut is effectively processed by the liver and delivered to systemic circulation for normal body growth. In turn, the liver synthesizes bile acids (BAs) and other mediators, like IgA, which influence intestinal microbial composition and barrier integrity, thereby maintaining intestinal homeostasis [8]. Bile acids are involved in energy homeostasis by regulating the metabolism of glucose and lipids and also help in conjugation and detoxification process as well as maintenance of intact intestinal epithelia. Bile acids also regulate microbial composition via antimicrobial peptides production; in turn, microbiota influences the bile acid pool in the intestine as they are involved in secondary bile acid production [9]. IgA secreted from the liver and intestine prevents growth and invasion of pathogenic bacteria to maintain normal gut-liver homeostasis [7]. In normal physiological conditions, translocation of gut bacteria and their metabolites is tightly regulated by the intestinal epithelial barrier, and if any reaches the liver, it is eliminated by hepatic Kupffer cells. Any breach in barrier integrity resulting from intestinal inflammation allows microbiota to pass through the portal vein to potentially trigger hepatic immune cells to enact an inflammatory response (from hepatic stellate cells and Kupffer cells), which may result in necrotic inflammation and hepatic fibrosis contributing to worsening fibrosis and thus liver disease progression [10]. Accumulating evidence suggests gut dysbiosis, bacterial endotoxin, and increased intestinal permeability are hallmark features of CLD and positively correlate with disease severity. These factors play a crucial role in the pathogenesis of not only CLD but have also been shown to promote HCC through various mechanisms (**Figure 1**).

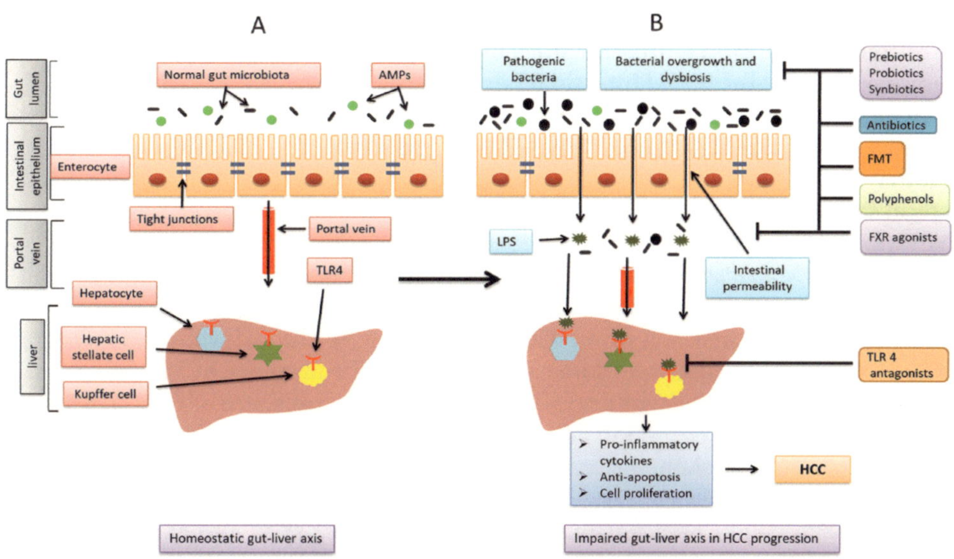

Figure 1.
An overview of homeostatic and impaired gut-liver axis in HCC progression. (A) In homeostatic condition gut lumen contains normal gut flora which is restricted by tightly closed intestinal epithelial cells to prevent its translocation to the liver. (B) Increased bacterial overgrowth in gut lumen and increased intestinal permeability promotes HCC progression through binding of LPS to toll-like receptor 4 (TLR4) which are present on Kupffer cells, hepatocytes, and HSC to elicit the release of pro-inflammatory cytokines and activation of proliferative and anti-apoptotic signals. Prebiotics, probiotics, synbiotics, FMT, and polyphenols can be used to restore eubiosis, while the use of antibiotics can potentially eliminate pathogenic bacteria and endotoxin release. FXR agonists can attenuate intestinal permeability and prevent bacterial translocation. TLR4 antagonists prevent binding of LPS to TLR4 and suppress cancer-promoting signals.

4. Gut dysbiosis

Dysbiosis defines any change in the typical gut microbial composition found in health. Several lines of evidence suggest that gut bacterial dysbiosis is a pathogenic factor in the progression of HCC whatever the trigger for CLD (e.g., alcohol, non-alcoholic steatohepatitis (NASH), viral hepatitis, etc.). The role of gut dysbiosis in the propagation of progressive CLD is likely triggered by the formation of microbial metabolites such as LPS, bacterial DNA, and deoxycholic acid, which causes chronic inflammation in the portal circulation and thus the liver. In cirrhotic patients overgrowth of the pathogenic bacteria such as *Enterobacteriaceae*, *Veillonellaceae*, and *Streptococcaceae* and decreased *Lachnospiraceae* have been observed to correlate with the child-turcotte-pugh (CTP) score, clinically used to assess the severity of cirrhosis [11]. Moreover, in cirrhotic patients studies have found an increase in both the oral and gut levels of the same microbial species suggesting invasion from the mouth to intestine [12]. It is therefore postulated oral bacterial overgrowth may have a profound effect on intestinal bacterial communities and thus CLD pathogenesis and HCC development. This concept is supported by a recent study that showed a high level of oral microbiota *Oribacterium* and *Fusobacterium* in HCC patients [13]. The alteration in gut microbiota composition in HCC is summarized in **Table 1**.

Microbial gene signatures that relate to energy production, nickel/iron transport, and amino acid transport appear to be altered in HCC patients when compared to healthy controls [13]. Moreover, when compared to cirrhotic patients, fecal samples from HCC patients have shown increased growth of phylum *Actinobacteria* and 13 genera including *Gemmiger* and *Parabacteroides* [14]. They also found a decrease in butyrate-producing bacteria and an increase in LPS-producing bacteria in HCC patients when compared to healthy controls [14]. A study conducted by *Ponziani* et al. in NAFLD-related HCC showed increased fecal *Bacteroides* and *Ruminococcaceae*, whereas reduced *Akkermansia* and *Bifidobacterium* were negatively correlated with intestinal inflammatory marker fecal calprotectin level [15]. This study also showed increased intestinal permeability in these patients accompanied by an increase in plasma level of IL8, IL13, CCL3, CCL4, and CCL5, showing the evidence that alteration in gut microbiota profile is associated with systemic inflammation that may contribute to HCC pathogenesis [15]. In another study, *E. coli* growth in fecal samples was significantly elevated in HCC patients compared to matched cirrhotic patients [16]. Interestingly, inoculation of AFB1 and/or *Helicobacter hepaticus* in *Helicobacter*-free C3H/HeN mice was associated with HCC progression [17]. This observation may suggest that neither direct bacterial translocation nor hepatocyte injury is necessary for HCC development. In clinical studies utilizing liver HCC tumor biopsy tissue, some authors report the presence of *Helicobacter* ssp. DNA, whereas other investigators failed to correlate the presence of *Helicobacter* ssp. DNA with HCC progression [18]. In DEN-treated rats, fecal and cecal samples show an increase of pathogenic bacterial species like *E. coli*, *Atopobium*, *Collinsella*, *Eggerthella*, and *Corynebacterium*; in contrast there was a decline in the numbers of beneficial bacteria like *Lactobacillus* spp., *Bifidobacterium* spp., and *Enterococcus* spp. [19]. Although the exact mechanism by which gut microbiota promotes HCC has not been firmly established, studies in murine models indicated LPS-TLR4 axis plays a crucial role in the progression of HCC [19, 20]. Zhang et al. suggest that gut dysbiosis merely promotes HCC by increasing LPS levels and that conversely probiotics may suppresses tumor growth [19]. Similarly, Dapito et al. propose that gut microbiota only has a role in the promotion of HCC rather than its initiation [20]. The ability of pathogenic bacteria to disrupt TJs protein thereby increasing intestinal permeability has also been postulated as another mechanism by which microbiota may promote CLD and HCC [21]. However further preclinical and clinical studies

Authors	Sample type	Changes in fecal microbiota composition	Clinical implication in HCC
Ren et al. [14]	Feces	*Klebsiella i*	• Increase in lipopolysaccharide-producing bacteria promotes HCC progression • Decrease in butyrate-producing bacteria promotes intestinal mucosal injury which contributes to HCC development
Ponziani et al. [15]	Feces	*Bacteroides* ↑ *Ruminococcaceae* ↑ *Enterococcus* ↑ *Phascolarctobacterium* ↑ *Oscillospira* ↑ *Bifidobacterium* ↓ *Blautia* ↓	• Increase in Gram-negative bacteria promotes HCC progression • Decrease in beneficial bacteria was correlated with intestinal inflammation favoring local microenvironment for HCC development
Grat et al. [16]	Feces	*Escherichia coli* ↑	• Increase in *pathogenic E. coli* contributes to HCC progression
Huang et al. [18]	HCC liver biopsy	*Helicobacter pylori* ↑	• Helicobacter linked to hepatocarcinogenesis by colonizing the liver
Zhang et al. [19]	Feces	*Escherichia coli* ↑ *Atopobium cluster* ↓ *Prevotella* ↓ *Bacteroides* ↑ *Lactobacillus* spp. ↑ *Bifidobacterium* spp. ↑ *Enterococcus* spp. ↓	• Alteration in gut microbiota profile promoted tumor formation in DEN-induced HCC rats
Yoshimoto et al. [38]	Feces	*Clostridium* cluster XI and XIVa ↑	• Increase in deoxycholic acid -producing bacteria accelerated HCC progression in DMBA-HFD-induced HCC rats • Deoxycholic acid is a risk factor for obesity-induced HCC development

Table 1.
Gut microbiota dysbiosis in HCC.

are needed to establish the causal link between gut microbiota and HCC progression and to further delineate the molecular mechanisms involved.

5. Inflammation as a key player: triggered by LPS-TLR4 mediated pathway

HCC is arising in an inflammatory environment of the CLD, and therefore, neutralizing inflammation with anti-inflammatory agents may reduce the incidence and recurrence of HCC. Much attention has been focused on the potential involvement of the toll-like receptors (TLR) signaling pathway in the development of liver inflammation and associated HCC progression. Gut-derived endotoxin initiates the innate immune system such as TLRs, which recognize bacterial products and are predominantly expressed throughout the gut-liver axis. In addition, TLR4 plays a central role through LPS (a component of Gram-negative bacteria)-induced hepatic inflammation, while TLR 2 senses component of Gram-positive bacteria such as peptidoglycan [22]. In this context, Yu et al. identified that increased activation of the TLR 4-LPS axis correlated with intestinal permeability in DEN-induced acute liver failure (ALF), which directly regulates pro-survival molecules and enhances hepatocyte proliferation [23]. Interestingly, in mice models the use of antibiotics and/or TLR4 genetic ablation prevented tumor growth and multiplicity [19, 23]. Dapito et al. showed a close link between gut microbiota and LPS-TLR 4 axis in HCC progression in a chimeric mice model [20]. This study also showed in DEN-CCl4 treated mice (with histological CLD) that low-dose LPS treatment triggered TLR4 activation and increased rate of tumor formation, whereas gut sterilization prevented HCC progression rather than regression of the established tumor [20]. Taken together these studies would therefore suggest that gut microbiota may not have a role in HCC initiation but may instead have a tumor-promoting effect through TLRs signaling pathways [20].

In respect of HCC promotion, multiple downstream targets of the LPS-TLR4 axis have been identified in both in vitro and in vivo studies. HSCs, Kupffer cells, and hepatocytes show TLR4 expression and thus are sensitive to LPS challenge [24]. Dapito et al. showed that TLR4 activation in HSCs, hepatocytes, and non-bone-marrow-derived resident cells promotes hepatocarcinogenesis by upregulating epiregulin (hepatomitogen) and inhibiting cleaved caspase 3 via NF-κB activation [20]. Moreover, Yu et al. showed hepatic Kupffer cells as the chief target for LPS-induced TLR4 activation by increasing pro-inflammatory cytokines such as TNF-α and IL-6 production [23]. Similarly, in vitro studies have shown evidence of LPS-TLR4-promoted HCC cell proliferation via NF-κB, MAPK, and STAT3 mediated signaling pathways [24]. LPS-TLR4 has also been shown to promote epithelial-to-mesenchymal transition (EMT) in HCC by upregulating NF-κB- and JNK/MAPK-mediated expression, while NF-κB and JNK/MAPK signaling blockade inhibited EMT occurrence [25]. Similarly, LPS-TLR4 axis is also known to enhance angiogenesis in HCC mice model via production of pro-angiogenic factors by HSCs in tumor stroma [26]. However further studies incorporating TLR4 deletion are needed to better understand its role in hepatocyte proliferation and distinguish paracrine signaling from HSCs and Kupffer cells in HCC progression.

6. Intestinal epithelial barrier dysfunction: role of tight junction proteins

Commensals and opportunistic pathogens are kept in check within the intestinal lumen by a single layer of intestinal epithelial cells (IEC) which spans almost 400 m^2 in surface area [27]. The gut barrier is highly dynamic in nature in which IEC is capable of self-renewal every 4–7 days with constant changes in intestinal luminal content. IEC are predominantly composed of absorptive enterocytes, which have metabolic and digestive functions. It also has secretory functions enacted by cell types such as enteroendocrine, goblet, and paneth cells which are specialized for maintaining digestive, immune, and epithelial barrier function [27]. Enteroendocrine cells connect the central and enteric neuroendocrine system via the secretion of various digestive hormones like gastrin, cholecystokinin, incretin, etc. The highly glycosylated mucins secreted by goblet cells form the first line of defense against microbial invasion and when compromised may predispose to disease as is evident in Mucin 2-deficient mice which are susceptible to colitis and inflammation-induced colorectal cancer [28, 29]. The intestinal barrier function is further strengthened by antimicrobial peptides (AMPs) including defensin, cathelicidin, and lysozyme [27]. These AMPs disrupt bacterial cell membranes and prevent adherence to gut mucosa.

Apart from IEC, the gut barrier is primarily maintained by tight junction (TJs) components (e.g., claudin, occludin, zonula occludens, and other junctional adhesion molecules (JAMs)) preserving intact epithelia which in turn regulate the paracellular movement of solutes, water, and other nutrients while restricting the entry of bacteria from the lumen to systemic circulation [30]. The mechanism of increased intestinal permeability is poorly understood. Growing evidence suggests that inflammation and TJ protein disruption are two of the key players driving increased intestinal permeability. In our previous study, we found increased systemic ZO-1 level in HCC patients reflecting increased intestinal permeability [31]. Moreover, plasma ZO-1 level was positively correlated with the inflammatory marker hs-CRP and with disease severity, suggesting inflammation drives intestinal permeability associated with HCC progression [31]. Bacterial overgrowth leads to increased production of pro-inflammatory cytokines such as TNF-α, IL-6, and IL-1β, which is mainly mediated through the TLR4-NF-kB signaling pathway, thereby promoting intestinal inflammation and HCC progression [19]. These pro-inflammatory cytokines have a direct effect on TJ proteins like claudin and ZO-1, leading to enhance intestinal permeability [32]. Furthermore, in both in vivo and in vitro models, LPS dose dependently increases intestinal permeability via upregulating TLR4-mediated CD14 expression in enterocytes [33]. Similarly, NLRP6-deficient mice show altered microbiota and enhanced colonic inflammation through the chemokine (C-C motif) ligand CCL5 [34]. This results in increased intestinal permeability to microbial products and thus increases hepatic inflammation and progression from NAFLD to NASH [34]. Moreover, enteric pathogens such as *Escherichia coli* and *Clostridium difficile* are increased in CLD and are capable of increased intestinal permeability by modulating TJ integrity [11, 21].

Bile acids are another key player for maintaining gut barrier function by promoting intestinal epithelial cell proliferation and microbiota composition [35]. There is clear evidence that bile acids have both direct antimicrobial effect and an indirect effect through FXR-induced AMPs and thus control growth and adhesion of intestinal bacteria. In fact, decreased bile acids pool in the intestine is associated with bacterial overgrowth and inflammation [36]. The study by Kakiyama et al. showed that cirrhosis reduced bile acids entering the intestine causing bacterial dysbiosis by reducing beneficial bacteria such as Gram-positive *Blautia and Ruminococcaceae* and increasing pathogenic bacteria like *Enterobacteriaceae* [37]. In a NASH-induced CLD/HCC mouse model, increased Gram-positive *Clostridium* clusters (XI and XVIa) were positively correlated with increased serum deoxycholic acid (DCA) [38]. Notably, *Clostridium clusters* are capable of synthesis of secondary bile acid DCA via 7α-dehydroxylation of primary bile acids. DCA is a DNA-damaging agent and a known pro-carcinogen shown to affect various cancer signaling pathways. In this context, a study by *Yoshimoto* et al. revealed DCA activates a senescent-associated secretory phenotype in HSCs, thereby producing various pro-inflammatory and pro-tumorigenic factors promoting HCC development in mice, while antibiotic treatment and/or blocking DCA production prevented HCC development [38]. Similarly, in a HCC mouse model induced by steatohepatitis-inducing high-fat diet (STHD-01), increased hepatic and fecal bile acids concentrations were observed [39]. In this model, DCA activated mTOR and promoted HCC development. However, following antibiotic treatment, there was a decrease in HCC progression suggesting an interrelationship between BA metabolism, gut microbiota, and HCC development [39].

Bile acids maintain homeostatic IEC proliferation via EGFR- and FXR-dependent pathways, which helps the continuous regeneration of enterocytes and maintain intact epithelia [40]. Several studies demonstrate that the intestinal bile acid pool also regulates TJ protein distribution and expression. In Caco-2 cell monolayers, incubation with dihydroxy bile acids decreased transepithelial resistance (TER) and was accompanied by increased phosphorylation and redistribution of occludin [41]. In human colonic biopsies, DCA induces Cr-EDTA permeability altering TER and increasing translocation of *E. coli*. Several in vivo studies have also elucidated the role of bile acids in the regulation of TJ permeability [42]. In HFD mice increased intestinal bile acid pool was associated with increased intestinal permeability with decreased expression of TJ proteins ZO-2 and JAM-A [43]. Similarly, in bile duct ligated (BDL) rats where intestinal BA delivery was prevented, there was increased bacterial translocation and increased intestinal permeability with decreased expression of claudin-1 and occludin. Conversely, the above effects were ameliorated by FXR activation [44]. These studies highlighted the protective role of FXR in the maintenance of intestinal barrier integrity; however, it is unclear whether these effects were from direct activation of FXR on TJ proteins or indirect effects from altered mucosal immune cells. In addition to FXR, another bile acid receptor TGR5 also modulates barrier permeability and TJ protein expression. In TGR5 null mice, increased intestinal permeability due to alteration of TJ protein expression develops colitis [45]. Therefore, the quantity and composition of BA pool in the intestine represent an important factor in the regulation of gut microbial community and gut barrier integrity.

7. Therapeutic approach controlling gut microbiota, gut dysbiosis, and inflammation to prevent HCC

7.1 Prebiotics, probiotics, and synbiotics

Traditionally, HCC is cured based on the available treatment options such as surgical treatment, chemotherapy, and local ablation therapy; however, patients are facing many problems including the poor hepatic reserve [46]. Furthermore, the possible therapeutic interventions targeting the gut-liver axis in HCC are summarized in **Table 2**.

Prebiotics are non-absorbant and nondigestible food ingredients which promote growth or activity of beneficial bacteria like *Bifidobacteria* and *Lactobacilli* and inhibit the growth of potentially pathogenic bacteria [47]. Currently, prebiotics like lactulose, lactitol, fructo-oligosaccharides, and galacto-oligosaccharides are commercially available [48]. Synthetic disaccharides like lactulose and lactitol are extensively used for the treatment of hepatic encephalopathy in CLD patients as ammonia detoxifying agents [48]. Also, these disaccharides are metabolized by colonic bacteria to produce lactic acid and acetic acid due to which pH in the gut lumen is decreased [49]. Low pH enhances the growth of non-urease-producing *lactobacilli* and inhibits pathogenic urease-producing bacteria [50]. Chen et al. showed that in chronic viral hepatitis patients, lactitol administration significantly decreased plasma endotoxin levels and increased the growth of beneficial *Lactobacilli* and *Bifidobacteria* species [51]. In contrast, Bajaj et al. reported lactulose administration in patients with HE did not improve dysbiosis and increased growth of Gram-negative bacteria such as *Enterobacteriaceae and Bacteroidaceae* [52]. This indicates the pattern of gut microbiota abundance is the major determinants of disease severity [52]. In HCC patients administration of lactulose (30 mL/day) for 14 days significantly reduced ALT and bilirubin levels, while antioxidant enzyme SOD, anti-inflammatory markers IFN-γ and IL-4, and blood cells CD4(+)/CD8(+) were found to be increased suggesting its ability to reduce inflammation and restore oxidation/antioxidant system imbalance [53]. Similarly in partial hepatectomized rats, administration of lactulose induces liver regeneration by

Authors	Intervention class	Medication	Desired effect in HCC
Zong et al. [53]	Prebiotics	Lactulose	• Lactulose treatment to HCC patients increased antioxidant enzymes and anti-inflammatory markers while improving tumor immunity and overall prognosis
Zhang et al. [19]	Probiotics	VSL#3	• VSL#3 treatment to DEN-induced HCC rats reduced tumor number and multiplicity by ameliorating hepatic and intestinal inflammation and improving intestinal permeability and restoring eubiosis
El-Nezami et al. [63]	Probiotics	*Lactobacillus rhamnosus LC 705* and *Propionibacterium freudenreichii subsp. shermani*	• Treatment to AFB1-induced HCC patients reduced aflatoxin-DNA adduct excretion in urine
Li et al. [46]	Probiotics	Prohep	• Treatment with Prohep to DEN-induced HCC mice reduced tumor size and angiogenic factors *VEGFA* and *TEK*
Kumar et al. [62]	Probiotics	Combination of probiotic fermented milk and chlorophyllin	• Treatment to AFB1-induced HCC rats reduced DNA damage, oncogenic signal, and tumor incidence
Yoshimoto et al. [38]	Antibiotics	4Abx (ampicillin, metronidazole, vancomycin, neomycin)	• Treatment with 4Abx in DMBA-HFD-induced HCC rats reduced tumor number and tumor size
Abdel-Hamid et al. [67]	Antibiotics	Clarithromycin and azithromycin	• Treatment to DEN-CCL4/acetylaminofluorene-induced HCC rats induced intrinsic and extrinsic apoptosis and inhibited HCC progression
Dapito et al. [20]	Antibiotics	Rifaximin	• Rifaximin treatment to DEN-CCL4 induced HCC rats reduced tumor number
Nguyen et al. [93]	TLR4 antagonists	TAK-242	• TAK-242 treatment to transgenic HCC mice reduced tumor burden and ameliorated hepatic steatosis and fibrosis
Nkontchou et al. [117]	Nonselective β-blockers	Propranolol	• Long-term treatment with propranolol reduced HCC incidence in HCV-related cirrhosis patients
Chang et al. [118]	Nonselective β-blockers	Propranolol	• Treatment with propranolol reduced mortality risk and improved survival in unresectable/metastatic HCC patients
Bishayee et al. [121]	Natural compound	Resveratrol	• Resveratrol treatment to DEN-induced HCC rats reduced hepatic nodules and prevented HCC progression
Ji et al. [124]	Natural compound	Quercetin	• Quercetin treatment to DEN-acetylaminofluorene-induced HCC rats reduced number of nodules
Teng et al. [125]	Natural compound	Curcumin	• Treatment with curcumin to HBV-related transgenic HCC mice reduced hepatic nodules and suppressed HCC progression

Table 2.
Therapeutic intervention targeting the gut-liver axis in HCC.

inducing hydrogen and abrogating oxidative stress (heme oxygenase-1, SOD-2) and inflammation (IL-6 and TNF-α) [54]. Moreover, mixed diets of galacto-oligosaccharides and fructo-oligosaccharides to infants were increased the growth of *Bifidobacterium*; however, this formulation has not been tried in patients with liver disease [55].

Probiotics are live microorganisms which when administered in adequate amounts confer a health benefit for the host [56]. Probiotic supplementation was also shown to restore intestinal dysbiosis in CLD patients [48]. Furthermore, mice treated with probiotic such as VSL#3 significantly reduces *Clostridium* spp. and modified gut microbiota [57]. In cirrhotic patients, VSL#3 supplementation for nearly 6 months was shown to reduce the risk of hospitalization and improved CTP and MELD score [58]. Similarly, in NASH-associated obese children, treatment with VSL#3 over the period of 4 months reduces fatty liver and improved lipid profile and insulin sensitivity [59]. The other probiotics such as *Lactobacillus salivarius* LI01 and *Pediococcus pentosaceus* LI05 reduced inflammation, protected the intestinal barrier, prevented bacterial translocation, restored eubiosis, and attenuated hepatic fibrosis in CCl_4-induced cirrhotic rats [60]. Similarly, *Lactobacillus* GG (LGG) supplemented with standard diet in cirrhosis patients show significantly reduced blood endotoxemia and TNF-α, thereby restoring eubiosis [61]. However, in HCC, probiotic usage is meager, and only a few studies have identified the therapeutic potential. VSL#3 (contains three strains of *Bifidobacteria*, four strains of *Lactobacilli*, and one strain of *Streptococcus thermophilus*) treatment to DEN-induced rat hepatocarcinogenesis has shown to attenuate HCC progression, reduce tumor number and multiplicity, ameliorate hepatic and intestinal inflammation, and thus restore gut dysbiosis [19]. Li et al. identified that subcutaneous administration of Prohep (a novel probiotic mixture of *Lactobacillus rhamnosus GG*, *Escherichia coli Nissle 1917*, and heat-inactivated VSL#3) reduced the tumor size and HCC growth [46]. Prohep improves beneficial bacteria such as *Prevotella* and *Oscillibacter* and control tissue inflammation as evidenced by decreased T helper 17 cells in the gut, thereby attenuating the progression of HCC [46]. Moreover, in aflatoxin B1-induced HCC rats, treatment with probiotic fermented milk and chlorophyllin significantly reduced tumor incidence by decreasing the expression of cyclin D1, bcl-2, and c-myc proto-oncogenes [62]. Similarly, aflatoxin-induced HCC patients treated with dietary supplementation of probiotics (using viable *Lactobacillus rhamnosus LC 705* and *Propionibacterium freudenreichii subsp. shermani)* decreased the urinary excretion of aflatoxin-DNA adduct (AFB-N7 guanine) and improved HCC [63]. Thus, probiotic supplementation could be beneficial to cirrhotic patients with the potential to progress to HCC.

Synbiotics are combined form of prebiotics and probiotics, which contains four fermentable fibers (symbiotic 2000) and four freeze-dried non-urease-producing lactic acid bacteria. Synbiotic administration to cirrhotic patients results in decreased plasma endotoxin and ammonia levels and increased fecal *Lactobacillus* spp. [64]. Interestingly 50% of these patients have improved child-turcotte-pugh score compared to placebo [64]. Moreover, in NAFLD patients synbiotic supplementation has shown to have beneficial effects by improving lipid profile, glucose homeostasis, hepatic marker enzymes, and inflammatory markers [65]. Synbiotic (FloraGuard) administration also has a protective role in alcohol-induced liver injury in rats [66]. In addition, the synbiotic treatment restored ethanol-induced intestinal permeability and increased the growth of beneficial bacteria *Bifidobacterium* spp. and *Lactobacillus* spp. [66]. Currently, studies are lacking for the use of synbiotics in chronic liver diseases or HCC prevention.

8. Antibiotics

Several studies have postulated that antibiotic treatment may cause gut microbiota dysbiosis. It may represent effective strategies to prevent the tumor-promoting gut microbiota, its metabolites DCA, and pro-inflammatory signal inducer LPS which all have a role in the progression of CLD and HCC. In DEN-CCl_4- and DMBA-HFD-induced HCC mice model, the oral antibiotics ampicillin, metronidazole, neomycin, and vancomycin significantly reduced the tumor number and size [20, 38]. In addition, this antibiotic combination also reduced the liver fibrosis and improved liver histology in cirrhosis. Moreover, the effectiveness of antibiotics administration was enhanced when given at late-stage HCC in mice rather than earlier stage [20]. In another study conducted in DEN-induced HCC rats, clarithromycin and azithromycin suppressed HCC progression through extrinsic and intrinsic apoptotic pathways, whereas erythromycin aggravated HCC and did not show antitumorigenic effect [67]. Vancomycin is an antibiotic used to treat a bacterial infection, which effectively prevented the mouse model of HCC; however, long-term administration to CLD patients develops potential side effects [38]. Many studies have concluded that norfloxacin and rifaximin treatments to cirrhotic patients have beneficial effects [68]. In a double-blind placebo-controlled clinical trial, long-term oral administration of norfloxacin to cirrhotic patients markedly reduces Gram-negative bacteria in the fecal matters and lowers the spontaneous bacterial peritonitis (SBP) [69]. Furthermore, CCl_4-induced cirrhotic animals showed decreased SBP and inflammation following norfloxacin treatment [70]. Norfloxacin was identified as a promising antibiotic in regulating gut microbiota overgrowth and prevention of BT in both cirrhotic humans and rodents; indeed its effect on HCC patients remains unidentified. Rifaximin is a broad spectrum oral antibiotic having potential bactericidal activity against aerobic and anaerobic Gram-negative bacteria [71]. It is an excellent choice of drug to cure HE in advanced cirrhotic patients [72]. The study conducted by *Vlachogiannakos* et al. showed treatment with rifaximin for 4 weeks significantly decreased portal pressure and LPS levels in decompensated cirrhotic patients [73]. Long-term treatment with rifaximin reduces SBP occurrence, variceal bleeding, HRS, and HE with an overall improvement in survival rate in cirrhotic patients [74]. Similarly, in murine DEN-CCl_4-induced HCC mouse model, rifaximin treatment was shown to ameliorate HCC progression [20]. Although rifaximin is clinically used for prevention of HE and other complications in cirrhotic patients, its role in HCC prevention in humans is further warranted.

9. Fecal microbiota transplantation (FMT)

Fecal microbiota transplantation is currently being used for the treatment of *Clostridium difficile* infection [75]. The enteric dysbiosis was restored to normal gut flora following FMT from healthy donor to *Clostridium difficile*-infected patients [75]. Moreover, in mice with gut dysbiosis induced by antibiotics and chemotherapy, treatments were reversed by FMT [76]. In experimental cirrhosis with hepatic encephalopathy, FMT improves liver function and HE grade by limiting inflammation and improving tight junction integrity [77]. In this context, Bajaj et al. reported that FMT in cirrhotic patients with recurrent HE improves cognition, restores dysbiosis, and improves MELD score compared to standard care in those patients [78]. A number of clinical trials are ongoing in patients with NASH and cirrhosis for the efficacy of FMT [79, 80]. Vrieze et al. reported in patients with severe metabolic syndrome that treatment with FMT from a healthy donor improves liver biochemistry, peripheral insulin resistance, and restoration of eubiosis [81]. Furthermore, in alcoholic hepatitis patients, FMT treatment significantly reduced liver disease severity and HE occurrence [82]. FMT recipients also showed an increase in beneficial bacteria like *Actinobacteria* and *Bifidobacterium longum* and decrease in *Pseudomonas* and *E. coli* with an increase in bile secretion [82]. Collectively these findings indicated that FMT may restore gut dysbiosis and reduce complications in cirrhotic patients and thus attenuate HCC development. However, scarce literature supporting the beneficial effect of FMT and long-term study is needed to prove permanent colonization in altered gut microbiota environment in cirrhotic patients. Moreover, there is a chance of inducing viral infection and transmission of other pathogens through FMT which may have deleterious effect and immunosuppression in advanced liver disease patients [83, 84].

10. TLR agonist or antagonist

Numerous studies have shown that LPS-TLR4 is a key inflammatory pathway in the progression of CLD and has a tumor-promoting effect on HCC [20, 23, 85]. Therefore blocking this pathway might represent a promising treatment approach in controlling cirrhosis and HCC progression. Several TLR4 antagonists have been developed toward controlling LPS-activated TLR4-mediated inflammatory responses which include polymyxin B [86], glycolipids interfering CD14-LPS interaction [87], eritoran [88], resatorvid (TAK242) [89], and thalidomide [90]. In BDL-induced cirrhotic rats, intravenous administration of TAK-242 significantly reduces plasma transaminases and inflammatory cytokines [91]. It also ameliorates acetaminophen-induced acute liver failure [92]. Similarly, in transgenic HCC mice (Hep*Pten*$^{-}$), TAK-242 treatment for 28 days significantly reduced tumor burden and ameliorated HCC progression [93]. Eritoran tetrasodium protects against liver ischemia/reperfusion injury by inhibiting inflammatory response induced by high-mobility group box protein B1 (HMGB1) [94]. Similarly in D-galactosamine- and LPS-induced acute liver failure, treatment with eritoran significantly reduces inflammation and hepatic marker enzymes [95]. Eritoran treatment also decreases proliferation and induces apoptosis in tumor cells in a chemically induced mouse model of colorectal carcinoma [96]. Although resatorvid and eritoran showed the beneficial effect in improving the survival of murine sepsis model, it failed to do so in patients with severe sepsis [97]. Several TLRs have been upregulated in HCC [98]. In addition, TLRs are also abundantly expressed on immune cells which recognize various pathogens such as HBV which upon activation induces an innate immune response [99]. All the TLRs are activated by two independent pathways: MyD88-dependent (except TLR3) and MyD88-independent (TLR3 and TLR4) pathway [100]. Activation of TLR3-TRIF signaling pathway leads to apoptotic activity independently and, in turn, also activates IRF3 transcription factor to produce interferons [100]. TLR3 agonist BM-06 (synthetic dsRNA) significantly inhibited HCC cell proliferation, increased apoptosis, and decreased cell invasion and migration with increased antiviral IFN level [101]. Activation of TLR9 leads to phosphorylation of NF-κB with increased production of pro-inflammatory cytokine TNF-α, IL-6, and IL-10 [102]. Mohamed et al. showed that inhibition of TLR7 and TLR9 with antagonist IRS-954 or chloroquine significantly reduces HCC cell proliferation, angiogenesis with increased apoptosis [103]. This was further supported by tumor xenograft and DEN-induced rat HCC model in which chloroquine treatment reduces HCC incidence [103]. Although growing evidence shows TLRs as an important mediator of HCC progression, the molecular mechanism for disease progression is not completely understood. Therefore, further research needs to be done for the use of TLR agonist or antagonist as a drug target for HCC prevention since TLRs are also involved in both cancer-promoting mechanism and immune-modulator which is responsible for an innate immune response against tumor cells and HBV and HCV infection [99, 104–106].

11. Prokinetics

Bacterial overgrowth due to impaired gut motility has been reported in cirrhotic patients [107]. Cisapride, a prokinetic drug, has shown beneficial effects not only by regulating intestinal motility but also inhibiting bacterial overgrowth and preventing bacterial translocation in both rodent models and liver cirrhotic patients [108, 109]. Cisapride in combination with norfloxacin significantly reduces the incidence of SBP in high-risk cirrhotic patients [110]. Although the mechanism of impaired gastrointestinal motility in cirrhotic patients is unclear, increased adrenergic activity may be responsible for the altered motility.

12. Nonselective beta-blockers (NSBB)

Nonselective β-blockers are prevalently used in decompensated chronic liver disease patients to reduce morbidity and mortality. It is used as bleeding prophylaxis in cirrhotic patients with esophageal varices. NSBB also antagonizes β-adrenoceptors. The β-adrenergic receptor pathway is involved in maintaining normal physiological functions. The catecholamines such as epinephrine and norepinephrine are the key ligands for β-adrenoceptors (β1 and β2). Furthermore, increased expression of β-adrenoceptors was observed in HCC cell membranes compared to healthy liver cells; however, the mechanisms remain unclear [111]. Catecholamines exhibit pro-carcinogenic effects in gastric, pancreatic, and breast cancer, which is antagonized by NSBB. Its beneficial effects to reduce the risk of HCC have also been identified by the very recent observational and experimental trials [112]. Moreover, in ovarian and breast cancer patients, NSBB treatment was shown to reduce cancer formation and growth. In cirrhotic patients, increased catecholamines results in disease severity, and thus, NSBB treatment may be potent to inhibit carcinogenesis in cirrhosis [113]. A recent study by Leithead et al. showed NSBB is safe and may confer benefit in patients with ascites complicating the end-stage liver disease [114]. In addition, Reiberger et al. observed that NSBB treatment ameliorates intestinal permeability and reduces BT in cirrhotic patients [115]. In a recent study, Wang et al. showed propranolol induces apoptosis and suppresses proliferation of liver cancer cells [116]. Of note, long-term treatment with propranolol in patients with HCV-related cirrhosis reduces the incidence of HCC [117]. Similarly, in patients with unresectable/metastatic HCC cohort, propranolol treatment significantly reduces mortality risk and improved overall survival suggesting β-blockers might be another therapeutic approach in HCC prevention [118].

13. Natural compounds

Treatment with natural compounds and food ingredients like polyphenols represents another therapeutic approach in the restoration of eubiosis, modulation of gut microbiota, reduction of inflammation, prevention of cirrhosis, and thus the progression of HCC. Many experimental data have shown evidence that flavonoids are proficient to alter gut microbial composition and restoration of eubiosis in chronic liver diseases. Proanthocyanidin improves beneficial microbiota *Bacteroides* such as *Lactobacillus* spp. and *Bifidobacterium* spp. composition and reduces intestinal inflammation and oxidative damage, thereby attenuating experimental colon cancer. Resveratrol, a flavonoid, is shown to modulate intestinal microbiota with a profound increase in *Bifidobacterium* spp. and *Lactobacillus* spp. and reduce systemic and colonic inflammation in rats [119]. Resveratrol also shown to have anticancer activity in HCC cell lines; inhibit proliferation, viability, invasion, and metastasis; and induce apoptosis [120]. Its anticancer property was also studied in DEN-induced hepatocarcinogenesis [121]. We found resveratrol treatment to cirrhotic mice attenuated systemic inflammation and ammonia levels and altered neuronal TJ proteins, thereby preventing secondary complications such as HE in cirrhosis [122]. Quercetin, a bioactive flavonoid, was shown to inhibit human HCC cell proliferation, migration, and invasion and trigger apoptosis both in vivo and in vitro [123]. Its profound antitumor effect was also shown in xenograft and DEN-induced HCC rodent models [124]. Curcumin, a powerful antioxidant, has a wide range of bioactive properties. Previous studies have shown evidence that curcumin has HCC chemoprevention in preclinical models as well as patients with HCC [125, 126]. Moreover, nimbolide from the leaf of the neem tree (*Azadirachta indica*) is another potential natural compound having antioxidant, anti-inflammatory, antibacterial, antiviral, and anticancer properties [127]. In vitro study in HCC cell line (HepG2) shows that nimbolide induces cell apoptosis by abrogating NF-κB and Wnt signaling pathway [128]. Currently, our lab is focusing on anticancer effects of nimbolide and its molecular mechanisms in an experimental hepatocarcinogenesis. Of note, these natural compounds have a wide variety of biological activities on gut microbiota and may preserve gut barrier integrity, microbial metabolites, TJ integrity, and mucosal immunology. Indeed, further human studies are warranted to see the effect of natural compounds on gut microbial modulation and prevention of HCC.

14. Targeting gut epithelial barrier to prevent HCC

Gut epithelial barrier acts as a fence for translocation of gut microbiota and its metabolite into the systemic circulation which is the major driving factor for CLD progression and HCC development [129]. Therefore, primarily targeting or restoring the gut epithelial barrier is an interesting therapeutic approach in HCC pathogenesis. Compelling evidence has shown that targeting gut microbiota (restoring eubiosis) directly or receptor-mediated pharmacological intervention using TLR4 antagonist or FXR agonist might improve epithelial barrier function [130, 131]. FXR is a BA receptor which is widely expressed throughout the gut-liver axis. Decreased BA is associated with intestinal bacterial overgrowth, increased gut permeability, and bacterial translocation in rodents [38]. FXR controls hepatic inflammation, promotes liver regeneration, and suppresses HCC formation mainly through enterokine FGF19 [132]. FXR null mice have an intestinal barrier dysfunction and high occurrence of HCC, whereas reactivation of FXR inhibited HCC through FGF15-cyp7a1 axis [133]. In this context, FXR agonist obeticholic acid (OCA) prevents gut barrier dysfunction and BT in cholestatic rats [131]. Furthermore, in CCl_4-induced cirrhotic rats, OCA treatment significantly reduces BT and inhibits intestinal inflammation by restoring intestinal TJ proteins such as ZO-1 and occludin and antimicrobial peptides [134]. OCA treatment also improves hepatic inflammation and decreased portal pressure in BDL cirrhotic rats [135]. Consequently, OCA treatment may prevent HCC by limiting intestinal inflammation and improving gut barrier dysfunction in advanced liver disease.

Increased TNF-α production in mesenteric lymph nodes by monocyte is the major factor responsible for increased intestinal permeability in cirrhosis and HCC [19, 136]. TNF-α decreases ZO-1 expression through NF-κB and MLCK activation [137]. TNF-α also downregulated occludin expression in Caco-2 enterocyte by targeting PI3k/Akt signaling [138]. In BDL rats, treatment with infliximab (IFX, a monoclonal antibody against TNF) significantly reduced portal pressure and attenuated inflammation [139]. Therefore modulating intestinal TJs protein with anti-TNF-α therapy may restore intestinal integrity. However, due to the immunosuppressive activity of TNF inhibitors, it may lead to systemic infection in cirrhosis patients. Hence, detailed knowledge for local inhibition is required for improvement in gut barrier dysfunction without affecting innate immune response.

Retinoic acid can modulate TJs proteins. In a mice model of colitis characterized by gut permeability, treatment with retinoic acid enhances barrier function by upregulating TJs proteins claudin-1, claudin-4, and ZO-1 [140]. However, the effect of retinoic acid in the preservation of intestinal integrity has not been tested in cirrhosis and HCC. Modulation of the epithelial barrier with probiotics seems to be beneficial. In this regard, *Zhang* et al. showed probiotics VSL#3 (combination of *S. thermophilus*, four *Lactobacillus* species, and three *Bifidobacterium* species) treatment restores intestinal permeability and dysbiosis and prevented HCC progression in rats [19]. Similarly, probiotics like *E. coli Nissle1971* (ECN) was also shown to enhance intestinal TJs integrity by upregulating ZO-1 expression in the mouse model of DSS-induced colitis [141].

In addition, treatment with red wine polyphenol promoted barrier function by significantly increasing mRNA expression of TJ proteins occludin, claudin-5, and ZO-1 in cytokine-stimulated HT-29 colon epithelial cells [142]. Resveratrol also preserves TJ barrier integrity and diminishes intestinal permeability by upregulating occludin, ZO-1, and claudin-1expression and thus abrogating intestinal inflammation and oxidative stress both in vivo and in vitro [143]. Similarly in NAFLD mice model, treatment with resveratrol enhances barrier function by increasing mRNA expression of TJ proteins ZO-1, occludin, and claudin-1 in the intestinal mucosa [144]. Curcumin also modulates intestinal barrier integrity and attenuates paracellular permeability and organization of TJs [145]. Thus, targeting TJ proteins, which maintain intact intestinal epithelia, is another area of therapeutic approach for the control of intestinal permeability in cirrhosis and HCC.

15. Clinical value

HCC is the end-stage liver disease, which mostly develops on the background of cirrhosis. As discussed above, the gut-liver axis plays a significant role in the progression of CLD and ultimately HCC and would be a potentially significant therapeutic target in the prevention of HCC. There have been several preclinical and human studies demonstrating an association between gut dysbiosis and HCC progression. However, from the animal studies, it is unclear whether gut microbiota initiates HCC or acts with other precipitating factors like chronic inflammation in the progression of HCC. Modulation of gut dysbiosis with prebiotics and probiotics, FMT, or preventing bacterial overgrowth with antibiotics may therefore prevent HCC. Moreover, in cirrhotic patients these interventions appeared to prevent secondary complications and improved survival. We may therefore speculate that the above interventions might prevent HCC development in high-risk cirrhotic patients. Moreover, we should consider trialing these therapies in HCC patients with unresectable tumors, which might improve survival time and secondary complications. Furthermore interventions that restore intestinal barrier integrity may prevent gut BT and may consider another line of therapy in HCC.

16. Conclusion

In conclusion, there is growing evidence to suggest gut microbiota may play a significant role in the progression of CLD and thus HCC, which is likely to involve multiple pathways ranging from gut dysbiosis, endotoxemia, inflammation, loss of TJ integrity, and intestinal permeability. It is therefore suggested that the use of agents that have the potential to target microbial dysbiosis and restore intestinal epithelial barrier integrity may prevent bacterial translocation and ultimately delay HCC progression. However, whether bacterial overgrowth and/or intestinal permeability act independently or synergistically as causal pathogenic factors to influence the inflammatory milieu so closely associated with HCC progression remains unclear. Further research is therefore warranted to better understand the molecular pathways involved and guide the development of novel therapeutic interventions that can be taken to clinical trial to limit CLD/HCC progression through the targeting of dysbiosis and its effect on inflammation and intestinal permeability.

Conflict of interest statement

The authors declare that they have no conflict of interest.

Abbreviations

ALT	alanine transaminase
AMPs	antimicrobial peptides
AST	aspartate transaminase
BAs	bile acids
BDL	bile duct ligation
CCL	chemokine ligand
CCl_4	carbon tetrachloride
CD	cluster of differentiation
CLD	chronic liver disease
CTP	child-turcotte-pugh
DCA	deoxycholic acid
DEN	diethylnitrosamine
DMBA	2,4-dimethoxybenzaldehyde
ERK	extracellular signal-regulated kinase
FMT	fecal microbiota transplantation
HCC	hepatocellular carcinoma
HFD	high-fat diet
HSCs	hepatic stellate cells
IBD	inflammatory bowel disease
IEC	intestinal epithelial cell
IL	interleukin
JNK	c-Jun N-terminal kinase
LBP	lipopolysaccharide binding protein
LPS	lipopolysaccharides
MAMPs	microbe-associated molecular patterns
MAPK	mitogen-activated protein kinase
MELD	model for end-stage liver disease
NAFLD	nonalcoholic fatty liver disease
NASH	nonalcoholic steatohepatitis

NF-κB	nuclear factor kappa-light-chain-enhancer of activated B cells
NLRP	nucleotide-binding oligomerization domain, leucine-rich repeat- and pyrin domain-containing
NSBB	nonselective beta-blockers
OCA	obeticholic acid
PRRs	pattern recognition receptor
SCFAs	short-chain fatty acids
STHD	steatohepatitis-inducing high-fat diet
TB	total bilirubin
TGR5	takeda G-protein-coupled receptor 5
TLR	toll-like receptors
TNF-α	tumor necrosis factor alpha
TJs	tight junctions
WHO	World Health Organization
ZO	zonula occluden

Author details

Amit Kumar Ram[1†], Gavin Wright[2†] and Balasubramaniyan Vairappan[1*†]

1 Liver Diseases Research Lab, Department of Biochemistry, Jawaharlal Institute of Postgraduate Medical Education and Research (JIPMER), Pondicherry, India

2 Basildon University Hospital, Essex, United Kingdom

*Address all correspondence to: balasubramaniyan.v@jipmer.edu.in

†These authors have contributed equally to this work.

References

[1] Ozakyol A. Global epidemiology of hepatocellular carcinoma (HCC epidemiology). Journal of Gastrointestinal Cancer. 2017;**48**(3):238-240

[2] Rooks MG, Garrett WS. Gut microbiota, metabolites and host immunity. Nature Reviews. Immunology. 2016;**16**(6):341-352

[3] Nagpal R, Yadav H. Bacterial translocation from the gut to the distant organs: An overview. Annals of Nutrition and Metabolism. 2017;**71**(Suppl 1):11-16

[4] Schnabl B, Brenner DA. Interactions between the intestinal microbiome and liver diseases. Gastroenterology. 2014;**146**(6):1513-1524

[5] Sekirov I, Russell SL, Antunes LCM, Finlay BB. Gut microbiota in health and disease. Physiological Reviews. 2010;**90**(3):859-904

[6] Conlon MA, Bird AR. The impact of diet and lifestyle on gut microbiota and human health. Nutrients. 2014;**7**(1):17-44

[7] Thaiss CA, Zmora N, Levy M, Elinav E. The microbiome and innate immunity. Nature. 2016;**535**(7610):65-74

[8] Bäckhed F, Ley RE, Sonnenburg JL, Peterson DA, Gordon JI. Host-bacterial mutualism in the human intestine. Science. 2005;**307**(5717):1915-1920

[9] Schneider KM, Albers S, Trautwein C. Role of bile acids in the gut-liver axis. Journal of Hepatology. 2018;**68**(5):1083-1085

[10] Wiest R, Garcia-Tsao G. Bacterial translocation (BT) in cirrhosis. Hepatology. 2005;**41**(3):422-433

[11] Chen Y, Yang F, Lu H, Wang B, Chen Y, Lei D, et al. Characterization of fecal microbial communities in patients with liver cirrhosis. Hepatology. 2011;**54**(2):562-572

[12] Qin N, Yang F, Li A, Prifti E, Chen Y, Shao L, et al. Alterations of the human gut microbiome in liver cirrhosis. Nature. 2014;**513**(7516):59

[13] Lu H, Ren Z, Li A, Zhang H, Jiang J, Xu S, et al. Deep sequencing reveals microbiota dysbiosis of tongue coat in patients with liver carcinoma. Scientific Reports. 2016;**6**:33142

[14] Ren Z, Li A, Jiang J, Zhou L, Yu Z, Lu H, et al. Gut microbiome analysis as a tool towards targeted non-invasive biomarkers for early hepatocellular carcinoma. Gut. 2019;**68**(6):1014-1023

[15] Ponziani FR, Bhoori S, Castelli C, Putignani L, Rivoltini L, Del Chierico F, et al. Hepatocellular carcinoma is associated with gut microbiota profile and inflammation in nonalcoholic fatty liver disease. Hepatology. 2019;**69**(1):107-120

[16] Grąt M, Wronka KM, Krasnodębski M, Masior Ł, Lewandowski Z, Kosińska I, et al. Profile of gut microbiota associated with the presence of hepatocellular cancer in patients with liver cirrhosis. Transplantation Proceedings. 2016;**48**(5):1687-1691

[17] Fox JG, Feng Y, Theve EJ, Raczynski AR, Fiala JLA, Doernte AL, et al. Gut microbes define liver cancer risk in mice exposed to chemical and viral transgenic hepatocarcinogens. Gut. 2010;**59**(01):88-97

[18] Huang Y, Fan X-G, Wang Z-M, Zhou J-H, Tian X-F, Li N. Identification of helicobacter species in human

liver samples from patients with primary hepatocellular carcinoma. Journal of Clinical Pathology. 2004;**57**(12):1273-1277

[19] Zhang H-L, Yu L-X, Yang W, Tang L, Lin Y, Wu H, et al. Profound impact of gut homeostasis on chemically-induced pro-tumorigenic inflammation and hepatocarcinogenesis in rats. Journal of Hepatology. 2012;**57**(4):803-812

[20] Dapito DH, Mencin A, Gwak G-Y, Pradere J-P, Jang M-K, Mederacke I, et al. Promotion of hepatocellular carcinoma by the intestinal microbiota and TLR4. Cancer Cell. 2012;**21**(4):504-516

[21] Berkes J, Viswanathan VK, Savkovic SD, Hecht G. Intestinal epithelial responses to enteric pathogens: Effects on the tight junction barrier, ion transport, and inflammation. Gut. 2003;**52**(3): 439-451

[22] Pradere J-P, Dapito DH, Schwabe RF. The Yin and Yang of toll-like receptors in cancer. Oncogene. 2014;**33**(27):3485-3495

[23] Yu L-X, Yan H-X, Liu Q, Yang W, Wu H-P, Dong W, et al. Endotoxin accumulation prevents carcinogen-induced apoptosis and promotes liver tumorigenesis in rodents. Hepatology. 2010;**52**(4):1322-1333

[24] Wang L, Zhu R, Huang Z, Li H, Zhu H. Lipopolysaccharide-induced toll-like receptor 4 signaling in cancer cells promotes cell survival and proliferation in hepatocellular carcinoma. Digestive Diseases and Sciences. 2013;**58**(8):2223-2236

[25] Jing Y-Y, Han Z-P, Sun K, Zhang S-S, Hou J, Liu Y, et al. Toll-like receptor 4 signaling promotes epithelial-mesenchymal transition in human hepatocellular carcinoma induced by lipopolysaccharide. BMC Medicine. 2012;**10**:98

[26] Lu Y, Xu J, Chen S, Zhou Z, Lin N. Lipopolysaccharide promotes angiogenesis in mice model of HCC by stimulating hepatic stellate cell activation via TLR4 pathway. Acta Biochimica et Biophysica Sinica. 2017;**49**(11):1029-1034

[27] Peterson LW, Artis D. Intestinal epithelial cells: Regulators of barrier function and immune homeostasis. Nature Reviews. Immunology. 2014;**14**(3):141

[28] Van der Sluis M, De Koning BAE, De Bruijn ACJM, Velcich A, Meijerink JPP, Van Goudoever JB, et al. Muc2-deficient mice spontaneously develop colitis, indicating that MUC2 is critical for colonic protection. Gastroenterology. 2006;**131**(1):117-129

[29] Velcich A, Yang W, Heyer J, Fragale A, Nicholas C, Viani S, et al. Colorectal cancer in mice genetically deficient in the Mucin Muc2. Science. 2002;**295**(5560):1726-1729

[30] Balda MS, Matter K. Tight junctions at a glance. Journal of Cell Science. 2008;**121**(Pt 22):3677-3682

[31] Ram AK, Pottakat B, Vairappan B. Increased systemic zonula occludens 1 associated with inflammation and independent biomarker in patients with hepatocellular carcinoma. BMC Cancer. 2018;**18**:572

[32] Capaldo CT, Nusrat A. Cytokine regulation of tight junctions. Biochimica et Biophysica Acta (BBA) - Biomembranes. 2009;**1788**(4):864-871

[33] Guo S, Al-Sadi R, Said HM, Ma TY. Lipopolysaccharide causes an increase in intestinal tight junction permeability in vitro and in vivo by inducing enterocyte membrane

expression and localization of TLR-4 and CD14. The American Journal of Pathology. 2013;**182**(2):375-387

[34] Henao-Mejia J, Elinav E, Jin C, Hao L, Mehal WZ, Strowig T, et al. Inflammasome-mediated dysbiosis regulates progression of NAFLD and obesity. Nature. 2012;**482**(7384):179-185

[35] Inagaki T, Moschetta A, Lee Y-K, Peng L, Zhao G, Downes M, et al. Regulation of antibacterial defense in the small intestine by the nuclear bile acid receptor. Proceedings of the National Academy of Sciences. 2006;**103**(10):3920 3925

[36] Gadaleta RM, van EKJ, Oldenburg B, Willemsen ECL, Renooij W, Murzilli S, et al. Farnesoid X receptor activation inhibits inflammation and preserves the intestinal barrier in inflammatory bowel disease. Gut. 2011;**60**(4):463-472

[37] Kakiyama G, Pandak WM, Gillevet PM, Hylemon PB, Heuman DM, Daita K, et al. Modulation of the fecal bile acid profile by gut microbiota in cirrhosis. Journal of Hepatology. 2013;**58**(5):949-955

[38] Yoshimoto S, Loo TM, Atarashi K, Kanda H, Sato S, Oyadomari S, et al. Obesity-induced gut microbial metabolite promotes liver cancer through senescence secretome. Nature. 2013;**499**(7456):97-101

[39] Yamada S, Takashina Y, Watanabe M, Nagamine R, Saito Y, Kamada N, et al. Bile acid metabolism regulated by the gut microbiota promotes non-alcoholic steatohepatitis-associated hepatocellular carcinoma in mice. Oncotarget. 2018;**9**(11):9925-9939

[40] Dossa AY, Escobar O, Golden J, Frey MR, Ford HR, Gayer CP. Bile acids regulate intestinal cell proliferation by modulating EGFR and FXR signaling. The American Journal of Physiology-Gastrointestinal and Liver Physiology. 2015;**310**(2):G81-G92

[41] Raimondi F, Santoro P, Barone MV, Pappacoda S, Barretta ML, Nanayakkara M, et al. Bile acids modulate tight junction structure and barrier function of Caco-2 monolayers via EGFR activation. The American Journal of Physiology-Gastrointestinal and Liver Physiology. 2008;**294**(4):G906-G913

[42] Münch A, Ström M, Söderholm JD. Dihydroxy bile acids increase mucosal permeability and bacterial uptake in human colon biopsies. Scandinavian Journal of Gastroenterology. 2007;**42**(10):1167-1174

[43] Murakami Y, Tanabe S, Suzuki T. High-fat diet-induced intestinal hyperpermeability is associated with increased bile acids in the large intestine of mice. Journal of Food Science. 2016;**81**(1):H216-H222

[44] Verbeke L, Mannaerts I, Schierwagen R, Govaere O, Klein S, Vander Elst I, et al. FXR agonist obeticholic acid reduces hepatic inflammation and fibrosis in a rat model of toxic cirrhosis. Scientific Reports. 2016;**6**:33453

[45] Cipriani S, Mencarelli A, Chini MG, Distrutti E, Renga B, Bifulco G, et al. The bile acid receptor GPBAR-1 (TGR5) modulates integrity of intestinal barrier and immune response to experimental colitis. PLoS One. 2011;**6**(10):e25637

[46] Li J, Sung CYJ, Lee N, Ni Y, Pihlajamäki J, Panagiotou G, et al. Probiotics modulated gut microbiota suppresses hepatocellular carcinoma growth in mice. Proceedings of the National Academy of Sciences. 2016;**113**(9):E1306-E1315

[47] Fotiadis CI, Stoidis CN, Spyropoulos BG, Zografos ED. Role of probiotics, prebiotics and synbiotics in

chemoprevention for colorectal cancer. World Journal of Gastroenterology. 2008;**14**(42):6453-6457

[48] Shukla S, Shukla A, Mehboob S, Guha S. Meta-analysis: The effects of gut flora modulation using prebiotics, probiotics and synbiotics on minimal hepatic encephalopathy. Alimentary Pharmacology and Therapeutics;**33**(6):662-671

[49] Pinzone MR, Celesia BM, Di Rosa M, Cacopardo B, Nunnari G. Microbial translocation in chronic liver diseases. International Journal of Microbiology. 2012. DOI: 10.1155/2012/694629. Available from: https://www.ncbi.nlm.nih.gov/pmc/articles/PMC3405644/

[50] Riggio O, Varriale M, Testore GP, Di Rosa R, Di Rosa E, Merli M, et al. Effect of lactitol and lactulose administration on the fecal flora in cirrhotic patients. Journal of Clinical Gastroenterology. 1990;**12**(4):433-436

[51] Chen C, Li L, Wu Z, Chen H, Fu S. Effects of lactitol on intestinal microflora and plasma endotoxin in patients with chronic viral hepatitis. The Journal of Infection. 2007;**54**(1):98-102

[52] Bajaj JS, Heuman DM, Hylemon PB, Sanyal AJ, White MB, Monteith P, et al. Altered profile of human gut microbiome is associated with cirrhosis and its complications. Journal of Hepatology. 2014;**60**(5):940-947

[53] Zong D-W, Guo C-Y, Cheng H-T, Hu H-T, Xiao J-C, Li H-L. Influence of lactulose on interventional therapy for HCC patients with hepatocirrhosis and hypersplenism. Asian Pacific Journal of Tropical Medicine. 2016;**9**(2):193-196

[54] Yu J, Zhang W, Zhang R, Ruan X, Ren P, Lu B. Lactulose accelerates liver regeneration in rats by inducing hydrogen. The Journal of Surgical Research. 2015;**195**(1):128-135

[55] Bakker-Zierikzee AM, Alles MS, Knol J, Kok FJ, Tolboom JJM, Bindels JG. Effects of infant formula containing a mixture of galacto- and fructo-oligosaccharides or viable bifidobacterium animalis on the intestinal microflora during the first 4 months of life. The British Journal of Nutrition. 2005;**94**(5):783-790

[56] Mack DR. Probiotics. Canadian Family Physician. 2005;**51**(11): 1455-1457

[57] Arthur JC, Gharaibeh RZ, Uronis JM, Perez-Chanona E, Sha W, Tomkovich S, et al. VSL#3 probiotic modifies mucosal microbial composition but does not reduce colitis-associated colorectal cancer. Scientific Reports. 2013;**3**:2868

[58] Dhiman RK, Rana B, Agrawal S, Garg A, Chopra M, Thumburu KK, et al. Probiotic VSL#3 reduces liver disease severity and hospitalization in patients with cirrhosis: A randomized, controlled trial. Gastroenterology. 2014;**147**(6):1327-1337.e3

[59] Alisi A, Bedogni G, Baviera G, Giorgio V, Porro E, Paris C, et al. Randomised clinical trial: The beneficial effects of VSL#3 in obese children with non-alcoholic steatohepatitis. Alimentary Pharmacology and Therapeutics. 2014;**39**(11):1276-1285

[60] Shi D, Lv L, Fang D, Wu W, Hu C, Xu L, et al. Administration of *Lactobacillus salivarius* LI01 or *Pediococcus pentosaceus* LI05 prevents CCl 4 -induced liver cirrhosis by protecting the intestinal barrier in rats. Scientific Reports. 2017;7(1):6927

[61] Bajaj JS, Heuman DM, Hylemon PB, Sanyal AJ, Puri P, Sterling RK, et al. Randomised clinical trial: Lactobacillus GG modulates gut microbiome, metabolome and endotoxemia in patients with cirrhosis. Alimentary

Pharmacology and Therapeutics. 2014;**39**(10):1113-1125

[62] Kumar M, Verma V, Nagpal R, Kumar A, Gautam SK, Behare PV, et al. Effect of probiotic fermented milk and chlorophyllin on gene expressions and genotoxicity during AFB_1-induced hepatocellular carcinoma. Gene. 2011;**490**(1-2):54-59

[63] El-Nezami HS, Polychronaki NN, Ma J, Zhu H, Ling W, Salminen EK, et al. Probiotic supplementation reduces a biomarker for increased risk of liver cancer in young men from southern China. The American Journal of Clinical Nutrition. 2006;**83**(5):1199-1203

[64] Liu Q, Duan ZP, Ha DK, Bengmark S, Kurtovic J, Riordan SM. Synbiotic modulation of gut flora: Effect on minimal hepatic encephalopathy in patients with cirrhosis. Hepatology (Baltimore, Md.). 2004;**39**(5):1441-1449

[65] Bakhshimoghaddam F, Shateri K, Sina M, Hashemian M, Alizadeh M. Daily consumption of synbiotic yogurt decreases liver steatosis in patients with nonalcoholic fatty liver disease: A randomized controlled clinical trial. The Journal of Nutrition. 2018;**148**(8):1276-1284

[66] Chiu W-C, Huang Y-L, Chen Y-L, Peng H-C, Liao W-H, Chuang H-L, et al. Synbiotics reduce ethanol-induced hepatic steatosis and inflammation by improving intestinal permeability and microbiota in rats. Food and Function. 2015;**6**(5):1692-1700

[67] Abdel-Hamid NI, El-Azab MF, Moustafa YM. Macrolide antibiotics differentially influence human HepG2 cytotoxicity and modulate intrinsic/extrinsic apoptotic pathways in rat hepatocellular carcinoma model. Naunyn-Schmiedeberg's Archives of Pharmacology. 2017;**390**(4):379-395

[68] Sidhu GS, Go A, Attar BM, Mutneja HR, Arora S, Patel SA. Rifaximin versus norfloxacin for prevention of spontaneous bacterial peritonitis: A systematic review. BMJ Open Gastroenterology. 2017;**4**(1):e000154

[69] Moreau R, Elkrief L, Bureau C, Perarnau J-M, Thévenot T, Saliba F, et al. Effects of long-term Norfloxacin therapy in patients with advanced cirrhosis. Gastroenterology. 2018;**155**(6):1816-1827.e9

[70] Gómez-Hurtado I, Gimenez P, García I, Zapater P, Francés R, González-Navajas JM, et al. Norfloxacin is more effective than Rifaximin in avoiding bacterial translocation in an animal model of cirrhosis. Liver International. 2018;**38**(2):295-302

[71] Koo HL, DuPont HL. Rifaximin: A unique gastrointestinal-selective antibiotic for enteric diseases. Current Opinion in Gastroenterology. 2010;**26**(1):17-25

[72] Patidar KR, Bajaj JS. Antibiotics for the treatment of hepatic encephalopathy. Metabolic Brain Disease. 2013;**28**(2):307-312

[73] Vlachogiannakos J, Saveriadis AS, Viazis N, Theodoropoulos I, Foudoulis K, Manolakopoulos S, et al. Intestinal decontamination improves liver haemodynamics in patients with alcohol-related decompensated cirrhosis. Alimentary Pharmacology and Therapeutics 2009;29(9):992-9

[74] Vlachogiannakos J, Viazis N, Vasianopoulou P, Vafiadis I, Karamanolis DG, Ladas SD. Long-term administration of rifaximin improves the prognosis of patients with decompensated alcoholic cirrhosis. Journal of Gastroenterology and Hepatology. 2013;**28**(3):450-455

[75] van Nood E, Vrieze A, Nieuwdorp M, Fuentes S, Zoetendal EG, de Vos WM, et al. Duodenal infusion of donor feces for recurrent *Clostridium difficile*. The New England Journal of Medicine. 2013;**368**(5):407-415

[76] Bastard QL, Ward T, Sidiropoulos D, Hillmann BM, Chun CL, Sadowsky MJ, et al. Fecal microbiota transplantation reverses antibiotic and chemotherapy-induced gut dysbiosis in mice. Scientific Reports. 2018;**8**(1):6219

[77] Wang W-W, Zhang Y, Huang X-B, You N, Zheng L, Li J. Fecal microbiota transplantation prevents hepatic encephalopathy in rats with carbon tetrachloride-induced acute hepatic dysfunction. World Journal of Gastroenterology. 2017;**23**(38):6983-6994

[78] Bajaj JS, Kassam Z, Fagan A, Gavis EA, Liu E, Cox IJ, et al. Fecal microbiota transplant from a rational stool donor improves hepatic encephalopathy: A randomized clinical trial. Hepatology (Baltimore, Md.). 2017;**66**(6):1727-1738

[79] Fecal Microbiota Transplantation for Decompensated Cirrhosis—Full Text View—ClinicalTrials.gov. 2018. Available from: https://clinicaltrials.gov/ct2/show/NCT03014505

[80] Fecal Microbiota Transplantation (FMT) in Nonalcoholic Steatohepatitis (NASH). A Pilot Study—Full Text View—ClinicalTrials.gov. 2018. Available from: https://clinicaltrials.gov/ct2/show/NCT02469272

[81] Vrieze A, Van Nood E, Holleman F, Salojärvi J, Kootte RS, Bartelsman JFWM, et al. Transfer of intestinal microbiota from lean donors increases insulin sensitivity in individuals with metabolic syndrome. Gastroenterology. 2012;**143**(4): 913-916.e7

[82] Philips CA, Pande A, Shasthry SM, Jamwal KD, Khillan V, Chandel SS, et al. Healthy donor fecal microbiota transplantation in steroid-ineligible severe alcoholic hepatitis: A pilot study. Clinical Gastroenterology and Hepatology. 2017;**15**(4):600-602

[83] Schwartz M, Gluck M, Koon S. Norovirus gastroenteritis after fecal microbiota transplantation for treatment of *Clostridium difficile* infection despite asymptomatic donors and lack of sick contacts. The American Journal of Gastroenterology. 2013;**108**(8):1367

[84] Gupta S, Allen-Vercoe E, Petrof EO. Fecal microbiota transplantation: In perspective. Therapeutic Advances in Gastroenterology. 2016;**9**(2):229

[85] Seki E, De Minicis S, Österreicher CH, Kluwe J, Osawa Y, Brenner DA, et al. TLR4 enhances TGF-β signaling and hepatic fibrosis. Nature Medicine. 2007;**13**(11):1324-1332

[86] Domingues MM, Inácio RG, Raimundo JM, Martins M, Castanho MARB, Santos NC. Biophysical characterization of polymyxin B interaction with LPS aggregates and membrane model systems. Biopolymers. 2012;**98**(4):338-344

[87] Piazza M, Rossini C, Della Fiorentina S, Pozzi C, Comelli F, Bettoni I, et al. Glycolipids and benzylammonium lipids as novel antisepsis agents: Synthesis and biological characterization. Journal of Medicinal Chemistry. 2009;**52**(4):1209-1213

[88] Barochia A, Solomon S, Cui X, Natanson C, Eichacker PQ. Eritoran tetrasodium (E5564) treatment for sepsis: Review of preclinical and clinical studies. Expert Opinion on Drug Metabolism and Toxicology. 2011;**7**(4):479-494

[89] Matsunaga N, Tsuchimori N, Matsumoto T, Ii M. TAK-242 (resatorvid), a small-molecule inhibitor of toll-like receptor (TLR) 4 signaling, binds selectively to TLR4 and interferes with interactions between TLR4 and its adaptor molecules. Molecular Pharmacology. 2011;**79**(1):34-41

[90] Patra MC, Choi S. Recent progress in the development of toll-like receptor (TLR) antagonists. Expert Opinion on Therapeutic Patents. 2016;**26**(6):719-730

[91] Oya S, Yokoyama Y, Kokuryo T, Uno M, Yamauchi K, Nagino M. Inhibition of toll-like receptor 4 suppresses liver injury induced by biliary obstruction and subsequent intraportal lipopolysaccharide injection. The American Journal of Physiology-Gastrointestinal and Liver Physiology. 2013;**306**(3):G244-G252

[92] Salama M, Elgamal M, Abdelaziz A, Ellithy M, Magdy D, Ali L, et al. Toll-like receptor 4 blocker as potential therapy for acetaminophen-induced organ failure in mice. Experimental and Therapeutic Medicine. 2015;**10**(1):241-246

[93] Nguyen J, Jiao J, Smoot K, Watt GP, Zhao C, Song X, et al. Toll-like receptor 4: A target for chemoprevention of hepatocellular carcinoma in obesity and steatohepatitis. Oncotarget. 2018;**9**(50):29495-29507

[94] McDonald K-A, Huang H, Tohme S, Loughran P, Ferrero K, Billiar T, et al. Toll-like receptor 4 (TLR4) antagonist eritoran tetrasodium attenuates liver ischemia and reperfusion injury through inhibition of high-mobility group box protein B1 (HMGB1) signaling. Molecular Medicine. 2015;**20**(1):639-648

[95] Kitazawa T, Tsujimoto T, Kawaratani H, Fukui H. Salvage effect of E5564, toll-like receptor 4 antagonist on d-galactosamine and lipopolysaccharide-induced acute liver failure in rats. Journal of Gastroenterology and Hepatology. 2010;**25**(5):1009-1012

[96] Kuo W-T, Lee T-C, Yu LC-H. Eritoran suppresses colon cancer by altering a functional balance in toll-like receptors that bind lipopolysaccharide. Cancer Research. 2016;**76**(16):4684-4695

[97] Opal SM, Laterre P-F, Francois B, LaRosa SP, Angus DC, Mira J-P, et al. Effect of eritoran, an antagonist of MD2-TLR4, on mortality in patients with severe sepsis: The ACCESS randomized trial. Journal of the American Medical Association. 2013;**309**(11):1154-1162

[98] Sun L, Dai JJ, Hu WF, Wang J. Expression of toll-like receptors in hepatic cirrhosis and hepatocellular carcinoma. The Genetics and Molecular Research. 2016;**15**(2). DOI: 10.4238/gmr.15027419

[99] Ma Z, Zhang E, Yang D, Lu M. Contribution of toll-like receptors to the control of hepatitis B virus infection by initiating antiviral innate responses and promoting specific adaptive immune responses. Cellular and molecular immunology. 2015;**12**(3):273-282

[100] Akira S, Sato S. Toll-like receptors and their signaling mechanisms. Scandinavian Journal of Infectious Diseases. 2003;**35**(9):555-562

[101] Chen L, Xu Y-Y, Zhou J-M, Wu Y-Y, Zhu Y-Y. TLR3 dsRNA agonist inhibits growth and invasion of HepG2.2.15 HCC cells. Oncology Reports. 2012;**28**(1):200-206

[102] Akira S, Takeda K. Toll-like receptor signalling. Nature Reviews. Immunology. 2004;**4**(7):499-511

[103] Mohamed FE, Al-Jehani RM, Minogue SS, Andreola F, Winstanley A, Olde Damink SWM, et al. Effect of toll-like receptor 7 and 9 targeted therapy

to prevent the development of hepatocellular carcinoma. Liver International. 2015;**35**(3):1063-1076

[104] Zou H, Wang W-K, Liu Y-L, Braddock M, Zheng M-H, Huang D-S. Toll-like receptors in hepatocellular carcinoma: Potential novel targets for pharmacological intervention. Expert Opinion on Therapeutic Targets. 2016;**20**(9):1127-1135

[105] So EY, Ouchi T. The application of toll like receptors for cancer therapy. International Journal of Biological Sciences. 2010;**6**(7):675-681

[106] Lopes JAG, Borges-Canha M, Pimentel-Nunes P. Innate immunity and hepatocarcinoma: Can toll-like receptors open the door to oncogenesis? World Journal of Hepatology. 2016;**8**(3):162-182

[107] Kalaitzakis E. Gastrointestinal dysfunction in liver cirrhosis. World Journal of Gastroenterology. 2014;**20**(40):14686-14695

[108] Pardo A, Bartolí R, Lorenzo-Zúñiga V, Planas R, Viñado B, Riba J, et al. Effect of cisapride on intestinal bacterial overgrowth and bacterial translocation in cirrhosis. Hepatology. 2000;**31**(4):858-863

[109] Madrid AM, Hurtado C, Venegas M, Cumsille F, Defilippi C. Long-term treatment with cisapride and antibiotics in liver cirrhosis: Effect on small intestinal motility, bacterial overgrowth, and liver function. The American Journal of Gastroenterology. 2001;**96**(4):1251-1255

[110] Sandhu BS, Gupta R, Sharma J, Singh J, Murthy NS, Sarin SK. Norfloxacin and cisapride combination decreases the incidence of spontaneous bacterial peritonitis in cirrhotic ascites. Journal of Gastroenterology and Hepatology. 2005;**20**(4):599-605

[111] Kassahun WT, Guenl B, Ungemach FR, Jonas S, Abraham G. Expression and functional coupling of liver β2 - adrenoceptors in the human hepatocellular carcinoma. Pharmacology. 2012;**89**(5-6):313-320

[112] Thiele M, Albillos A, Abazi R, Wiest R, Gluud LL, Krag A. Non-selective beta-blockers may reduce risk of hepatocellular carcinoma: A meta-analysis of randomized trials. Liver International. 2015;**35**(8):2009-2016

[113] Dietrich P, Moleda L, Kees F, Müller M, Straub RH, Hellerbrand C, et al. Dysbalance in sympathetic neurotransmitter release and action in cirrhotic rats: Impact of exogenous neuropeptide Y. Journal of Hepatology. 2013;**58**(2):254-261

[114] Leithead JA, Rajoriya N, Tehami N, Hodson J, Gunson BK, Tripathi D, et al. Non-selective β-blockers are associated with improved survival in patients with ascites listed for liver transplantation. Gut. 2015;**64**(7):1111-1119

[115] Reiberger T, Ferlitsch A, Payer BA, Mandorfer M, Heinisch BB, Hayden H, et al. Non-selective betablocker therapy decreases intestinal permeability and serum levels of LBP and IL-6 in patients with cirrhosis. Journal of Hepatology. 2013;**58**(5):911-921

[116] Wang F, Liu H, Wang F, Xu R, Wang P, Tang F, et al. Propranolol suppresses the proliferation and induces the apoptosis of liver cancer cells. Molecular Medicine Reports. 2018;**17**(4):5213-5221

[117] Nkontchou G, Aout M, Mahmoudi A, Roulot D, Bourcier V, Grando-Lemaire V, et al. Effect of long-term propranolol treatment on hepatocellular carcinoma incidence in patients with HCV-associated cirrhosis. Cancer Prevention Research (Philadelphia, Pa.). 2012;**5**(8):1007-1014

[118] Chang P-Y, Chung C-H, Chang W-C, Lin C-S, Lin H-H, Dai M-S,

et al. The effect of propranolol on the prognosis of hepatocellular carcinoma: A nationwide population-based study. PLoS One. 2019;**14**(5):e0216828

[119] Larrosa M, Yañéz-Gascón MJ, Selma MV, González-Sarrías A, Toti S, Cerón JJ, et al. Effect of a low dose of dietary resveratrol on colon microbiota, inflammation and tissue damage in a DSS-induced colitis rat model. Journal of Agricultural and Food Chemistry. 2009;**57**(6):2211-2220

[120] Gao F, Deng G, Liu W, Zhou K, Li M. Resveratrol suppresses human hepatocellular carcinoma via targeting HGF-c-met signaling pathway. Oncology Reports. 2017;**37**(2):1203-1211

[121] Bishayee A, Dhir N. Resveratrol-mediated chemoprevention of diethylnitrosamine-initiated hepatocarcinogenesis: Inhibition of cell proliferation and induction of apoptosis. Chemico-Biological Interactions. 2009;**179**(2):131-144

[122] Vairappan B, Sundhar M, Srinivas BH.Resveratrol restores neuronal tight junction proteins through correction of ammonia and inflammation in CCl4-induced cirrhotic mice. Molecular Neurobiology. 2019;**56**(7):4718-4729

[123] Lee RH, Cho JH, Jeon Y-J, Bang W, Cho J-J, Choi N-J, et al. Quercetin induces antiproliferative activity against human hepatocellular carcinoma (HepG2) cells by suppressing specificity protein 1 (Sp1). Drug Development Research. 2015;**76**(1):9-16

[124] Ji Y, Li L, Ma Y-X, Li W-T, Li L, Zhu H-Z, et al. Quercetin inhibits growth of hepatocellular carcinoma by apoptosis induction in part via autophagy stimulation in mice. The Journal of Nutritional Biochemistry. 2019;**69**:108-119

[125] Teng C-F, Yu C-H, Chang H-Y, Hsieh W-C, Wu T-H, Lin J-H, et al. Chemopreventive effect of phytosomal curcumin on hepatitis B virus-related hepatocellular carcinoma in a transgenic mouse model. Scientific Reports. 2019;**9**(1):10338

[126] Tang Y. Curcumin targets multiple pathways to halt hepatic stellate cell activation: Updated mechanisms in vitro and in vivo. Digestive Diseases and Sciences. 2015;**60**(6):1554-1564

[127] Wang L, Phan DDK, Zhang J, Ong P-S, Thuya WL, Soo R, et al. Anticancer properties of nimbolide and pharmacokinetic considerations to accelerate its development. Oncotarget. 2016;**7**(28):44790-44802

[128] Kavitha K, Vidya Priyadarsini R, Anitha P, Ramalingam K, Sakthivel R, Purushothaman G, et al. Nimbolide, a neem limonoid abrogates canonical NF-κB and Wnt signaling to induce caspase-dependent apoptosis in human hepatocarcinoma (HepG2) cells. European Journal of Pharmacology. 2012;**681**(1-3):6-14

[129] Wiest R, Lawson M, Geuking M. Pathological bacterial translocation in liver cirrhosis. Journal of Hepatology. 2014;**60**(1):197-209

[130] Toffanin S, Cornella H, Harrington A, Llovet JM. HCC is promoted by bacterial translocation and TLR-4 signaling: A new paradigm for chemoprevention and management. Hepatology. 2012;**56**(5):1998-2000

[131] Verbeke L, Farre R, Verbinnen B, Covens K, Vanuytsel T, Verhaegen J, et al. The FXR agonist obeticholic acid prevents gut barrier dysfunction and bacterial translocation in cholestatic rats. The American Journal of Pathology. 2015;**185**(2):409-419

[132] Piglionica M, Cariello M, Moschetta A. The gut-liver axis in hepatocarcinoma: A focus on the nuclear receptor FXR and the enterokine FGF19.

Current Opinion in Pharmacology. 2018;**43**:93-98

[133] Degirolamo C, Modica S, Vacca M, Tullio GD, Morgano A, D'Orazio A, et al. Prevention of spontaneous hepatocarcinogenesis in farnesoid X receptor–null mice by intestinal-specific farnesoid X receptor reactivation. Hepatology. 2015;**61**(1):161-170

[134] Úbeda M, Lario M, Muñoz L, Borrero M-J, Rodríguez-Serrano M, Sánchez-Díaz A-M, et al. Obeticholic acid reduces bacterial translocation and inhibits intestinal inflammation in cirrhotic rats. Journal of Hepatology. 2016;**64**(5):1049-1057

[135] Mookerjee RP, Mehta G, Balasubramaniyan V, Mohamed FEZ, Davies N, Sharma V, et al. Hepatic dimethylarginine-dimethylaminohydrolase1 is reduced in cirrhosis and is a target for therapy in portal hypertension. Journal of Hepatology. 2015;**62**(2):325-331

[136] Parlesak A, Schäfer C, Schütz T, Bode JC, Bode C. Increased intestinal permeability to macromolecules and endotoxemia in patients with chronic alcohol abuse in different stages of alcohol-induced liver disease. Journal of Hepatology. 2000;**32**(5):742-747

[137] Ma TY, Iwamoto GK, Hoa NT, Akotia V, Pedram A, Boivin MA, et al. TNF-α-induced increase in intestinal epithelial tight junction permeability requires NF-κB activation. The American Journal of Physiology-Gastrointestinal and Liver Physiology. 2004;**286**(3):G367-G376

[138] Mankertz J, Amasheh M, Krug SM, Fromm A, Amasheh S, Hillenbrand B, et al. TNFα up-regulates claudin-2 expression in epithelial HT-29/B6 cells via phosphatidylinositol-3-kinase signaling. Cell and Tissue Research. 2009;**336**(1):67-77

[139] Balasubramanian V, Mehta G, Jones H, Sharma V, Davies NA, Jalan R, et al. Post-transcriptional regulation of hepatic DDAH1 with TNF blockade leads to improved eNOS function and reduced portal pressure In cirrhotic rats. Scientific Reports. 2017;**7**(1):17900

[140] Osanai M, Nishikiori N, Murata M, Chiba H, Kojima T, Sawada N. Cellular retinoic acid bioavailability determines epithelial integrity: Role of retinoic acid receptor α agonists in colitis. Molecular Pharmacology. 2007;**71**(1):250-258

[141] Ukena SN, Singh A, Dringenberg U, Engelhardt R, Seidler U, Hansen W, et al. Probiotic *Escherichia coli* Nissle 1917 inhibits leaky gut by enhancing mucosal integrity. PLoS One. 2007;**2**(12):e1308

[142] Nunes C, Freitas V, Laranjinha J. Modulation of tight junctions in intestinal epithelial cells by red wine polyphenols. Free Radical Biology and Medicine. 2018;**120**:S149

[143] Mayangsari Y, Suzuki T. Resveratrol ameliorates intestinal barrier defects and inflammation in colitic mice and intestinal cells. Journal of Agricultural and Food Chemistry. 2018;**66**(48):12666-12674

[144] Chen M, Hou P, Zhou M, Ren Q, Wang X, Huang L, et al. Resveratrol attenuates high-fat diet-induced non-alcoholic steatohepatitis by maintaining gut barrier integrity and inhibiting gut inflammation through regulation of the endocannabinoid system. Clinical Nutrition. 2019. DOI: 10.1016/j.clnu.2019.05.020

[145] Wang J, Ghosh SS, Ghosh S. Curcumin improves intestinal barrier function: Modulation of intracellular signaling, and organization of tight junctions. The American Journal of Physiology-Cell Physiology. 2017;**312**(4):C438-C445

Chapter 11

Splenectomy in Liver Cirrhosis with Splenomegaly and Hypersplenism

Adianto Nugroho

Abstract

Spleen is a "mysterious" organ since with unique functions, and might be related to other pathology in the human body. Splenomegaly and hypersplenism can manifest following the development of portal hypertension in liver cirrhosis through fibrogenesis, immune and microenvironment dysregulation. Cirrhotic patients are generally considered as immunocompromised and prone to infections. Splenectomy in cirrhotic patients has produced concern over decrease immunity and elevated risk of infection, namely overwhelming post splenectomy pneumococcal sepsis. This review discus the splenectomy effect to the liver and how it can play a role in cirrhotic patients with portal hypertension without readily available access to liver transplantation.

Keywords: splenectomy, liver cirrhosis, hypersplenism, splenomegaly, liver transplantation

1. Introduction

The spleen is a unique organ with many functions, including its crosstalk with the liver in cirrhotic patients. This review aims to answer a clinical question "Should splenectomy be done in liver cirrhosis with hypersplenism and splenomegaly?".

2. The spleen

The spleen is an organ full of mystery, as stated by Galen. From the ancient times until the Renaissance, descriptions of the gross anatomy of the spleen were relatively accurate, yet the physiology of this organ remains incomplete and inaccurate. Even until today, much of spleen's function are still yet to be discovered [1].

Spleen comprised of two distinct compartments, both functional and morphological, namely red pulp and white pulp. The red pulp filters blood to remove foreign material and damaged erythrocytes. It also serves as iron, erythrocytes and platelets storages. With one fourth of body's lymphocytes stores in the spleen, it is the largest secondary organ which initiate immune response to blood-borne antigens [2]. It exerts important effects on local and systemic immune responses, which have the potential to affect different tissues and organs [3]. The white pulp, composed by periarteriolar lymphoid sheath (PALS), the follicles and the marginal zones, are the one responsible for this so called immune functions [2].

In addition, the spleen also produces opsonins, a substances that bind to the foreign antigen, which in turn enhance their uptake and phagocytosis by macrophages. Furthermore, the B-lymphocytes within the germinal centers of the spleen are also sites for the production of antibody activated by foreign antigen. The realization of this important immunological function has promoted the desire for splenic preservation [4].

3. Liver cirrhosis and the spleen

The association between the liver and spleen are shown in three different categories. Both organ, anatomically important in the portal circulation. Histologically, they share similar possession of reticuloendothelial structures, participating in substance exchange and cellular migration. And immunologically, both organs plays essential roles in immune homeostasis and pathogen clearance [2].

The first recorded encounter between spleen and cirrhosis could be trace back to Carl Freiderich Quittenbaum (1793–1852) of Rostock, Germany, who removed the spleen of a woman with cirrhosis and ascites "more from the patient's urgent entreaty rather than the surgeon's judgment." Unfortunately the woman lived only 6 h after the surgery [5].

The palpable spleen has long been considered as an obvious signs of liver cirrhosis, frequently occurs in parallel with hypersplenism, to be the major cause of cytopenia and thrombocytopenia. This condition are relatively sub-fatal, even in the absence of a bleeding varices. During the progression of liver cirrhosis, the spleen-derived immune cells and cytokines may travel into the injured liver via portal blood flow. Together with the portal hypertension and congestion, this will result in splenomegaly and hypersplenism. Furthermore, the chemokines, DAMPs like HMGB1, or exosomes, are also release into the circulation, which will trigger the activation and/or migration of splenocytes. This mechanism are known as the liver and spleen crosstalk pathways during liver cirrhosis [2].

Spleen size in patients with cirrhosis varies by the etiology of the disease. While in healthy adults, the size of the spleen in usually less than 12 cm, in cirrhotic patients it is relatively larger, as shown in the study by Kashani et al. This study revealed that the mean spleen size in the alcohol group (13.1 ± 2.5 cm) was significantly smaller than in the hepatitis C (15.0 ± 3.4 cm) and nonalcoholic steatohepatitis (15.2 ± 3.0 cm) groups (95% confidence intervals of the mean difference, 0.6 to 3.3 and 0.8 to 3.4 cm, respectively), sonographically [6].

4. Splenectomy effects to the liver

Cirrhotic patients are generally considered as immunocompromised, mainly due to the development of bacterial infection and community-acquired infections. Since the spleen is the largest lymphoid organs with large amount of T and B cells, macrophages, and dendritic cells, splenectomy in cirrhotic patients has produced concern over decrease immunity and elevated risk of infection, namely overwhelming post splenectomy pneumococcal sepsis.

However, a study by Hirakawa et al., showed the possibility of reducing suppressive cell fractions and enhancement of the effector cell population and functions by means of splenectomy, thus ameliorate the impaired immune status of cirrhotic patients [7].

Yamada et al. demonstrated that splenectomy improved hepatic functional reserves and nutritional metabolism, together with improvement in thrombocytopenia and leukopenia in cirrhotic patients. Splenectomy is thought to induce a decrease in platelet pooling or breakdown in the spleen of thrombocytopenic patients, and as a result, increase blood platelet counts. Bilirubinemia secondary to hypersplenism, which is caused by an increase in bilirubin production, that overloads the capacity of the liver to metabolize bilirubin, are also reduced after splenectomy [8].

In a study by Ueda et al. of rats undergoing major liver resection with or without splenectomy, early stage splenic red pulp TGF-β1 production and secretion into the portal blood exert an inhibitory effect on liver regeneration. Splenectomy reversed this inhibition and enhanced the regeneration of hepatocytes [9].

Study by Huang et al., unveiled serum cytokine profiles in HBV-related cirrhosis patients with PH and hypersplenism, indicating a potential role of the hypertensive spleen in the progression of liver disease. Furthermore, the changes in cytokine levels following splenectomy maybe potential advantageous to reduce liver fibrosis and accelerate liver regeneration as well as reduce the risk of HCC [10].

Splenectomy also enhanced the repopulation of adoptively transferred bone marrow cell in cirrhotic liver and decreased collagen deposition through the upregulation of MM9 expression in transferred bone marrow cells, as suggested by Iwamoto et al. [11], and improved the efficiency of adipose tissue-derived mesenchymal cell transplant into the liver by enhancing liver SCF-1 and HGV expressions [12].

Considering all of the above mention mechanism, targeting spleen for the treatment of liver cirrhosis can be achieved through [2]:

- amelioration of cirrhosis' fatal complications such as bleeding esophageal or gastric varices
- efficiently improving liver function and the prognosis of esophageal varices
- increasing the efficacy of liver transplantation and improving the prognosis of HCC
- supplementary treatment for anti-HCV therapy in combination with interferons and other pharmaceuticals.

5. Technical and perioperative consideration for splenectomy in cirrhotic liver

Surgery in a patient with liver disease carries specific and higher risks, compare to those with normal populations. Perioperative care including assessment and optimalization is the key to a safe surgery. Many cirrhosis patients present themselves with a relative contraindications that preclude surgery.

The predictors for complications including Child-Pugh class B or C, ascites, etiology of cirrhosis other than PBC, elevated creatinine, preoperative infection, COPD, preoperative upper GI bleeding, invasiveness of surgical procedure, intraoperative hypotension, and ASA status 4–5. While the predictors of mortality including male gender, Child-Pugh class B or C, ascites, etiology of cirrhosis other than PBC, preoperative infection, ASA status 4–5 and respiratory surgery. The presence of 1 risk factors carries a 9.3% risk of complications, and this increase with the more numbers of risk factors. A total of 7–8 risk factors carries a 100% risk of complications [13].

Friedman proposed the following list of contraindication to elective surgery in patients with liver disease, including acute viral hepatitis, alcoholic hepatitis, acute liver failure, acute renal failure, severe coagulopathy, hypoxemia and cardiomyopathy [14].

Regarding the preferred method for splenectomy, recently laparoscopic has become technically feasible, safe and effective procedure for hypersplenism secondary to cirrhosis, and contributes to less blood loss, shorter length of stay and less impairment of liver function. However, this methods are generally more costly and might not readily available in every hospital. Thus the choice of splenectomy method must be personally selected for each patient, surgeon and hospital [15].

6. Splenectomy as a bridge to liver transplant

It is already a general consensus that liver transplantation is the preferred treatment options for patient with end stage liver disease. However, the waiting time for liver transplantation is also long due to the shortage of donor organs, even in living donor liver transplantation setting. Moreover, in some countries, liver transplantation still not a feasible option for all patients.

One among many alternatives is by doing a splenectomy prior to liver transplantation in patient with liver cirrhosis and subsequent splenomegaly-hypersplenism. A study by Kong et al., studied 833 patient patients underwent liver transplantation, of which 88 patients had splenectomy before liver transplantation. They found that postoperative infection and 90-days mortality in the splenectomy and non-splenectomy group were not statistically difference. Furthermore, the post-transplant thrombocytopenia and early allograft dysfunctions is significantly lower in splenectomy group compare to non-splenectomy group. They suggested that pre-transplantation splenectomy is recommended in cases with risky patients without appropriate source of liver for LT. Taking into consideration the possibility of more difficult operation due to adhesion when transplantation is being done. One thing to note is that as a "re-operation" the splenectomy is often as- sociated with more difficult dissection due to adhesions [16].

7. Summary

Splenectomy is beneficial in reversal of the pathologic process through live regeneration and pre-transplant splenectomy could be an alternative in patients without appropriate source of liver for liver transplantation. However, perioperative considerations should be thoroughly assessed to allow a safe surgery.

Conflict of interest

"The authors declare no conflict of interest."

Notes/thanks/other declarations

Part of this article was presented in APASL Congress, Bali, March 2020.

Author details

Adianto Nugroho
Department of Surgery, HPB Section, Digestive Division, Fatmawati Central General Hospital, Jakarta, Indonesia

*Address all correspondence to: adiyusuf97@gmail.com

References

[1] Paraskevas, G.K., Koutsouflianiotis, K.N., Nitsa, Z. *et al.* Knowledge of the anatomy and physiology of the spleen throughout Antiquity and the Early Middle Ages. *Anat Sci Int* 2016; **91,** 43-55

[2] Cesta MF. Normal structure, function, and histology of the spleen. *Toxicol Pathol*. 2006;34(5):455-465.

[3] Li, L, Duan, M, Chen, W *et al.* The spleen in liver cirrhosis: revisiting an old enemy with novel targets. *J Transl Med* 2017;**15,** 111

[4] Stricland A, Lloyd D. The spleen and indications for splenectomy. Surgery 2007;25(2): 98-101

[5] Morgenstern L. A history of splenectomy. In: Hiat JR, Phillips EH, Morgenstern L, ed. Surgical disease of the spleen. Springer, 1997.

[6] Kashani A, Salehi B, Anghesom D, Kawayeh AM, Rouse GA, Runyon BA. Spleen size in cirrhosis of different etiologies. *J Ultrasound Med*. 2015; 34(2):233-238.

[7] Hirakawa Y, Ogata T, Sasada T, Yamashita T, Itoh K, Tanaka H and Okuda K: Immunological consequences following splenectomy in patients with liver cirrhosis. Exp Ther Med 18: 848-856, 2019

[8] Yamada S, Morine Y, Imura S, et al. Liver regeneration after splenectomy in patients with liver cirrhosis. *Hepatol Res*. 2016;46(5):443-449.

[9] Ueda S, Yamanoi A, Hishikawa Y, et al. Transforming growth factor-b1 released from the spleen exerts a growth inhibitory effect on liver regen- eration in rats. Lab Invest. 2003;83(11):1595-603.

[10] Huang N, Ji F, Zhang S, et al. Effect of Splenectomy on Serum Cytokine Profiles in Hepatitis B Virus-Related Cirrhosis Patients with Portal Hypertension. *Viral Immunol*. 2018;31(5):371-378.

[11] Iwamoto T, Terai S, Mizunaga Y, et al. Splenectomy enhances the anti-fibrotic effect of bone marrow cell infusion and improves liver function in cirrhotic mice and patients. *J Gastroenterol*. 2012;47(3):300-312.

[12] Tang WP, Akahoshi T, Piao JS, et al. Splenectomy enhances the therapeutic effect of adipose tissue-derived mesenchymal stem cell infusion on cirrhosis rats. *Liver Int*. 2016;36(8):1151-1159

[13] Rai R, Nagral S, Nagral A. Surgery in a patient with liver disease. *J Clin Exp Hepatol*. 2012;2(3):238-246

[14] Friedman L.S. Surgery in the patient with liver disease. Trans Am Clin Climatol Assoc. 2010;121:192-205

[15] Zhan XL, Ji Y, Wang YD. Laparoscopic splenectomy for hyper-splenism secondary to liver cirrhosis and portal hypertension. *World J Gastroenterol* 2014; 20(19): 5794-5800

[16] Kong, L., Li, M., Li, L. *et al.* Splenectomy before adult liver transplantation: a retrospective study. *BMC Surg 2017;* **17,** 44

Chapter 12

Histopathology of Wilson Disease

Nese Karadag Soylu

Abstract

Wilson Disease (WD) is a genetic metabolic disease of copper metabolism. The implicated gene is ATP7B, encodes a P-type ATPase which transports copper. The resultant defective metabolism of copper results in copper accumulation in multiple tissues especially liver, eye and central nervous system. WD occurs worldwide, usually between 5 and 35 years; a wider age range is also reported. Clinical presentations are diverse and include combinations of hepatic, neurological, ophthalmic and psychiatric manifestations. Other organs or tissues may also be affected. Biochemical abnormalities such as serum ceruloplasmin and 24-h urinary copper excretion are important for the diagnosis but are not always abnormal in WD. The liver histopathology has several different patterns from mild nonspecific changes to acute fulminant hepatitis and cirrhosis. Copper histochemistry is helpful in diagnosis. Genetic testing is another diagnostic tool. It is important to diagnose WD because it is fatal when overlooked, curable when diagnosed. The diagnosis should be keep in mind at all ages in patients with hepatic disease, neurological disease, or psychiatric symptoms.

Keywords: Wilson disease, copper, liver, histopathology, histochemistry

1. Introduction

Wilson Disease (WD) is an autosomal recessive genetic metabolic disease of copper metabolism. Its incidence is vary in different geographic areas with an average incidence of 1 in 30,000 individuals worldwide. Recent studies suggest a considerably higher prevalence of 1:1500–1:3000 for WD. It is caused by mutations in the ATP7B gene encoding a copper transporting P-type ATPase required for copper excretion into the bile [1, 2]. WD is first described by the American neurologist Samuel Alexander Kinnier Wilson in 1912. There are earlier case reports mostly by neurologist in mid 1800s [3]. Kayser and Fleischer mentioned the pigmented corneal rings, in 1902 and 1903 respectively In 1911, Wilson presented his monograph describing the "progressive lenticular degeneration". Bramwell, in 1916, was the first to realize the importance of liver pathology in WD. In 1948, Cumings described the copper abnormalities in WD and in 1952, Scheinberg and Gitlin showed that the ceruloplasmin levels were low in most of WD patients. In 1956, Walshe introduced the penicillamine as a chelating agent, the first effective treatment for the condition [3, 4]. This discovery of successful chelation therapy makes WD one of the most satisfying genetic diseases to be diagnosed and treated.

Originally WD was described as a neurodegenerative disease associated with cirrhosis of the liver. Later, WD was observed in children and adolescents with acute or chronic liver disease without any neurologic symptoms [5]. Now, WD is considered a multi-systemic disorder, in which hepatic, neurological and psychiatric symptoms are often associated with renal, endocrine, osteoarticular, corneal and myocardial disturbances, all related to abnormal copper metabolism ending with systemic accumulation of the copper [6, 7].

Ultrastructural findings of WD have also been studied. The mitochondrial changes are the most distinctive and pathogenetically significant and include heterogeneity of size and shape, increased matrix density, separation of inner from outer membranes, enlarged intercristal spaces and various types of inclusions. Importantly, ultrastructural mitochondrial changes in WD cannot be considered pathognomonic; although exceedingly rare with cholestatic liver disease, such changes are found with mtDNA depletion disorders [4, 8].

WD has considerable variation in clinical presentations, the most common ones being liver disease and neuropsychiatric disturbances [9]. There is considerable phenotypic variation in WD: Some patients present with hepatic disease during the first decade of life, some with neurological degeneration in adolescence or adult life, with or without overt liver disease. In a study by Ferenci et al., the severity of liver disease did not show correlation with the mutation status. Rather, they reported that the prevalence of cirrhosis increased with age in pediatric patients. They found that hepatic disease was more common among females, whereas neurological presentation occurred more frequently in males [10]. The wide range of disease patterns cannot be explained just by different mutations. Environmental, epigenetic, and other genetic factors are also contribute pathogenesis of WD [6, 10].

Classically low serum copper and low ceruloplasmin levels with high urinary copper content make a triad which is usually associated with WD diagnosis. But this triad may be absent or incomplete in 3% of genetically confirmed WD cases [7].

Early diagnosis of WD is important. But it is also important to make the diagnosis of WD prior to transplantation. Because organ transplant networks make special provision for acute liver failure (ALF) due to WD when considering the urgency of transplantation and the terminology relating to acute presentations of liver disease become relevant when listing a case of WD [11].

A large variability in the age of onset and in the clinical presentation of WD exists. Hepatic manifestations of WD at presentation can be extremely variable, and range from asymptomatic hepatomegaly, isolated splenomegaly, persistent or intermittent elevation of serum aminotransferases, jaundice, fatty liver or pseudo-autoimmune hepatitis, acute hepatitis, compensated or decompensated cirrhosis to acute liver failure (ALF). The varied clinical manifestations of WD due to pathological copper accumulation in different organs, even in the early course of the disease, often pose a diagnostic challenge [7].

The main therapeutic strategy is using chelating agents, particularly D-penicillamine. Liver transplantation (LT) is reserved for patients unresponsive to medical therapy or with fulminant hepatic failure. LT for neurological complications is highly controversial and generally cannot be recommended [8].

2. Pathogenesis and clinical manifestations

Copper is an essential element for cellular function. Dietary copper is absorbed in the stomach and duodenum and reaches the liver by the portal vein [1]. Intestinal uptake is regulated by the Menkes ATPase (ATP7A). The ATP7A gene is expressed in most tissues except the liver. Menkes disease, an X-linked copper deficiency disorder, results from mutations in this gene. The abnormal gene in Wilson disease is ATP7B (the Wilson ATPase) which shows 56% homology to ATP7A [8]. It is expressed mainly in the liver but its expression is not restricted to liver cells. This data suggests that ATP7B dysfunction might be responsible for the systemic disturbances of copper trafficking in the whole human body [1, 6]. The hepatic protein ATP7B encodes a copper-transporting P-type ATPase, transporting copper into the secretory pathway for incorporation into apoceruloplasmin, forming ceruloplasmin. ATP7B moves copper into the trans-Golgi network, where ceruloplasmin peptide acquires its complement of copper, assumes its folded state and is then released into the circulation [12]. Excess is excreted eventually into the bile. Without the normal complement of copper, the peptide folds differently and has a decreased circulating half-life, leading to a low level of serum ceruloplasmin. Biliary excretion of copper is necessary for its homeostasis. When ATPB7 is defective, excess copper accumulates in the hepatocytes. Eventually the excess copper exceeds the storage capacity causing hepatocellular injury and release of copper into the circulation. Most WD patients have a low level of circulating ceruloplasmin which is a direct result of defective copper handling in hepatocytes as a result of mutation of the ATP7B gene. Free copper is extremely toxic and can produce irreversible cellular damage. The functional consequences of pathogenic ATP7B mutation are increased intracellular copper levels. This produces oxidative stress and free radical formation as well as mitochondrial dysfunction, which results in cell death in the liver, brain, kidneys, heart, eyes, and joints. As this disease damages multiple systems at one time, it poses a diagnostic challenge [2]. Over 600 gene alteration in ATP7B were recognized [6, 12]. The most common ones are single-nucleotide missense and nonsense mutations, chased by insertions/deletions, and, rarely, splice site mutations. H1069Q is the most common mutation around the world, seen in most of the WD carriers in Europe and USA, with some absence for this mutation in some countries [6]. Correlation of phenotype with specific mutations (genotype) is difficult in Wilson disease because the vast majority of affected individuals are compound heterozygotes, possessing one copy each of two different mutations. Differences in clinical features of various mutations between siblings and even identical twins suggests that other genes or environmental factors are important [6, 8]. In a study by Ferenci et al., it was suggested that the HSD17B13:TA allele may modulate the phenotype and outcome of WD by reducing the transition from copper induced hemolysis to fulminant WD. Furthermore, it is associated with milder histological changes [10]. When testing for mutations of the WD gene ATP7B becomes inexpensive and rapid, genetic testing may become the starting point for diagnostic investigation [1].

WD has a myriad of clinical presentations, hepatic, neurological, ophthalmic and psychiatric, that mimic other conditions. WD may present at any age. Although most patients present between ages 5 and 35, the age range is much wider. There are cases reported as early as 9 months and as late as the eighth decade [1, 2, 13]. So far, the oldest patient in English literature is a 77- year-old Turkish woman [14].

Approximately one half of the patients with WD present with liver disease. In the majority of cases, WD manifests its presence during childhood or teenage years in the form of liver symptoms [7]. Hepatic symptoms and presentations of WD are very variable from asymptomatic cases to cases with overt cirrhosis or with ALF. Liver disease may mimic all forms of common liver conditions. All children with an apparent diagnosis of autoimmune hepatitis should also be investigated for WD, and adults with a presumptive diagnosis of autoimmune hepatitis failing to respond rapidly and appropriately to corticosteroid therapy must be carefully evaluated for WD. In terms of the rate of progression of the disease, cirrhosis is usually diagnosed in the second decade of life, although some individuals do not develop cirrhosis, even after the fourth decade of life [15]. Hepatic manifestations usually present earlier than neurological symptoms by 5 years. The most common hepatic signs and symptoms are jaundice, hepatomegaly and abdominal pain [1]. In a subset of patients focal liver lesions may show up, showing with a wide run of imaging highlights. The lion's share of focal liver lesions in patients with WD are benign nodules, but there are reports that have depicted malignant liver tumors or dysplastic nodules in these patients. Although rare in WD compared to other liver diseases, hepatocellular carcinoma occurs in patients of all ages. Cholangiocarcinoma may also occur in WD [8].

Neurologic manifestations include tremor, gait disturbances, choreiform movements, Parkinsonism or akinetic rigid syndrome i.e., partial parkinsonism, dysarthria, pseudobulbar palsy, rigid dystonia, seizures, migraine headaches, and insomnia. In WD cohorts, neurological presentation is associated with a significantly longer time from onset of symptoms to diagnosis than hepatic presentation, ranging from 2.5 to 6 years. In large case series, mean age at onset of neurologic problems extends from 15 to 21 a long time of age, a decade after onset of liver disease, but a number of patients have been analyzed with a starting neurologic onset earlier than age 10 [7]. Psychiatric manifestations encompass depression, neuroses, personality changes, psychosis and poor performance at school. It was reported that 30—40% of patients have psychiatric symptoms at diagnosis and 20% had seen a psychiatrist prior to their WD diagnosis [12]. WD should be ruled out in any teenager with unexplained cognitive, psychiatric, or movement disorder [13]. Neuropsychiatric signs are the predominant presentation in adults but also may be present in up to 50% of teenagers. WD should also be included in the differential diagnosis work-up of unclear neuropsychiatric syndromes in patients after age 60 years [9].

Ocular findings include the Kayser–Fleischer (KF) ring, due to copper accumulation in Desçemet's membrane, and sunflower cataracts, due to copper accumulation in the lens. They are diagnosed by slit lamp examination. In known cases of hepatic WD, the rings are present in just over half of patients. KF rings are usually absent in children with liver disease. KF rings are rarely observed in other conditions such as in patients with chronic cholestatic diseases, monoclonal gammopathies, multiple myeloma, arci senilis, and pulmonary carcinoma and are thus not specific for WD [1, 7]. Of note, KF rings are not so easy to diagnose without experience, some authors suggest that anterior segment Scheimpflug imaging (Pentacam, Oculus) could be more helpful to diagnose or confirm KF rings by ophthalmologists with little experience in patients with WD. In general it is said that when neurological symptoms are present, KF rings is present in almost all WD patients at disease diagnosis [7]. But there are reports of cases with neurological involvement without KF rings [8].

Other presentations and clinical findings are intermittent bouts of jaundice caused by haemolysis, gynaecomastia, amenorrhoea, repeated spontaneous abortion, cardiac complications including ECG abnormalities, ventricular fibrillation, cardiomyopathy, orthostatic hypotension, urolithiasis, renal tubular disease, hypoparathyroidism, pancreatitis and rhabdomyolysis [8].

3. Laboratory findings

Elucidation of some straightforward biochemical tests have been appeared to be both touchy and decently particular for WD. Two such records incorporate a proportion of alanine aminotransferase (ALT) by aspartate aminotransferase (AST), and a proportion of alkaline phosphatase (ALP) by total bilirubin (TB). An ALT/AST proportion of more than 2.2 contains a sensitivity of 94% and a specificity of 86%; the ALP/TB proportion of less than 4 encompasses a sensitivity of 94% and a specificity of 96% [4].

In Wilson disease, the 24-hour urine copper excretion is usually >100 μg (1.6 μmol) and almost always exceeds 40 μg (0.6 μmol). When penicillamine 500 mg is administered by mouth at the beginning and 12 h later during a 24-hour urine collection, copper excretion >25 μmoles (1587 μg) per 24 h is taken as diagnostic. This test has been validated only in children, and its sensitivity is not as great as originally thought [8].

Ceruloplasmin is the major carrier for copper in the blood. Testing for serum ceruloplasmin is often done when searching for the cause of unexplained liver disease. There are physiologic variations in the serum level of ceruloplasmin. It is very low in early infancy to the age of 6 months, peak at higher than adult levels in early childhood, and then decrease to the normal adult range [1]. A serum ceruloplasmin level < 200 mg/L (<20 mg/dL) has been considered consistent with WD, and diagnostic if associated with KF rings. Except WD, conditions such as marked renal or enteric protein loss, severe end stage liver disease of any etiology, neurologic diseases copper deficiency, and Menkes disease can show low ceruloplasmin levels [1, 7, 13].

Total serum copper (which incorporates non–ceruloplasmin bound copper or "free copper" and copper joined in ceruloplasmin) is ordinarily diminished in extent to the diminished serum ceruloplasmin. However, in patients with WD with extreme liver damage, serum copper may be inside the ordinary extend or uniquely hoisted within the setting of ALF due to the discharge of copper from liver tissue stores and the increase in free copper in the blood [13]. A novel approach is the direct specification of labile copper (non-Cp-bound copper), called interchangeable copper (CuEXC). It permits to calculate the "relative replaceable copper" (REC) which alludes to the proportion of CuEXC to total copper. REC was assessed as a convenient diagnostic appliance for WD with a high sensitivity and specifity allows the calculation of relative interchangeable copper (REC) that compares to the proportion between CuEXC and total serum copper. It is represented that REC is a great diagnostic biomarker with a specifity and specificity near to 100% for the determination of WD when its value is >18.5%. It allows a separation of Wilsonian liver disease from other types of liver disorders such as autoimmune, infectious. Moreover, REC can make a great aid to family screening, because it is possible to make a distinction between WD patients and heterozygous carriers or healthy subjects. The CuEXC value at diagnosis indicates of extrahepatic involvement and its seriousness [7]. But further studies are needed to evaluate its diagnostic accuracy in children with liver disease [13].

The urine copper shows to the sum of non-ceruloplasmin bound copper within the circulation. Urinary copper concentration is measured per 24 h since there's noteworthy changeability within the copper substance of spot urine collections for them to be utilized. The customary level taken as demonstrative of WD is >100 μg/24 h (>1.6 μmol/24 h) in symptomatic patients [1]. In asymptomatic children or children with mild liver disease, urinary copper values are often normal [13]. However, high urinary copper values may be seen in other sorts of liver disorders (e.g., autoimmune hepatitis, unremitting active liver disease, or cholestasis and in specific during acute liver failure of any etiology). Heterozygotes may too have borderline levels [7].

The diagnosis is not fundamentally straightforward indeed even when the disease is effectively being considered. In a patient within the age-range 5–50 years who has liver disease or characteristic neurological symptoms, finding serum caeruloplasmin underneath 5 mg/dL is profoundly compatible with WD; association too a Kayser–Fleischer (KF) ring affirms the diagnosis. In nearly one-third of patients, serum caeruloplasmin can be within normal limits. As a sole, serum caeruloplasmin is not an adequate diagnostic test for WD. KF rings are diagnostic, but they can also be seen in patients who have persistent cholestasis of other etiology. Lack of KF rings happens in around 50% of adult patients with liver disease and hence does not run the show out WD. KF rings may not be determined even when there's neurological involvement.

4. Histopathology and histochemistry

Liver biopsy is typically performed when clinical and laboratory findings are not diagnostic or for evaluation of unexplained liver disease or abnormal liver tests. Another aim is to determine the degree of hepatic inflammation and for hepatic copper quantitation [1]. The spectrum of hepatic pathological changes occurring in WD is very broad, ranging from elementary changes typical of a toxic pathology, to inflammatory changes typical of viral or autoimmune etiology [6]. The main features are microvesicular and macrovesicular steatosis, glycogenated hepatocyte nuclei, inflammation, and variable hepatocellular anisonucleosis [16, 17].

The manifestations of liver involvement have a varied spectrum depending on the stage of the disease. In the earlier steps, hepatocyte injury may at first manifest as simple steatosis (**Figure 1**) with frequent association of glycogenated nuclei. Steatosis, Mallory-Denk bodies (MBDs), lipogranulomas and glycogenated nuclei have been represented as characteristic morphologic findings in liver biopsies with WD. This picture frequently imitates alcoholic and non-alcoholic fatty liver disease [6]. The distinction from nonalcoholic steatohepatitis (NASH) depends upon the demonstration of accumulated copper in the hepatocytes by histochemical stains. Lipofuscin accumulates in periportal areas, and some of the granules are large, irregular in shape and vacuolated. The intermediate stage of the disease shows

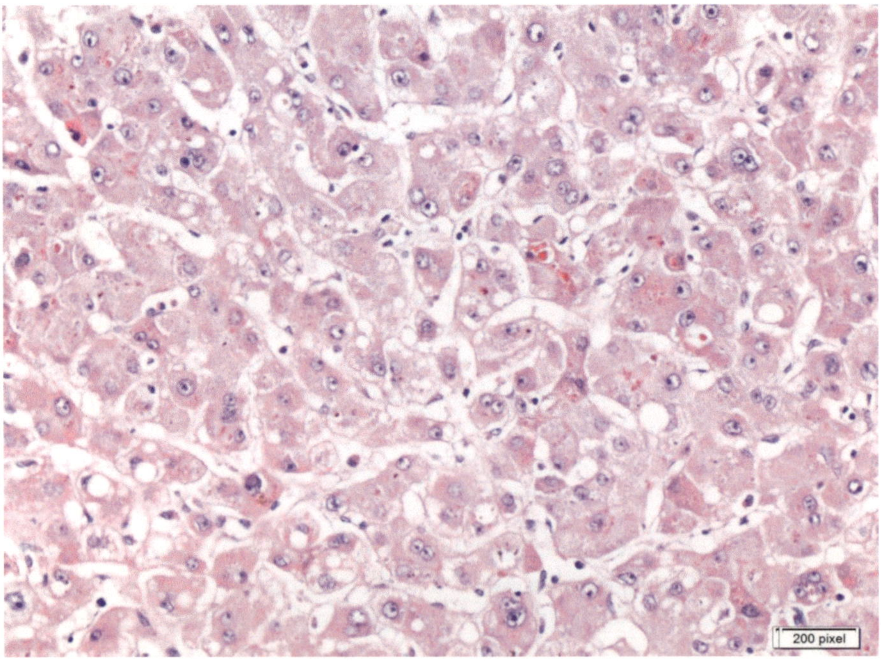

Figure 1.
Steatosis and anisonucleosis in a hepatectomy specimen (H&E).

histological features similar to those of chronic hepatitis of any etiology including viral or autoimmune hepatitis, with the arrival of the portal and periportal inflammation composed of lymphocytes and plasma cells, which results in the destruction of the limiting plate, and parenchymal necrosis followed by bridging fibrosis [4]. Because of low-titer autoantibodies (mainly antinuclear antibodies) are commonly found in patients with WD, differential diagnosis with autoimmune hepatitis (AIH) can be more complicated. Also, cases of WD and concomitant AIH have been reported [13]. More than 50% of cases may show the presence of intra-cytoplasmic eosinophilic MBDs (**Figure 2**). The literature suggests that steatosis, glycogenated nuclei and MBDs in periportal hepatocytes are features that may be used to distinguish the chronic hepatitis of WD from other more common etiologies [1]. In the cirrhotic stage which is usually macronodular but can be mixed or even micronodular, the histologic features are non-specific, and usually little or no inflammation is present. Some cases may show mild steatosis or features of steatohepatitis. Clusters of large hepatocytes with a granular eosinophilic cytoplasm (oncocytic or oxyphil cells), resulting from an increased number of mitochondria, are often seen but this is not specific for WD [8]. The distribution of copper is quite variable, with some of the cirrhotic nodules containing a lot and others containing little or none. Defining widespread copper deposits by histochemistry can help for the diagnosis. It should be noted that the distribution of copper is variable: some nodules with prominent staining, others with minimal or none (**Figure 3**). This could generate false negative impression in biopsy specimens, and it has been suggested that two liver cores may be needed for copper detection and diagnosis. Cases which present with ALF or fulminant hepatitis, the histology includes portal and parenchymal inflammatory infiltrate, associated with hepatocyte injury, swelling and necrosis. There may be massive or submassive necrosis. Copper can be demonstrated in hepatocytes and when there has been significant necrosis, in Kupffer cells and portal macrophages [1, 8]. In contrast, copper is rarely demonstrable in Kupffer cells or portal macrophages in the cirrhotic stage [8].

Excess copper storage in the hepatocytes is a relevant sign of WD, and determination of hepatic copper content in the liver biopsy, is important in the diagnosis of WD. This may be accomplished by utilizing special histochemical stains for copper

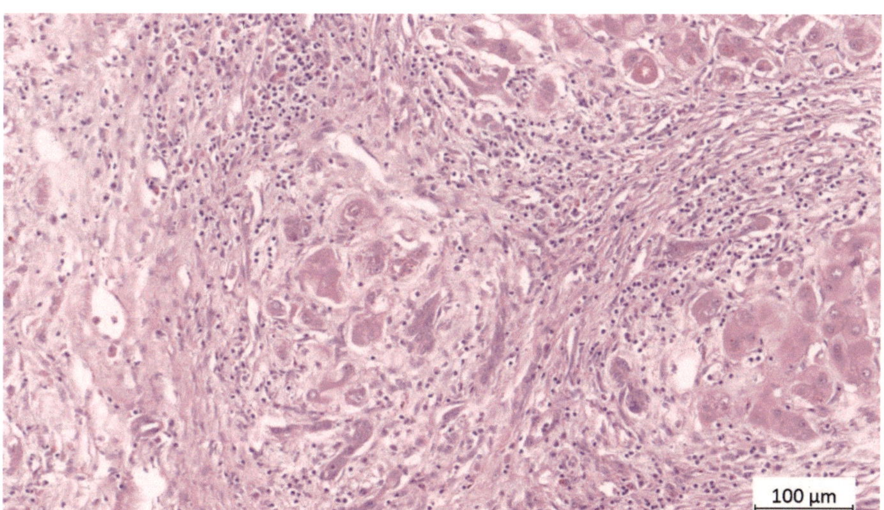

Figure 2.
Mallory-Denk bodies in a hepatectomy specimen (H&E).

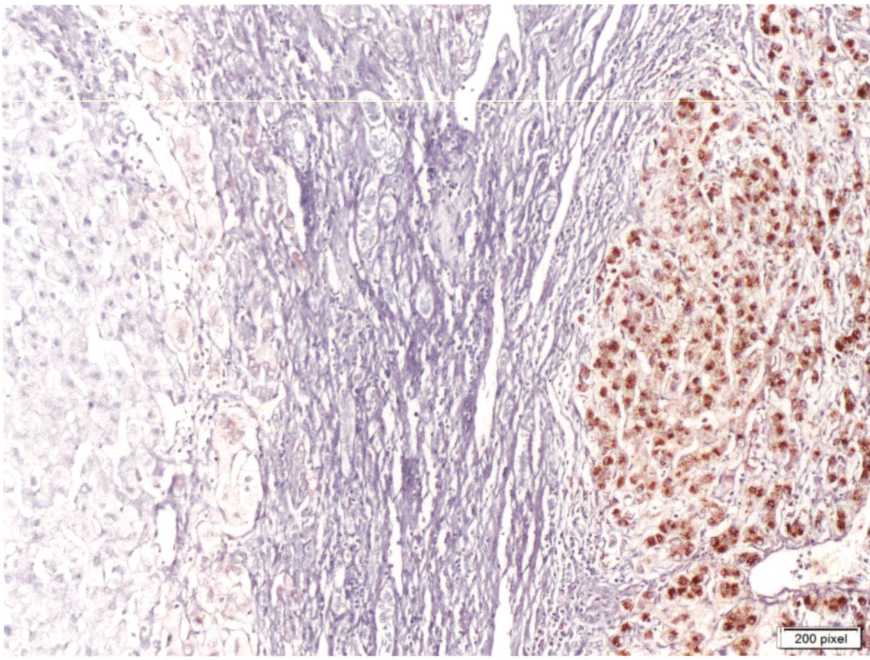

Figure 3.
Heterogenous copper accumulation in a hepatectomy specimen (Rhodanine).

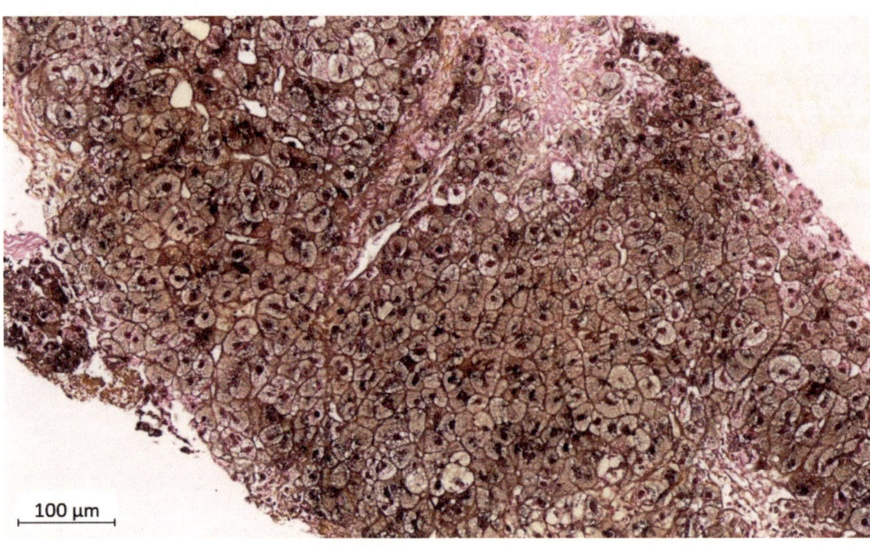

Figure 4.
Diffuse cytoplasmic staining pattern (Timm).

which are rhodanine, rubeanic acid and Timm's silver stains, and for copper related protein of which are orcein, aldehyde fuchsin and Victoria blue. None of these stains is fully sensitive nor specific. Orcein reveals the accumulation of metallothioneins, the proteins involved in excess copper sequestration. Positive staining appears as large irregular granules dark-brown in color. In the Timm's stained slides, if there is mild accumulation copper shows up small black or greenish-black granules in the intracytoplasmic perinuclear area or canalicular side of hepatocytes, and when there is heavy accumulation, the whole cytoplasm of the hepatocyte stuffed with coarse granules. With rhodanine stain copper accumulation appears as

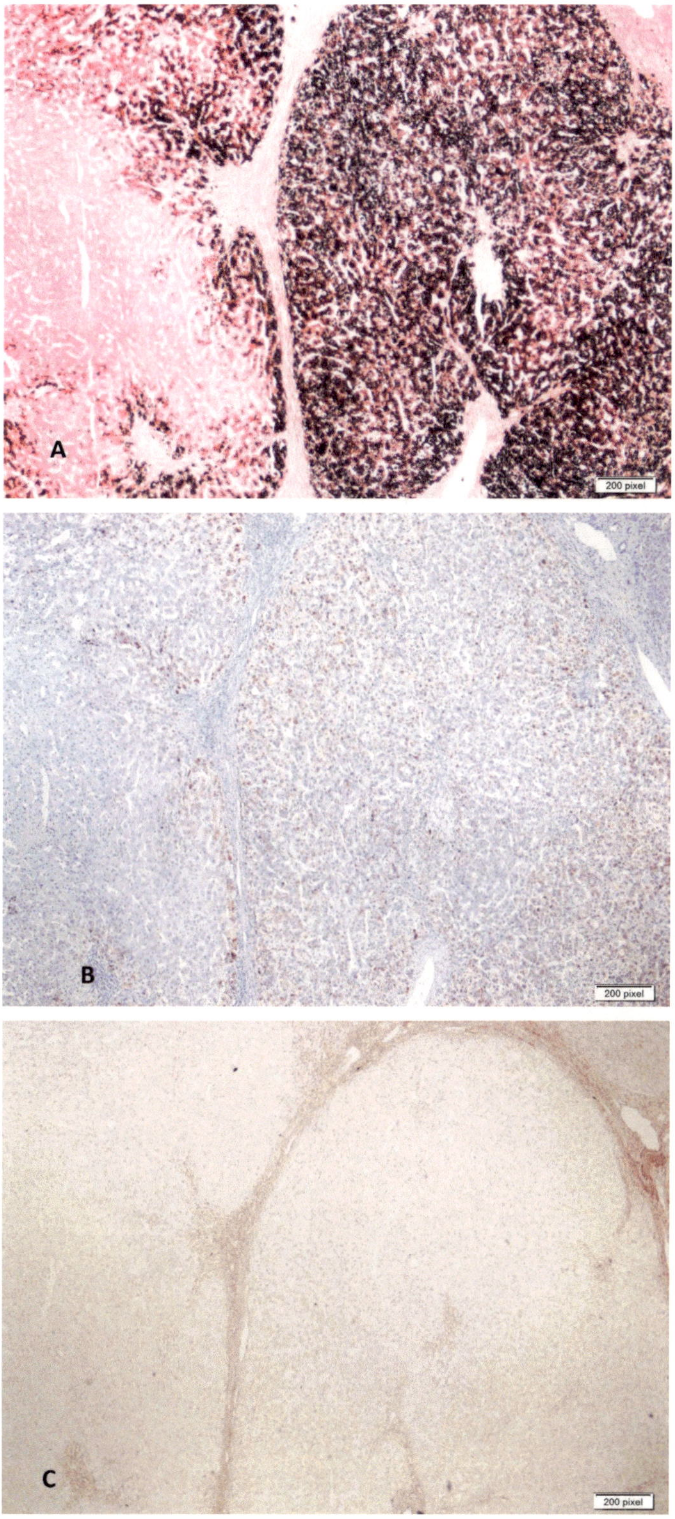

Figure 5.
Different sensitivities of copper stains in the same case (A. Timm, B. Rhodanine, C. Orcein).

small red granules [1, 6, 8]. Out of granular staining, diffuse cytoplasmic staining pattern (**Figure 4**) can be seen with copper stains, which is frequently reported in WD [18].

The most effective method is vary in different reports. In our study with transplant hepatectomies, we found that positivity rates of Timm, rhodanine and orcein are 85%, 82%, and 48% respectively (**Figure 5A-C**). We thought that pannodular (prominent diffuse staining of nodule), staining is a powerfull indicator of WD. In this context, we suggested that pannodular staining is a more convincing staining pattern for the histopathologic diagnosis of WD and against other diseases with copper accumulation [16]. In our routine practice we do Timm's stain for every liver biopsy and hepatectomy. Next to evaluating copper accumulation for diagnosis WD disease, it can help to define late stage fibrosis [18]. It should be keep in mind, copper accumulation can be seen in other diseases such as cholestatic liver diseases, alcoholic liver disease and idiopathic copper toxicosis [6]. In chronic cholestasis and non WD cirrhosis, copper staining is usually limited to periseptal areas with a patchy/focal distribution (**Figure 6**). It is suggested that that in the absence of advanced fibrosis (or WD), a positive rhodanine stain for copper argues strongly in favor of chronic biliary diseases and against other liver diseases [19]. Of note, marked hepatic copper overload mimicking WD has been described in children with MDR3 deficiency [8]. It is important to remember that negative staining for both copper and copper-associated protein does not exclude the diagnosis of WD.

In equivocal cases, measurement of liver copper content is recommended as the next step for diagnosis of WD. A 5-fold increase of hepatic copper concentration is considered as diagnostic for diagnosis of hepatic WD [5]. In a more strict definition, a copper content >250 μg/g dry weight (normal value <50 mg/g dry weight) in adult patients without cholestasis is accepted as diagnostic for WD. Probably depending on sampling error due to nonhomogeneous copper distribution in the liver, lower values are reported in up to 20% of patients with WD. The exactness of liver copper estimation is moved forward with an optimal measured biopsy sample (ideally >1 cm long, min. 0.5 cm) that ought to be put on a little piece of paper for drying,

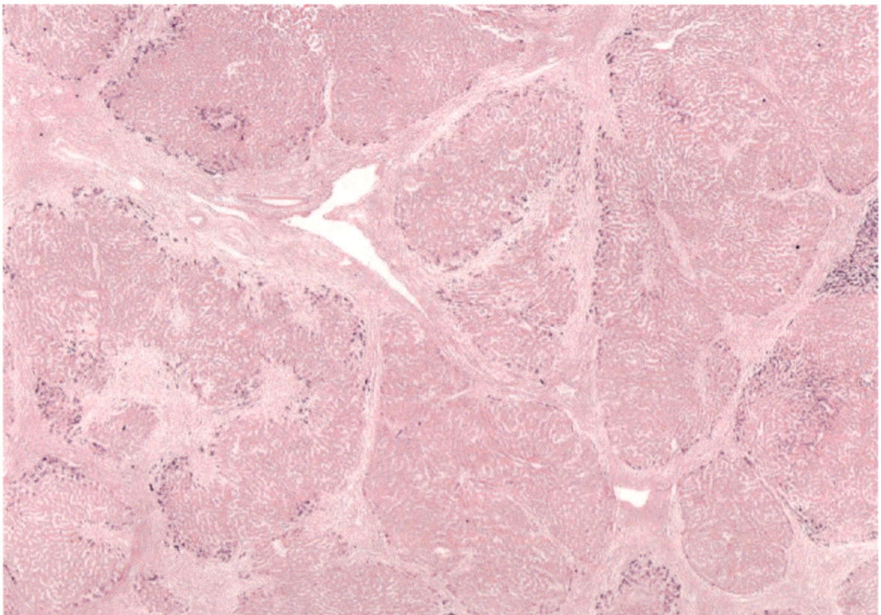

Figure 6.
Periseptal copper accumulation in a non WD cirrhosis (Timm).

and in a dry plastic copper-free holder for atomic absorption analysis on fresh tissue [13]. Hepatic copper levels in advanced stage chronic biliary diseases in adults and children often exceed 250 mg/100 g of dried liver, sometimes reaching levels higher than those observed in WD [19]. In spite of the fact that utilize of dried tissue has been proposed for tissue copper quantitation, the utilize of formalin-fixed, paraffin-embedded (FFPE) tissue is said fair as valuable. Utilizing FFPE tissue specimens evacuates the specialized troubles related to dried unfixed tissue, as well as gives the same tissue for histopathological and quantitative assessments. Since copper accumulation may well be non homogenious indeed even in most progressed cases of WD, the availability of light microscopy on the same tissue being evaluated for copper may well be a really valuable tool in mostly tending to this potential examining inclination tissue quantitation of copper is subject to [17]. Although liver copper content is a useful parameter, but a value below 250 μg/g does not exclude WD. Diagnosis requires the combination of a variety of clinical and biochemical tests [5].

5. Conclusion

WD is a curable disease, but early diagnosis is essential to stop the progression to cirrhosis or worsening of the neurological and psychiatric conditions. As a treatable disease, WD should be detected by any health professionals at any care level. If WD is not recognized and adequately treated, the progression of liver disease to cirrhosis and liver failure can be rapid or irreversible brain damage can occur. Unfortunately, even though of all advances, the diagnosis of WD shows up frequently compelling, due to the variability of its clinical manifestation and to the complexity of the microscopic findings within the liver biopsy. Liver histopathology, in reality, does not show a unique morphology, but it may appear in different patterns. From a pathologist's perspective, when evaluating the liver biopsies, WD should be included in the differential diagnosis especially in pediatric age and also cryptogenic adult cases.

Thanks

The author would like to thank to Dr. Emine Samdanci as a team member of hepatopathology and to Dr. Seyma Eren and Dr. Meryem Uludag for photography.

Author details

Nese Karadag Soylu
Department of Pathology, Medical School, Inonu University, Malatya, Turkey

*Address all correspondence to: nesekaradag@yahoo.com

References

[1] Guindi M. Wilson disease. Seminars in Diagnostic Pathology. 2019;36: 415-422. DOI: 10.1053/j.semdp.2019.07.008

[2] Chaudhury S, Patkar P. Wilson's Disease: An Update. Med J DY Patil Vidyapeeth. 2018;11:92-3.11 (2018): 92-3. DOI: 10.4103/MJDRDYPU.MJDRDYPU_139_17

[3] Barbosa ER, Machado AAC, Cançado ELR, Deguti MM, Scaff M. Wilson's disease: a case report and a historical review. Arq Neuropsiquiatr. 2009;67(2b): 539-43. DOI: 10.1590/S0004-282X2009000300036

[4] Madakshira MG, Das A, Umair M, Dutta U. Liver histology and histochemistry in Wilson disease. Autops Case Report [Internet]. 2018;8(3): e2018026. DOI: 10.4322/acr.2018.026

[5] Ferenci P, Steindl-Munda P, Vogel W, et al. Diagnostic Value of Quantitative Hepatic Copper Determination in Patients With Wilson's Disease. Clin Gastroenterol Hepatol. 2005; 3: 811-8. DOI: 10.1016/s1542-3565(05)00181-3

[6] Gerosa C, Fanni D, Congiu T, Piras M, Cau F, Moi M, Faa G. Liver pathology in Wilson's disease: From copper overload to cirrhosis. Journal of Inorganic Biochemistry. 2019;193: 106-111. DOI: 10.1016/j.jinorgbio.2019.01.008

[7] Poujois A, Woimant F. Challenges in the diagnosis of Wilson disease. Ann Transl Med. 2019;7(Suppl 2):: S56. DOI: 10.21037/atm.2019.02.10

[8] Quaglia A, Roberts EA, Torbenson M. Disorders of copper metabolism. In: Burt AD, Ferrell LD, Hübscher SG, editors. MacSween's Pathology of the Liver. 7th ed. Elsevier; 2018. p. 200-206. ch3

[9] Žigrai M, Vyskoči M, Tóthová A, Vereš P, Bluska P, Valkovič P. Late-Onset Wilson's Disease. Front Med (Lausanne). 2020;(7): 26. DOI: 10.3389/fmed.2020.00026

[10] Ferenci P, Stremmel W, Czlonkowska A, et al. Age and sex but not ATP7B genotype effectively influence the clinical phenotype of Wilson. Hepatology. 2019;69: 1464-76. DOI: 10.1002/hep.30280

[11] Shribman S, Webb G, Taylor R, Warner TT, Duckworth A, Gimson A, et al. Liver transplantation for late-onset presentations of acute liver failure in Wilson's disease: the UK experience over 2 decades. JHEP Rep. 2020;2(3): 100096. DOI: 10.1016/j.jhepr.2020.100096

[12] Poujois A, Woimant F. Wilson's disease: A 2017 update. Clinics and Research in Hepatology and Gastroenterology. 2018;42: 512—520. DOI: 10.1016/j.clinre.2018.03.007

[13] Socha P, Janczyk W, Dhawan A, et al. Wilson's Disease Wilson's disease in children: a Position paper by the Hepatology Committee of the European Society for Paediatric Gastroenterology, Hepatology and Nutrition. J Pediatr Gastroenterol Nutr. 2018;66:334-344. DOI: 10.1097/MPG.0000000000001787

[14] Sohtaoglu M, Ergin H, Özekmekçi S, et al. Patient with late-onset Wilson disease: deterioration with penicillamine. Mov Disord. 2007;22:290-1. DOI: 10.1002/mds.21201

[15] Sini M, Sorbello O, Sanna F, et al. Histologic evolution and long-term outcome of Wilson's disease: results of a single-center experience. Eur J Gastroenterol Hepatol. 2013;25(1): 111-7. DOI: 10.1097/MEG.0b013e328358f7

[16] Karadag N, Tolan K, Samdanci E, et al. Effect of Copper Staining in Wilson

Disease: A Liver Explant Study. Exp Clin Transplant. 2017;15(5): 542-546. DOI: 10.6002/ect.2015.0319

[17] Hafezi-Bakhtiari S, Adeyi OA. Metabolic Disorders of the Liver. Diagnostic Histopathol. 2014;20: 125-133. DOI: 10.1016/j.mpdhp.2014.01.012

[18] Miyamura H, Nakanuma Y, Kono N. Survey of copper granules in liver biopsy specimens from various liver abnormalities other than Wilson's disease and biliary diseases. Gastroenterol Jpn. 1988;23: 633-638. DOI: 10.1007/BF02782948

[19] Mounajjed T, Oxentenko AS, Qureshi H, Smyrk TC. Revisiting the topic of histochemically detectable copper in various liver diseases with special focus on venous outflow impairment. Am. J. Clin. Pathol. 2013;139: 79-86. DOI: 10.1309/AJCPDZR4OHDQNG3L

Chapter 13

Towards the Study of Liver Failure: Protocol for a 90% Extended Hepatectomy in Mice

Maria J. Lizardo Thiebaud, Eduardo Cervantes-Alvarez and Nalu Navarro-Alvarez

Abstract

Studies have shown that extended hepatectomy mimics post-hepatectomy liver failure (PHLF) and could also be used to study other small-for-flow syndromes. Extended hepatectomy can be defined as the removal of more than 70% of liver volume. At the molecular level, there seems to be a delayed entrance to the cell cycle, and thus liver dysfunction ensues. Therefore, there is an imperious need to study the mechanisms of such delay to understand how it can be regulated. While the classical 70% hepatectomy model to study liver regeneration has been previously described thoroughly, there are no protocols describing the surgical procedure for a 90% extended hepatectomy (90% EHx). Therefore, we here describe a detailed and reproducible protocol for such model, defining specific aspects that must be considered as well as the most common complications and troubleshooting strategies.

Keywords: liver regeneration, 90% extended hepatectomy, liver failure

1. Introduction

Liver regeneration is the process by which lost tissue is replaced through compensatory hyperplasia of the remaining healthy tissue [1–3]. The regenerative capacity of the liver has been studied since the early nineteenth century [4], when scientists observed changes in liver tissue after surgical procedures. By using portosystemic shunts, they first speculated that overall flow was important for liver regeneration, and not specifically portal blood flow. Later on, a combined model including lobectomies and shunts was used as the main model for liver regeneration [4]. Finally, the acknowledgment that portal blood flow was crucial for liver homeostasis gave rise to the "humoral theory," and with this, the race to find factors in the portal blood that promoted liver regeneration began [4].

Most of what we currently know about liver regeneration is thanks to the results obtained with surgical models. These models are the most precise, since timing and volume removal can be controlled. In fact, the surgical technique for a 2/3 hepatectomy in rats as a model for liver regeneration has been described and perfected since first published by Higgins and Anderson in 1931 [5–7]. With advances in anesthesia and analgesia, the extension of the 2/3 hepatectomy provides a useful model for the study of liver regeneration and liver failure [8–10].

IntechOpen

Studies have shown that extended hepatectomy in rats and mice mimics post-hepatectomy liver failure (PHLF), as well as other small-for-flow syndromes observed in humans, including the small-for-size syndrome (SFSS) seen after transplantation [8, 11–14].

PHLF is a syndrome that can result following liver resection for the removal of a tumor or in the context of living donor liver transplantation (LDLT). PHLF is characterized by postoperative liver dysfunction, with clinical signs of hyperbilirubinemia, coagulopathy, portal hypertension, and ascites [15, 16]. PHLF represents the leading cause of mortality post-PHx (>60%), which varies from 0.5 to 8% depending on the extent of resection and the quality of the underlying parenchyma [5, 6, 17–19]. When assessing parameters for prediction of post-hepatectomy complications, the major liver resection has three times more chance of developing PHLF [20].

The precise mechanisms behind PHLF are poorly understood, but it appears to depend not only on the quality and the quantity of the remaining liver parenchyma [1] but on its ability to surmount the effects of surgical resection. Specifically, the tissue must be capable of limiting hepatocyte death, resisting metabolic stress, and preserving or recovering an adequate synthetic function [21 25]. For liver regeneration to occur, there must be homeostasis. Preventing liver failure thus enhances regeneration [17, 26].

Depending on the quality of the parenchyma, there is a predicted threshold of the future liver remnant. This threshold is used to plan extended resections [14, 16, 27]. In order for the liver to function correctly and to cover the minimum demands of the organism, the total liver volume (TLV) has to be at least 20%, or more than 0.5% of the patient's body weight [16, 18, 19, 28]; otherwise, failure can develop. Animal models have the same characteristics, and by using a percentage of liver volume removed, one can predict the development of liver failure. In fact, several studies have shown that in rodents, acute liver failure (ALF) may develop after 90% EHx [8–10]. At the molecular level, there appears to be a delay in the entrance to the cell cycle and as a consequence, liver dysfunction [10].

Due to the multifactorial processes involved in these syndromes, animal models are important tools to improve our understanding of the pathogenesis of ALF and also for the development of new therapeutic approaches. Considering the above, challenging the hepatostat with surgical removal of extensive liver volume, 90% EHx is a helpful model for the study of acute liver failure in the context of liver surgery [19]. Therefore, we here describe a reproducible and detailed protocol for the establishment of a surgical liver failure model in rodents through 90% extended hepatectomy.

2. Experimental design

When using animals as models, many factors have to be considered as delineated as follows.

2.1 Anatomy

The anatomy of the liver in mice differs substantially from that of the humans (**Figure 1a** and **b**). It measures approximately 1.5–2 × 1 cm and weighs 1–1.5 g [9]. It is constituted of four main lobes, the right lobe (RL), the left lobe (LL), the median lobe (ML), and the omental or caudate lobe (CL). The RL is divided in the right superior lobule (RSL) and right inferior lobule (RIL) (**Figure 1a** and **b**). The ML is partially divided in half by the gallbladder, whereas the CL is further divided in anterior and posterior lobules (**Figure 1a** and **b**). Each segment has an attributed

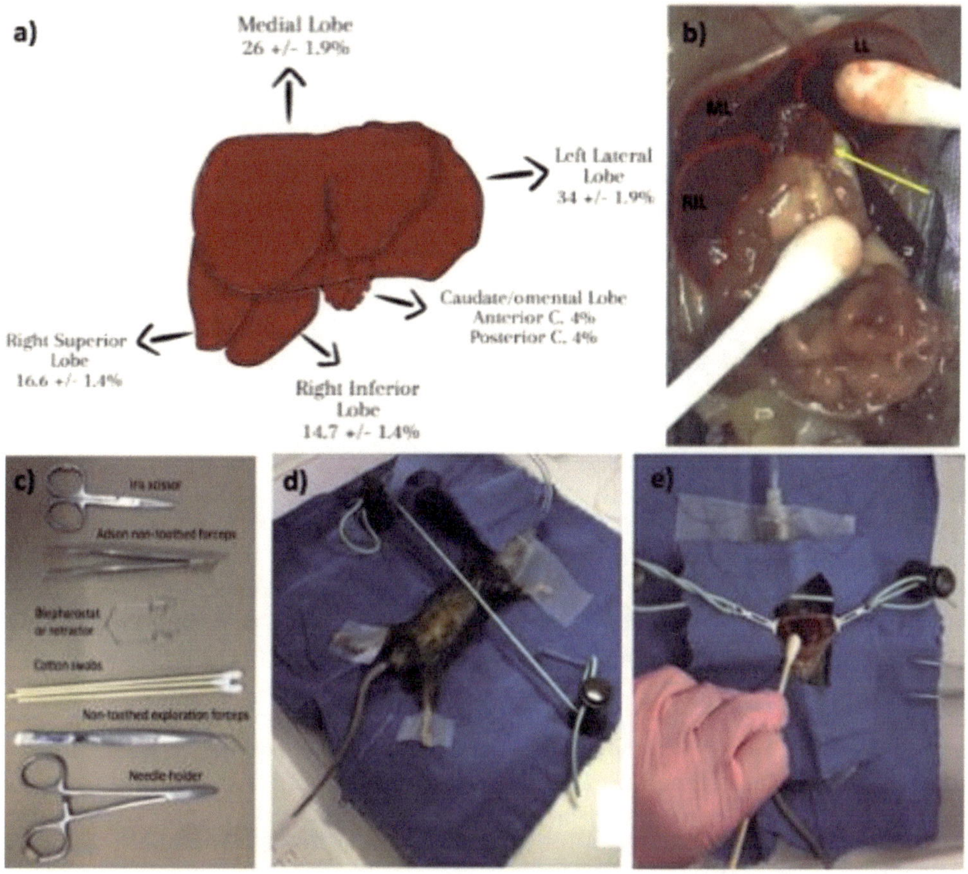

Figure 1.
(a) Anatomy of the mouse liver with the relative volume of each lobe, modified from Martins et al. (2007). (b) Anatomy of the liver lobes as seen in vivo. The yellow arrow signals the caudate lobe. (c) The surgical instruments used in the procedure. (d) Positioning of the mouse on a surgical platform covered by sterile covers. The mouse is immobilized with tape. (e) View of abdominal cavity once it is open and appropriately uncovered. LL, left lobe; ML, medial lobe; RIL, right inferior lobe.

percentage of contribution to the total liver volume (TLV), which constitutes the basis for the planning of a partial (PHx) or extended hepatectomy (EHx). The ML represents 30% of the TLV, with a range between 24 and 28%. The LL represents 40% of the TLV, with a range between 32 and 36%. The RL represents 24% of the TLV, with the RSL and RIL contributing between 12% and 16% each. And lastly, the CL represents 6–8% of the TLV.

2.2 Sex, age, timing of surgery, health status, and nutrition of the subjects

In animals, it is known that age and sex affect the liver's regeneration capacity. Compared to young mice, older mice have a reduced capacity of regeneration due to decreased growth hormone levels [22]. In regard to sex, female hormones are known to affect most of the physiological processes in the body, and the regeneration is no exception [29]. Therefore, the preferred characteristics of the subjects are male mice with an age ranging from 8 to 14 weeks and a weight more than 20 g [1, 21–23].

The circadian rhythm and glucocorticoids have been demonstrated to have an effect on liver regeneration [30, 31]. Specifically, performing the surgery passed noon, there seems to be a delay in the regeneration process mediated through the differential transcription of wee1, which controls cell cycle proteins, thus disturbing the progression of the cycle. Externally, cortisol levels are known to affect DNA synthesis by altering the levels of important enzymes [32]. In fact, it has been shown that the combination of adrenalectomy and partial hepatectomy enhances liver regeneration [33]. Therefore, depending on the specific objective of the study, it is advisable to perform the surgeries in the morning.

The subject's nutrition and health status may affect liver regeneration, especially during the initial phases when hepatocytes are entering the cell cycle [22, 34]. Earlier studies have shown that metabolism affects liver regeneration. Indeed, insulin is one of the main cofactors for liver regeneration [35]. Despite the fact that insulin aids in the process, enhancing insulin secretion through glucose supplementation after partial hepatectomy has been shown to decrease liver regeneration [36]. This could be explained by the effect glycogen synthesis has in other metabolic pathways in the hepatocyte.

Following 70% of liver tissue removal, glycogen storage is reduced. The animal thus develops hypoglycemia, which can be severe enough to cause the animal's demise. To prevent that, supplementation becomes reasonable; however, extrinsic glucose affects hepatic fat accumulation. To compensate hypoglycemia, catabolic hormones are produced, which aid in proliferation of hepatic tissue. The hepatic tissue is oxidizing fatty acids meaning most of the machinery will be concentrated either in beta-oxidation or the cell cycle. Introducing carbohydrates (glucose, fructose, or sorbitol) to the diet is therefore detrimental [34]. The molecular mechanisms are still under study. If carbohydrates are combined with other nutrients, including lipids or/and amino acids, this effect can be prevented. In fact, supplementing lipids or amino acids increases the mitotic activity of cells in a regenerating liver [34].

Likewise, a long-term or short-term low-carbohydrate diet before surgery slows down the process of regeneration. A study where mice being fed with a very low-carbohydrate diet before surgery showed impaired proliferative capacity in hepatocytes. The diet consisted of 5.5% of carbohydrate and a 70% of fat without lowering caloric intake. Though a low-carbohydrate diet seems to accelerate fat accumulation in hepatocytes, other pro-regeneration activities were affected. A stall in the priming phase of liver regeneration was confirmed as key cytokine RNA levels in liver tissue were low, and there was a decrease in phosphorylation of second messengers of important mitogenic signaling cascades [37].

In other words, the unique metabolic state in which hepatocytes are found during liver regeneration is not to be altered. To favor the regenerative process, only beneficial substrates such as amino acids or lipids should be used. With the objective of preventing severe hypoglycemia, we recommend adding dextrose before and not after the surgery.

In the same line, it has been shown that selective bowel decontamination for gram-negative bacteria reduces the development of PHLF in a rat model [38]. The reasoning behind this is based on the fact that during hepatectomy there is significant bacterial translocation, which, when in check by the immune system, promotes liver regeneration. Keeping an appropriate sterile environment in the animal facility thus becomes an absolute requirement.

3. Materials

3.1 Animals

In general, this procedure describes extended hepatectomy performed in 8–14 weeks of age B57CL/6 male mice. All animal studies have been approved by the Universidad Panamericana's ethics committee (protocol #E1704) and have therefore been performed in accordance with the ethical standards laid down in the 1964 Declaration of Helsinki and its later amendments.

3.2 Anesthesia

The procedure may last less than 30 min in skillful hands, but it may lengthen depending on the complexity of the anatomy and the experience of the operator. Therefore, in choosing the anesthetic, the best choice is isoflurane (Sofloran Vet) since others have been shown to be hepatotoxic [7]. Not only is the recovery with isoflurane good, but it is also fast, which helps in evaluating the efficacy of the surgical procedure.

3.3 Analgesia

Analgesia is key to a good surgical procedure. Buprenorphine is the analgesic of choice since it has been proven to diminish pain efficiently [39]. About half an hour before beginning, a subcutaneous injection of buprenorphine is recommended at a dose of 0.05–1 mg/kg, followed by its administration every 8–12 h for the next 72 h. Meloxicam is a good alternative and has the advantage of being used as a single dose/day, compared to the twice daily administration of buprenorphine [39].

3.4 Materials, instruments, and equipment

3.4.1 Materials

- Isoflurane (Sofloran Vet)
- Sterile normal saline (NS) (Baxter ABB1306AE)
- Sterile normal saline with 10% dextrose (D10)
- Iodine (Germisin, Altamirano 027)
- 70% ethanol (Alcohol Luna)
- Sterile wooden cotton swabs (we usually require 4–5)

3.4.2 Sutures

- 4-0 silk suture for the viscera (SOFSILK S-182 USSC sutures)
- 5-0 vicryl for peritoneum closure (Vicryl JP493 Ethicon)
- 5-0 nylon (Mononylon Ethilon P698 Ethicon) for the skin

3.4.3 Standard surgical instruments

- Microsurgery scissors, also known as Iris scissor (Trauma, Lanceta), to cut the skin, peritoneum, and the stumps once they are tied (**Figure 1c**).
- Straight, non-toothed microdissecting forceps (Trauma or Weldon Instrumental, Lanceta) to hold the skin and peritoneum.
- Curved, non-toothed microdissecting forceps (Trauma, Lanceta), helps when doing the knots on the lobules.
- Retractors (a blepharostat can be used) (Braintree Scientific).

- Mayo-Hegar needle holder (Trauma, Lanceta) for suturing the peritoneum and skin.

3.4.4 Equipment

- Anesthesia machine/isoflurane vaporizer (SomnoSuite, Low-Flow Anesthesia System)
- Surgical bed (Surgisuite Multi-Function Surgical Platform, standard)

4. Methods: recipient anesthesia and peri- and postoperative care

Critical: Administer intraperitoneally or subcutaneously 500 μl of NS+D10 2 h before the surgery.

1. Sedate the mice using isoflurane 2–3% for induction and 1% for maintenance.
2. During the surgery, as well as postoperatively, the mouse has to be placed on a warm pad, to prevent hypothermia (**Figure 1d**). After surgery the mice are left in the warm pad until they are able to move and stand up without stimuli.
3. Buprenorphine must be administered 30 min before surgery and following a schedule (each 8–12 h) for the following 72 h.
4. To prevent dehydration 500 μl of normal saline should be administered intraperitoneally or subcutaneously.
5. During follow-up, we use a score to evaluate the status of the mouse as seen in **Table 1**. Though the score was validated in 70% hepatectomized mice, in our hands, it has worked well in establishing a prognosis in mice with an extended hepatectomy. A score of less than 5 at 6 h and 12 h has a bad prognosis. The values correlate with serum levels of IL-6, liver enzymes, and histological features of regeneration [40]. We also use this score for decision-making. Depending on the score, one can consider placing the mouse more time on a warming pad as well as euthanizing if the score does not increase after 12–24 h. While regeneration will progress as expected in 70 and 85% hepatectomy, a 90% hepatectomy is fulminant and causes acute liver failure and death within 24–48 h.

Category	0	1	2
Activity	Stay still Touch without response (TOR)	Stay still Touch with response (TWR, limp away)	Walks free
Fur	Wet abdomen and butt/ unkempt fur	Between	Dry and neat fur
Body posture	Hunched (TOR)	Moderate hunched (TWR)	Normal stretch
Breath	Deep		Normal (nonobservable)
Eyes	Half-close (TOR)	Half-close (TWR)	Open and alert

Table 1.
Mouse body condition score for the major liver resection (taken from Xu et al.).

4.1 Procedure for extended 90% hepatectomy (timing 40–50 min)

1. Weight the mouse.

2. Following anesthesia induction, the abdomen should be shaved; however, this can be done before anesthesia (**Figure 1d**).

3. Clean the dorsum of the mouse with ethanol before placing it on the surgical bed covered with sterile fields.

4. Cleaning of the abdomen must be done with iodine and ethanol 70%.

5. A midline incision is made in two planes (skin and peritoneum). Visibility is of critical importance during the procedure. Separation is done with a blepharostat or simple clips as described by Mitchell and Willenbring [31].

6. Start by visualizing the full anatomy of the liver (**Figure 1b** and **e**).

7. Once the liver is visualized, the falciform ligament may be cut.

Caution: The falciform ligament must be cut carefully and not too close to the diaphragm since the fascia can be cut, causing a hole in the pleural cavity.

8. Next, the first lobe to be removed will be the median lobe (**Figure 2a–c**). By using cotton swabs, mobilize the median lobe upward (toward the diaphragm), and place a silk suture under it (**Figure 2a**).

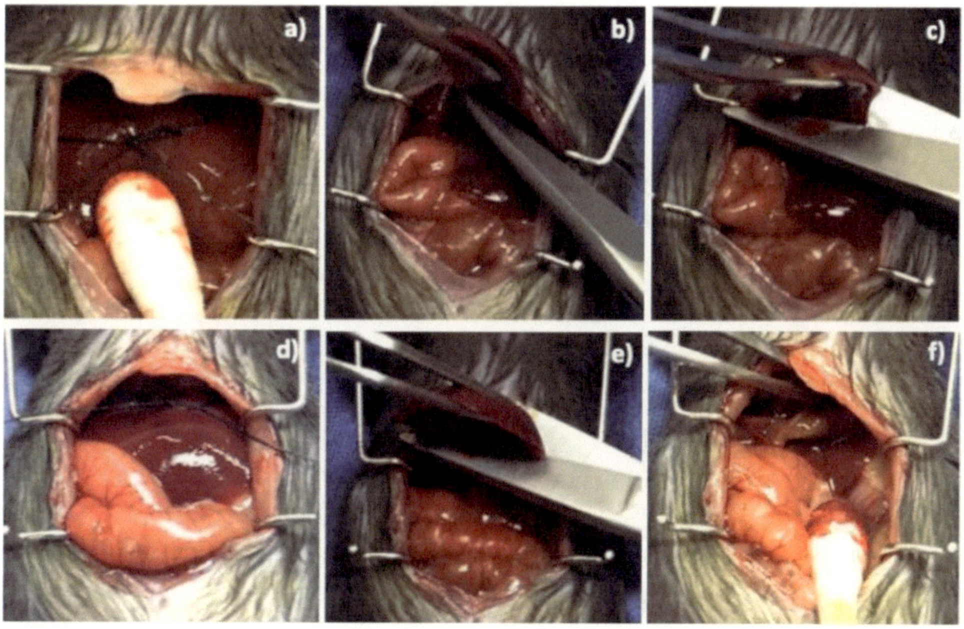

Figure 2.
For the removal of the ML, (a) the suture is accommodated leaving several centimeters from the base of the medial lobe. The lobules are cut separately. (b) The right ML is cut first as it is the most visible of the two. (c) The left ML is cut last, making sure not to perforate the gallbladder. (d) The suture is accommodated surrounding the LL. (e) The LL is excised. (f) The stump and a well-perfused caudate lobe are visualized.

Caution: Cotton swabs are used instead of forceps since the tissue is fragile and bleeds easily.

1. Once that is accomplished, return the lobe to its original position with the cotton swab.

2. There is no need of dissecting the different vessels.

3. Tie the knot at the base of the lobe, making sure to leave enough remnant in the stump as knots that are too close to the base can damage the circulation in the inferior vena cava and suprahepatic veins, compromising the rest of the lobes (**Figure 2a**).

Critical step: One good reference of how long the stump must be is the origin of falciform ligament or the gallbladder.

Troubleshooting: if the stump is too big, the functional volume will not be as accurate.

4. As the knot tends to slide downward, which increases the remnant tissue, one must make sure that the ends are well placed as described in step 10 before tying the knot.

Critical step: To accommodate the ends of the silk suture along the borders of the lobe, pull carefully the lobe downward with a cotton swab.

Critical step: Afterward, double-check the tightness of the knot manually.

1. Subsequently, the ends of the suture are cut.

2. Upon noticing a change of color in the sutured lobe, the lobe to be resected can be held with forceps and then cut with the microsurgery scissors (**Figure 2b** and **c**).

Caution: Care must be taken not to cut through the gallbladder as the bile is toxic to tissues of the abdominal cavity. A good advice is to cut the portions separately.

Caution: Once tied, the resection of the lobes needs to be done with extreme caution, since the knot can be cut unintentionally.

Critical step: Remember to always check for hemostasis.

3. The next lobe to be resected is the left lobe, as shown in (**Figure 2d–f**). Following the same technique as for the median lobe, lift the lobe toward the diaphragm with a cotton swab to place a silk suture under it, return the lobe to its original position, and tie the knots strong enough to avoid bleeding. Be careful not to section the liver.

Critical step: Always separate the left lateral lobe from the caudate lobe as sometimes there is a ligament that unites them both.

4. After tying the knots and cutting the edges, resect the lobe leaving only the required remnant (**Figure 2e–f**).

Caution: Once tied, the resection of the lobes needs to be done with extreme caution, since the knot can be cut unintentionally.

Troubleshooting: If the stump is too big, the functional volume will not be as accurate.

1. After resecting the median lobe and the left lateral lobe, the right inferior lobule is visible. To increase visualization, the intestines may be moved outside the abdominal cavity with a cotton swab. We recommend placing them within a wet gauze to prevent the intestines from drying (**Figure 3a**).

2. When visualized, the inferior right lobe is moved toward the inferior vena cava with a cotton swab to place the silk suture under it. The silk suture is accommodated parallel to the lobule (**Figure 3b**).

3. Once that is done, replace the lobule over the silk suture using a cotton swab.

Critical step: The knot must be made using very fine forceps as tying it tends to move the lobule out of the knot (**Figure 3c**).

1. Four to five knots have to be placed as described above.

2. The ends of the silk suture are cut.

3. Once the lobule changes color, one can proceed to cut it (**Figure 3d** and **e**).

Caution: When resecting the right lobe, one must place the suture with diligence, making sure not to touch the kidney.
Caution: Once tied, the resection of the lobes needs to be done with extreme caution, since the knot can be cut unintentionally.
Caution: Sites of bleeding need to be identified.

1. Notice that if one leaves the superior right lobule together with the caudate lobe, approximately 22–24% of hepatic volume can be left, thus becoming a partial hepatectomy of 82–86%.

2. The last lobule left to be removed is the superior right lobule (**Figure 4**). This is technically difficult since it is located deep within the vault of the diaphragm. The use of clips reduces the technical difficulty.

3. When using silk sutures, we recommend doing the knot outside the cavity (**Figure 4a**). Once this is done, with a swab the superior right lobule is moved toward the inferior vena cava (**Figure 4b**), rapidly placing the silk suture knot parallel to it. With the swab, one locates the lobule within the knot.

Critical step: As mentioned before, the knot must be tied using forceps with very fine tips and within the abdominal cavity (**Figure 4c** and **d**).

1. The first knot does not have to be tight; the second one must be tightened with the fingers, applying as much force as possible.

2. The lobule can be cut once it changes color (**Figure 4e**).

Caution: The resection of the lobes needs to be done with extreme caution, since the knot can be cut unintentionally.

3. After hemostasis is reassured (**Figure 4f**), the abdominal cavity can be closed.

Caution: Always check for perfusion of the caudate lobe, as seen in **Figure 4g**.

Critical step: We recommend suturing the peritoneum separately from the skin (**Figure 5**). This helps prevent evisceration as mice tend to remove the stitches.

1. The peritoneum is closed with an absorbable suture like 5-0 vicryl or PDS, using a running suturing technique to keep tension at the closure (**Figure 5b** and **c**).

2. The skin is closed with 4-0 nylon using a simple interrupted suturing technique or clips (**Figure 5d–f**).

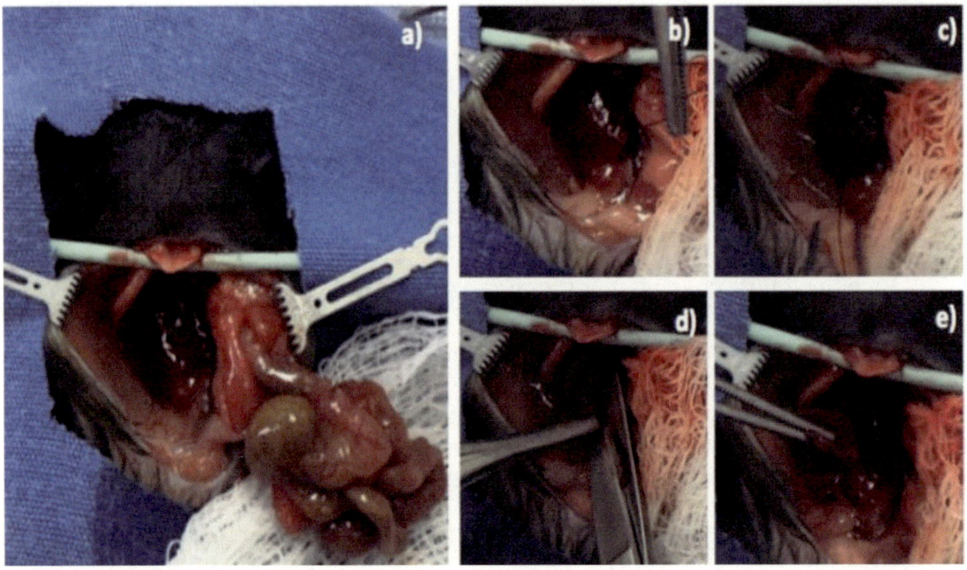

Figure 3.
(a) For the extirpation of the RL, evisceration must be made, and the intestine should be covered by a wet gauze. (b) The silk suture is placed beneath the RIL. (c) The knot is carefully tightened. (d) The lobe is excised. (e) A forceps can be used to remove the excised tissue.

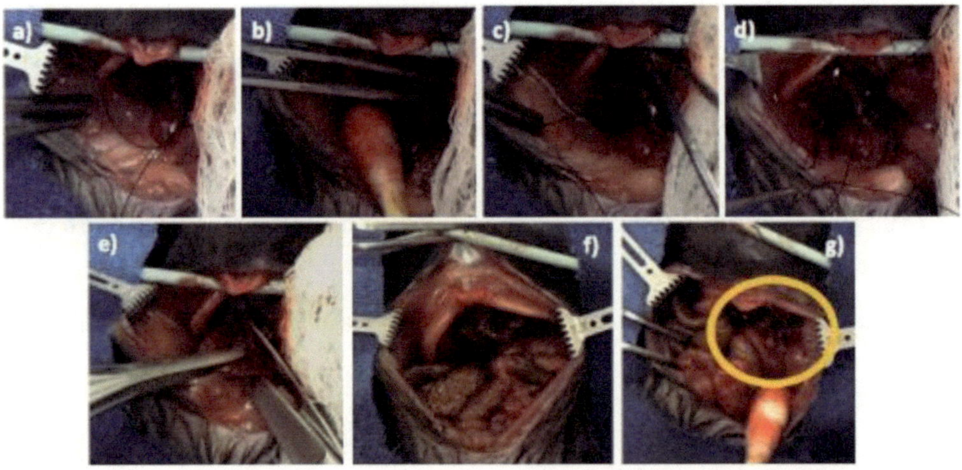

Figure 4.
For removal of the RSL, (a) the knot is made outside the peritoneal cavity and (b) is positioned carefully around the lobule with the help of the forceps. (c) The knot is tightened with the forceps inside the peritoneal cavity. (d) If the correct force is applied, the silk suture does not cut through the tissue, and no bleeding is seen. (e) The lobe is removed carefully. (f) The remaining stumps within the cavity is shown. (g) The only remaining lobe will be the caudate lobe.

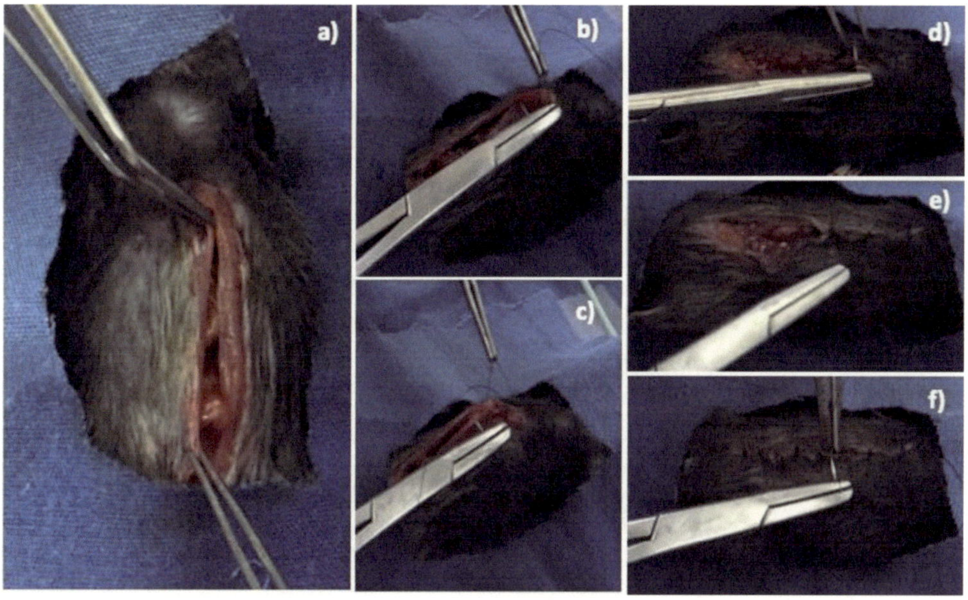

Figure 5.
(a) Apposition of the borders of the peritoneum is made before beginning the suture of the incision. (b) A simple continuous suture is made on the peritoneum lining. (c) The suture is performed from proximal to distal. (d) The skin is sutured with simple interrupted sutures, (e) from the xiphoid process to the pelvis area. (f) The space between the sutures must be even.

5. Troubleshooting

One important aspect of every surgical procedure is the anesthesia. Incorrect dosing can be fatal to the subject. Weighting the animal and calculating the anesthetic correctly are crucial.

Following the steps of the procedure, using the adequate number of silk suture, is important as thinner sutures can cut the tissue when tying the knot. This produces unwanted bleeding.

As to the knot, inadequate tying and incorrect placement may complicate the procedure. If the knot is not tight enough after excision of the tissue, the bleeding can be very profuse and difficult to stop. In competent hands, a second knot can be placed. This stops the bleeding. Sometimes, the bleeding is not noticed until the animal dies after 12–24 h of the procedure. The main cause of death is usually internal bleeding due to technical errors with the knot.

As mentioned before, if the knot is placed at the median lobe too proximate to the inferior vena cava, the perfusion of the remnant lobe is compromised. In this case, perfusion of the caudate lobe (**Figure 6**) indicates that the EHx becomes a full hepatectomy. The under-perfused tissue will not be able to enter the process of regeneration before acute liver failure establishes.

The stump volume is important in achieving a real EHx. If the stump volume is too big, not only will the animal be left with a caudate lobe, it will also be left with a partial lobe, whether it is the median, the left, or the right lobe. The only way to notice this is after the surgery, as the animal will show clinical features of liver failure. If liver failure does not develop, that means the model failed and more remnant tissue was left in place than the actual 10% that was supposed to be left for a 90% EHx.

A summary of the main complications and errors is found in **Table 2**.

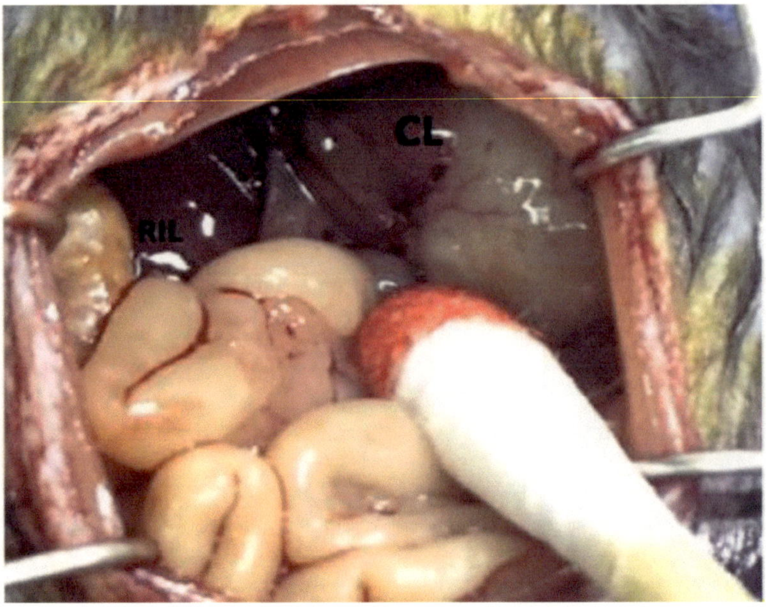

Figure 6.
After resection of the median lobe, when tying too high toward the inferior vena cava, the hepatic circulation is affected as seen in the color acquired by the CL.

Troubleshooting	Step	Problem	Possible reason	Solution
Death during procedure	17–25	Bleeding	Tightness of knot	Use forceps to tie knot first proximal to the tissue, deep within the cavity
Death in less than 24 h	8–25	Bleeding	Tightness of knot	Ensure tightness of knot manually
				Avoid cutting through the knot
More than 48-h survival	8–25	Survival	Stump volume	Cut enough tissue as to approximate the % of functional liver volume you want to resect
Bad perfusion of caudate lobe	8–13	Fulminant hepatic failure	Knot made too high upon the hilum of the median lobe	Use the gallbladder as reference for doing the stump; leave at least 2 mm of stump

Table 2.
Troubleshooting.

6. Quantifying results

6.1 Liver regeneration

To assess liver regeneration, the liver-to-body weight ratio (LBWR) can be calculated by considering the weight of the animal after the surgery and weight of the remnant lobe (the caudate lobe). The stumps are not considered in the ratio unless the stumps made were too big and have regenerated. The LBWR tells the volume of regenerated tissue in proportion to the body. As mentioned before, the liver has a hepatostat, and thus the body weight has to be considered.

For the assessment of mitosis in liver samples, a basic H&E or an immunohistochemistry against Ki-67 or bromodeoxyuridine (BrdU) can help count the number

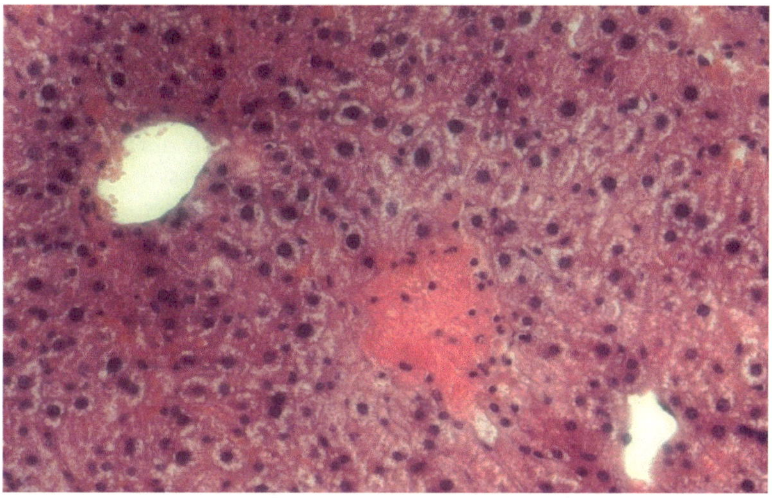

Figure 7.
Tissue slide stained with H&E showing steatosis and a necrotic area in a sample of the liver 24 h post-hepatectomy.

of replicating cells. Mitotic cells are identified by the condensation of the chromatin and loss of nuclear membrane. Identifying the late phases of mitosis is much easier. Quantifying the positivity of cells to Ki-67 reflect that these cells are in the cell cycle. Ki-67 is known to modulate most of the phases in the cell cycle but has its peak when the cell reaches the mitosis phase. Bromodeoxyuridine assay works by administering intramuscularly a dose (50 mg/kg) of BrdU to the animal before sacrifice. BrdU is an analogue of thymidine, and as such it becomes incorporated to the DNA. When an antibody against BrdU is used, cells that are in the S phase or beyond can be identified.

6.2 Liver failure

To assess liver failure in the live animal, the quantification of liver enzymes through colorimetric assays is helpful. Clinical assessment is sensible. As described above, the value of the mouse body condition score after the major liver resection can predict the outcome of the procedure [40]. A score less than or equal to 5 measured consecutively within 24 h post-hepatectomy correlated with increased levels of liver enzymes, pro-inflammatory cytokines, and decreased regeneration measured through ki-67 staining in liver tissue.

In the dead animal, the LBWR is key to assess the degree of regeneration, which is inversely proportional to liver dysfunction. Once the tissue is procured, microscopically, steatosis is a hallmark of liver failure (**Figure 7**). On the other hand, the calculation of the survival rate helps predict the hours an animal with liver failure is able to survive.

Biomarkers can be developed to assess the possibility of liver regeneration or liver failure. Nonetheless, the value of these biomarkers will depend on the existence of therapeutics to enable regeneration or prevent liver failure. Thus, there is a need of using surgical models to study these payoffs, which are two factual extremes of a method frequently used in clinical practice.

7. Conclusions

We have here described a reproducible mouse model for a 90% extended hepatectomy which mimics closely small-for-flow syndromes and thus an important acute liver failure scenario. Even though the obvious problem in this setting and the objective of this extended hepatectomy model is to severely reduce liver mass, which describes the term small for size, liver dysfunction is now increasingly recognized to occur due to a small-for-flow syndrome [41–43]. As Golriz and authors suggest, the appropriate term for this syndrome should be small for size and flow [44]. The critical turning point in the understanding of this phenomenon is that portal flow to the remaining liver mass or liver graft is excessive, leading to histopathological consequences including sinusoidal endothelial denudation, periportal hemorrhage, arterial vasospasm, portal vein thrombosis, and biliary strictures [45, 46]. Considering the physiopathology that originates this type of acute liver failure, it has been experimentally demonstrated that interventions aimed to reduce portal overpressure such as the use of vasoconstrictors or splenic artery ligation have positive effects on liver regeneration and hepatocellular viability [41, 42]. In the clinical setting, Kaido and authors have successfully lowered the limit of graft-to-recipient weight ratio to 0.6% in adult-to-adult living donor liver transplantation by maintenance of an intraoperative final portal pressure below 15 mmHg, which may involve ligation of portosystemic shunts or even splenectomy [43]; it is worth noting that traditionally the minimum ratio considered as safe for liver transplantation or resection is 0.8%, based on a study where probability of graft survival at 90 days is less than 54% [47].

Acknowledgements

This research has been funded by the Universidad Panamericana through the grant "Fomento a la Investigación UP 2017," under project code UP-CI-2017-CS-MX-02.2.

Conflict of interest

The authors declare no conflict of interest.

Nomenclature

BrdU	bromodeoxyuridine
CL	caudate lobe
D10	dextrose 10%
Ehx	extended hepatectomy
LBWR	liver-to-body weight ratio
LLL	left lateral lobe
ML	medial lobe
NS	normal saline
PHx	partial hepatectomy
PHLF	post-hepatectomy liver failure
RIL	right inferior lobe
RSL	right superior lobe
SFSS	small-for-size syndrome
TLV	total liver volume

Author details

Maria J. Lizardo Thiebaud[1], Eduardo Cervantes-Alvarez[2,3] and Nalu Navarro-Alvarez[1,2,4]*

1 Universidad Panamericana, School of Medicine, México City, Mexico

2 Department of Gastroenterology, Instituto Nacional de Ciencias Medicas y Nutrición, Salvador Zubirán, México City, Mexico

3 PECEM, Faculty of Medicine, Universidad Nacional Autónoma de México, Mexico City, Mexico

4 Department of Surgery, Massachusetts General Hospital, Center for Transplantation Sciences, Harvard Medical School, Boston, MA, United States

*Address all correspondence to: nnavarro@up.edu.mx

References

[1] Pahlavan PS, Feldmann RE, Zavos C, Kountouras J. Prometheus' challenge: Molecular, cellular and systemic aspects of liver regeneration. The Journal of Surgical Research. 2006;**134**(2):238-251

[2] Michalopoulos GK, DeFrances MC. Liver regeneration. Science. 1997;**276**: 60-66

[3] Taub R. Liver regeneration: From myth to mechanism. Nature Reviews. Molecular Cell Biology. 2004;**5**(10):836-847

[4] Mortensen KE, Revhaug A. Liver regeneration in surgical animal models—A historical perspective and clinical implications. European Surgical Research. 2011;**46**(1):1-18

[5] Martins PNA, Theruvath TP, Neuhaus P. Rodent models of partial hepatectomies. Liver International [Internet]. 2008;**28**(1):3-11. DOI: 10.1111/j.1478-3231.2007.01628.x

[6] Higgins G, Anderson R. Experimental pathology of the liver I restoration of the liver of the white rat following partial surgical removal. Archives of Pathology. 1932;**12**:186-202

[7] Greene AK, Puder M. Partial hepatectomy in the mouse: Technique and perioperative management. Journal of Investigative Surgery. 2003;**16**:99-103

[8] Makino H, Togo S, Kubota T, Morioka D, Morita T, Kobayashi T, et al. A good model of hepatic failure after excessive hepatectomy in mice. The Journal of Surgical Research. 2005;**127**(2):171-176

[9] Hori T, Ohashi N, Chen F, Baine AMT, Gardner LB, Jermanus S, et al. Simple and sure methodology for massive hepatectomy in the mouse. Annals of Gastroenterology. 2011;**24**(4):307-318

[10] Lehmann K, Tschuor C, Rickenbacher A, Jang JH, Oberkofler CE, Tschopp O, et al. Liver failure after extended hepatectomy in mice is mediated by a p21-dependent barrier to liver regeneration. Gastroenterology [Internet]. 2012;**143**(6):1609-1619.e4. DOI: 10.1053/j.gastro.2012.08.043

[11] Darnis B, Mohkam K, Schmitt Z, Ledochowski S, Vial JP, Duperret S, et al. Subtotal hepatectomy in swine for studying small-for-size syndrome and portal inflow modulation: Is it reliable? HPB. 2015;**17**(10):881-888

[12] Panis Y, McMullan DM, Emond JC. Progressive necrosis after hepatectomy and the pathophysiology of liver failure after massive resection. Surgery. 1997;**121**(2):142-149

[13] Van Den Broek MAJ, Olde Damink SWM, Dejong CHC, Lang H, Malagó M, Jalan R, et al. Liver failure after partial hepatic resection: Definition, pathophysiology, risk factors and treatment. Liver International. 2008;**28**(6):767-780

[14] Yagi S, Uemoto S. Small-for-size syndrome in living donor liver transplantation. Hepatobiliary & Pancreatic Diseases International [Internet]. 2012;**11**(6):570-576. DOI: 10.1016/S1499-3872(12)60227-6

[15] Kauffmann R, Fong Y. Post-hepatectomy liver failure. Hepatobiliary Surgery and Nutrition. 2014;**3**(5):238-246

[16] Lafaro K, Buettner S, Maqsood H, Wagner D, Bagante F, Spolverato G, et al. Defining post hepatectomy liver insufficiency: Where do we stand? Journal of Gastrointestinal Surgery. 2015;**19**(11):2079-2092

[17] Ray S, Mehta NN, Golhar A, Nundy S. Post hepatectomy liver

failure—A comprehensive review of current concepts and controversies. Annals of Medicine and Surgery [Internet]. 2018;**34**(2222):4-10. DOI: 10.1016/j.amsu.2018.08.012

[18] Dimitroulis D, Tsaparas P, Valsami S, Mantas D, Spartalis E, Markakis C, et al. Indications, limitations and maneuvers to enable extended hepatectomy: Current trends. World Journal of Gastroenterology. 2014;**20**(24): 7887-7893

[19] Viebahn CS, Yeoh GCT. What fires prometheus? The link between inflammation and regeneration following chronic liver injury. International Journal of Biochemistry and Cell Biology. 2008;**40**(5):855-873

[20] Nanashima A, Abo T, Arai J, Matsumoto H, Kudo T, Nagayasu T. Functional liver reserve parameters predictive for posthepatectomy complications. The Journal of Surgical Research [Internet]. 2013;**185**(1):127-135. DOI: 10.1016/j.jss.2013.05.021

[21] Wang Y, Ye F, Ke Q, Wu Q, Yang R, Bu H. Gender-dependent histone deacetylases injury may contribute to differences in liver recovery rates of male and female mice. Transplantation Proceedings. 2013;**45**(2):463-473

[22] Michalopoulos GK. Principles of liver regeneration and growth homeostasis. Comprehensive Physiology. 2013;**3**(1):485-513

[23] Enkhbold C, Morine Y, Utsunomiya T, Imura S, Ikemoto T, Arakawa Y, et al. Dysfunction of liver regeneration in aged liver after partial hepatectomy. Journal of Gastroenterology and Hepatology. 2015;**30**(7):1217-1224

[24] Helling TS. Liver failure following partial hepatectomy. HPB [Internet]. 2006;**8**(3):165-174. DOI: 10.1080/13651820510035712

[25] Palmes D, Budny TB, Dietl KH, Herbst H, Stratmann U, Spiegel HU. Detrimental effect of sinusoidal overperfusion after liver resectionandpartiallivertransplantation. Transplant International. 2005;**17**(12):862-871

[26] van Mierlo KMC, Schaap FG, Dejong CHC, Olde Damink SWM. Liver resection for cancer: New developments in prediction, prevention and management of postresectional liver failure. Journal of Hepatology [Internet]. 2016;**65**(6):1217-1231. DOI: 10.1016/j.jhep.2016.06.006

[27] Lin XJ, Yang J, Chen XB, Zhang M, Xu MQ. The critical value of remnant liver volume-to-body weight ratio to estimate posthepatectomy liver failure in cirrhotic patients. The Journal of Surgical Research [Internet]. 2014;**188**(2):489-495. DOI: 10.1016/j.jss.2014.01.023

[28] Guglielmi A, Ruzzenente A, Conci S, Valdegamberi A, Iacono C. How much remnant is enough in liver resection? Digestive Surgery. 2012;**29**(1):6-17

[29] Michalopoulos GK. Liver regeneration after partial hepatectomy: Critical analysis of mechanistic dilemmas. American Journal of Pathology [Internet]. 2010;**176**(1):2-13. DOI: 10.2353/ajpath.2010.090675

[30] Matsuo T, Yamaguchi S, Mitsui S, Emi A, Shimoda F, Okamura H. Control mechanism of the circadian clock for timing of cell division in vivo. Science (80-). 2003;**302**(5643):255-259

[31] Mitchell C, Willenbring H. A reproducible and well-tolerated method for 2/3 partial hepatectomy in mice. Nature Protocols. 2008;**3**(7):1167-1170

[32] Tsukamoto I, Kojo S. Effect of glucocorticoid on liver regeneration after partial hepatectomy in the rat. Gut. 1989;**30**(3):387-390

[33] Barbason H, Bouzahzah B, Herens C, Marchandis J, Sulon J, van Cantfort J. Circadian synchronization of liver regeneration in adult rats: the role played by adrenal hormones. Cell and Tissue Kinetics. 1989;**22**:451-460. Available from: papers2://publication/uuid/BF06944C-5B46-4AC2-B2DB-589386E42EE5

[34] Holecek M. Nutritional modulation of liver regeneration by carbohydrates , lipids , and amino acids : A review. Nutrition. 1999;**15**(10):784-788

[35] Block GD, Locker J, Bowen WC, Petersen BE, Katyal S, Strom SC, et al. Population expansion, clonal growth, and specific differentiation patterns in primary cultures of hepatocytes induced by HGF/SF, EGF and TGFoL in a chemically defined (HGM) medium. Journal of Cell Biology [Internet]. 1996;**132**(6):1133-1149. Available from: http://www.ncbi.nlm.nih.gov/pmc/articles/PMC2120765/pdf/jc13261133.pdf%5Cnpapers3://publication/uuid/E4364133-7E8D-4521-924A-30F44ED982C0

[36] Huang J, Rudnick DA. Elucidating the metabolic regulation of liver regeneration [Internet]. American Journal of Pathology. American Society for Investigative Pathology. 2014;**184**:309-321. DOI: 10.1016/j.ajpath.2013.04.034

[37] Chen H, Lin Y, Sun W, Cai Y, Li H. Liver regeneration is impaired in mice with acute exposure to a very low carbohydrate diet. Digestive Diseases and Sciences. 2017;**62**(5):1256-1264

[38] Ren W, Wang X, Zhang A, Li C, Chen G, Ge X, et al. Selective bowel decontamination improves the survival of 90% hepatectomy in rats. The Journal of Surgical Research [Internet]. 2015;**195**(2):454-464. DOI: 10.1016/j.jss.2015.01.024

[39] Tubbs JT, Kissling GE, Travlos GS, Goulding DR, Clark JA, King-Herbert AP, et al. Effects of buprenorphine, meloxicam, and flunixin meglumine as postoperative analgesia in mice. Journal of the American Association for Laboratory Animal Science. 2011;**50**(2):185-191

[40] Xu Y, Navarro-Alvarez N, Yang C, Markmann JF, Dong J, Yeh H. A reliable scoring system after major liver resection in mice. The Journal of Surgical Research [Internet]. 2016;**204**(1):75-82. DOI: 10.1016/j.jss.2016.03.066

[41] Carrapita J, Abrantes AM, Campelos S, Gonçalves AC, Cardoso D, Sarmento-Ribeiro AB, et al. Impact of splenic artery ligation after major hepatectomy on liver function, regeneration and viability. Scientific Reports [Internet]. 2016;**6**:1-12. DOI: 10.1038/srep34731

[42] Kim D-S, Ji WB, Han JH, Choi YY, Park H-J, Yu Y-D, et al. Effects of splanchnic vasoconstrictors on liver regeneration and survival after 90% rat hepatectomy. Annals of Surgical Treatment and Research. 2018;**94**(3):118

[43] Kaido T, Mori A, Ogura Y, Hata K, Yoshizawa A, Iida T, et al. Lower limit of the graft-to-recipient weight ratio can be safely reduced to 0.6% in adult-to-adult living donor liver transplantation in combination with portal pressure control. Transplantation Proceedings [Internet]. 2011;**43**(6):2391-2393. DOI: 10.1016/j.transproceed.2011.05.037

[44] Golriz M, Majlesara A, El Sakka S, Ashrafi M, Arwin J, Fard N, et al. Small for size and flow (SFSF) syndrome: An alternative description for posthepatectomy liver failure. Clinics and Research in Hepatology and Gastroenterology [Internet]. 2016;**40**(3):267-275. DOI: 10.1016/j.clinre.2015.06.024

[45] Asencio JM, Vaquero J, Olmedilla L, García Sabrido JL. " Small-for-flow"

syndrome: Shifting the " size" paradigm. Medical Hypotheses. 2013;**80**(5):573-577

[46] Demetris AJ, Kelly DM, Eghtesad B, Fontes P, Wallis Marsh J, Tom K, et al. Pathophysiologic observations and histopathologic recognition of the portal hyperperfusion or small-for-size syndrome. The American Journal of Surgical Pathology. 2006;**30**(8):986-993

[47] Kiuchi T, Kasahara M, Uryuhara K, Inomata Y, Uemoto S, Asonuma K, et al. Impact of graft size mismatching on graft prognosis in liver transplantation from living donors. Transplantation. 1999;**67**(2):321-327

Chapter 14

Liver Assist Devices for Liver Failure

Amrendra Kumar Mandal, Pavani Garlapati, Benjamin Tiongson and Vijay Gayam

Abstract

Historically, mortality rates for liver failure have been high, regardless of the type. With new advancements in liver transplantation (LTx), 1-year survival rates have improved up to 95% in most recent estimates. While some patients may live past the critical period, the majority of patients do not survive the interval period for awaiting LTx or liver regeneration. The function of the liver to detoxify and correct several biochemical parameters has been achieved to some extent through artificial liver support technology, although constant innovations are still being developed for the most optimal liver support device. The complex function of the liver makes it challenging since it does not only detoxify toxic by-products but also participates in numerous other synthetic and metabolic functions of the body. Liver support systems are divided into an artificial liver assist device (ALD) and a bioartificial liver assist device (BLD). ALDs include molecular adsorbent recirculating system (MARS), Prometheus, single-pass albumin dialysis, and selective plasma filtration therapy. These devices work as a blood purification system of the liver. On the other hand, BLD has hepatic cell lines incorporated in its equipment, which aims to function as a complex biological liver system providing support to its biochemical processes. Several clinical and randomized trials have conflicting results on the survival of the patients with acute liver failure (ALF), and the ideal liver support system still seems a far-off goal.

Keywords: liver failure, liver assist devices, bioartificial liver assist device, artificial liver assist device

1. Background

In the last decade, liver-related deaths have been steadily increasing. In 2016, it was responsible for more than one million deaths across the world [1]. ALF is defined as a rapid onset deterioration of liver function with coagulopathy and onset of encephalopathy of a previously healthy individual. It can be further classified into hyper-acute, acute, and sub-acute according to the O'Grady system of classification. The clinical manifestation includes jaundice, encephalopathy, and hematemesis or melena; however, unlike chronic liver disease, ascites and portal hypertension are rarely seen. The common etiologies include acute viral hepatitis, drug-induced liver injury, and ischemic hepatocellular injury. High mortality rates are associated with ALF [2]. Supportive therapy options are limited in the interim between the development of ALF until liver function improves/or the patient undergoes liver LTx. Due to limited organ availability for patients waiting for LTx, and the rapid deterioration of a patient with ALF, the mortality rate approaches approximately 50% [3, 4].

Numerous studies are ongoing in an attempt to delay or prevent the need for LTx in patients with ALF. Artificial hepatic assist devices, auxiliary liver transplantation, a liver dialysis system, and xenotransplantation are the most sought-after therapeutic options. Several liver assist devices (LAD) have been manufactured since the 1990s on the pathophysiological basis of albumin dialysis, the best-known being the following: the molecular adsorbent recirculating system (MARS), single-pass albumin dialysis system (SPAD), and the fractionated plasma separation and adsorption system –FPSA (Prometheus). These systems remove the albumin-bound toxins that accumulate in liver failure. Older techniques previously were not able to remove these toxins and maybe the reason for the ineffectiveness of traditionally designed devices. The knowledge gained from these provided a platform for a better understanding of newer LADs, to perform the liver's functions more effectively. LADs facilitate the removal of water-soluble substances, such as ammonia, urea, and other smaller proteins, such as some cytokines, by standard dialysis [3]. Removal of these cytokines and other identifiable inducers of hepatic encephalopathy (HE), such as amino acids (e.g., tryptophan or glutamine), reduces the grade of HE and consequently reduces complications of liver failure [5]. Furthermore, they function to remove conjugated or unconjugated bilirubin, protoporphyrin, bile acids, glycoside derivatives, phenols, short- and medium-chain fatty acids, such as octanoate, or heterocyclic organic compounds. In one study, removal of plasmatic nitric oxide (NO) and some pro-inflammatory and anti-inflammatory cytokines lead to the improvement of clinical conditions of HE, renal and respiratory function, and hemodynamic derangement and subsequent sequential organ failure [6].

LAD designed to treat patients with ALF are classified into two main categories: non-cell-based systems, including plasmapheresis, plasma exchange, albumin dialysis, and charcoal-based hemadsorption, and systems that incorporate hepatic tissue (bioartificial liver support systems) [7, 8].

In the last decade, a significant shift in the development of these devices has emerged. The utility and efficacy of these new LADs are currently being evaluated in the clinical setting.

1.1 Types of liver support systems

Liver support systems are divided broadly into two categories: biological and mechanical. Artificial or mechanical liver support consists of artificial and bio-artificial systems. Two artificial systems, the MARS, and the SPAD, clear selected toxins; however, they provide no synthetic support, nor do they improve survival in a randomized clinical trial (RCT) [9].

Biological systems combine the functional potential of hepatocyte incorporation with that of hemodialysis, enabling non-invasive, continuous treatment for patients with ALF. Regardless of their safety and cost-effectiveness, they do not improve portal hypertension or portosystemic shunting [9].

1.2 Artificial liver support devices

1.2.1 Molecular adsorbent recirculating system (MARS)

MARS was developed in 1990 and is the most widely published and clinically used artificial liver support system (**Figure 1**). The method is based on two basic

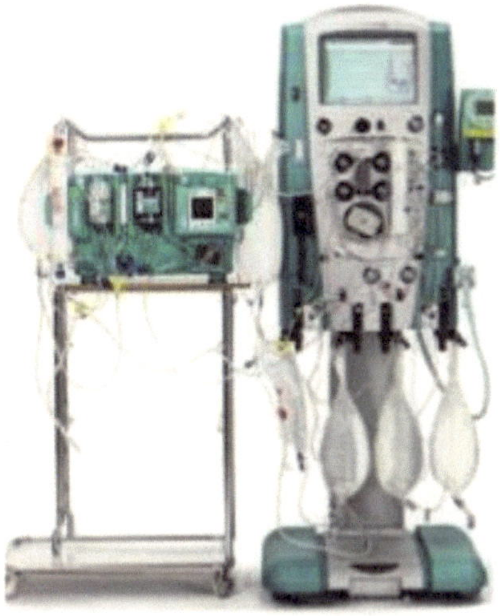

Figure 1.
Molecular adsorption recirculation system (MARS). Adapted from https://www.slideshare.net/tyfngnc/salon-a-17-kasim-2011-1410-1430-ender-egedik.

principles: protein-binding affinity and solute movement, which acts along the concentration gradient [10]. The combination of conventional dialysis against an albumin dialysate is utilized, followed by a traditional procedure of dialysis to remove the toxins from the dialysate [11]. It is composed of a blood circuit, an albumin circuit (containing 60 ml of 20% human albumin, charcoal column, and an anion exchange column with cholestyramine), and a traditional "renal" dialysate circuit as shown in **Figures 2–3**. Blood is passed through an albumin-incorporated high-flux dialysis membrane into which hydrophobic water-soluble and protein-bound toxins are released. The removal of toxins eventually takes place through the diffusion process, which depends on the free toxin level (mainly affected by the molar ratio of a toxin to albumin). The albumin dialysate is then recycled and is able to accept further toxins until both columns are saturated, eliminating the need for continuous infusion of albumin.

MARS can also eliminate cytokines and modify the inflammatory response involved in liver failure. Cytokines have been implicated in the development of HE, systemic inflammatory response syndrome (SIRS), vasodilation, and multiple organ failure. These proteins mediate hepatic inflammation, cholestasis, and liver cell necrosis and apoptosis [12]. Furthermore, studies have shown significant removal of some pro-inflammatory cytokines when using MARS, such as TNF-α, interleukin-6, and interleukin-1 β, and anti-inflammatory cytokines, such as interleukin-10 [13]. However, other studies were unable to demonstrate an effective change in the plasma cytokine concentration in patients with liver failure, possibly due to the high rate of its production [14]. Donati et al. showed 269 patients treated with MARS with no effect on cytokine plasma levels but a significant rise in hepatic growth factor concentration (enhances liver regeneration) [15]. In another study, Dominik et al. demonstrated some beneficial results in an in vitro study, where MARS improved the elimination of some cytokines with more extensive pore membranes, which could be attributed to optimizing the cytokine plasma profile of patients [16]. Ultimately, the precise roles of different cytokines in the pathophysiology of liver failure and the influence of MARS on cytokine profiles are yet to be understood and could be an exciting topic for further research.

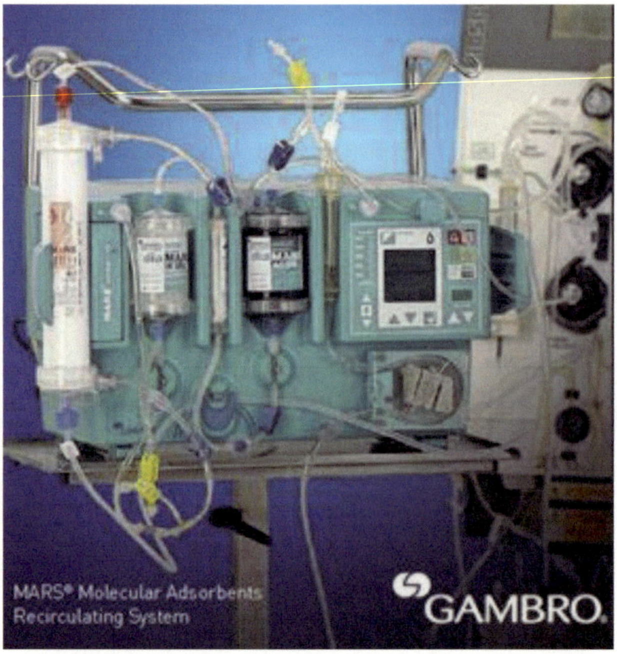

Figure 2.
Cartridges in MARS. Adapted from Tawada Healthcare / Gambro Equipment Supplier.

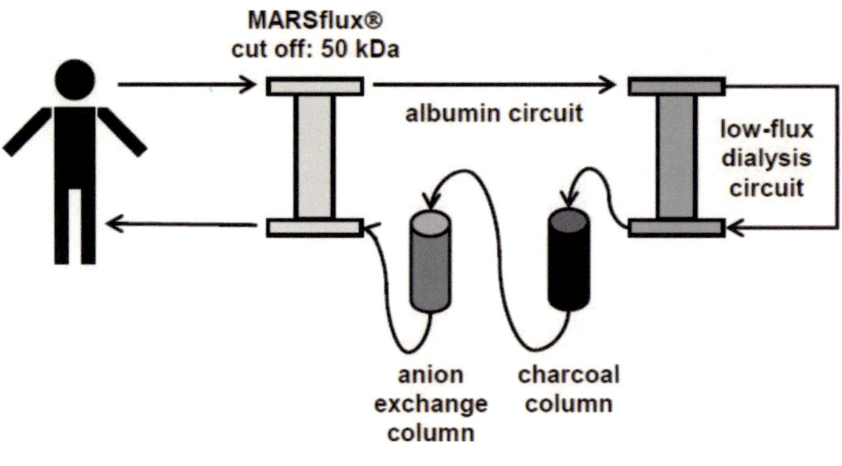

Figure 3.
Schema of the operating principle in MARS. Adapted from Karla et al. Extracorporeal liver support devices for Listed patients. Liver Transplantation 22839–8482016 AASLD.

Interestingly, some authors have been exploring other active substances that can also be eliminated by MARS. In one study, Gay et al. demonstrated that in patients with cholestasis and pruritus, the proteins dialyzed and then absorbed in the anion-exchange resin cartridge of MARS showed elimination of some biologically relevant proteins, such as secreted Ly6/uPAR-related protein-1 (SLURP1) or defensin human neutrophil peptide-1 (HNP-1), which are involved in the inflammatory and defensive processes [17].

When using MARS, particular attention should be given to the monitoring of some critical drugs during treatment, such as fluoroquinolones and meropenem, with dose adjustments done to ensure therapeutic levels.

Anticoagulation during MARS is also essential to consider issue since there is a delicate hemostatic balance that needs to be maintained in patients with liver failure who are at high risk of bleeding. The most used drug in practice is unfractionated heparin, but there are some concerns regarding hemorrhagic risk and heparin-induced thrombocytopenia. Also, some studies have explored the use of continuous extracorporeal systems without anticoagulation and have found a comparable circuit lifespan [18]. The anticoagulant-free approach may also be a reasonable option in patients with a high risk of bleeding. Citrate has been shown to be safe with longer treatment time, preventing filter loss [19]. However, its regular use needs to be validated in an RCT. Unfractionated heparin is the anticoagulant of choice in most clinical trials, but some studies have also used local citrate anticoagulation, with no reported adverse effects [19].

Technical issues have also been raised about the stability of the binding properties of albumin after passing the adsorber columns or about the clinical relevance of some stabilizers (such as octanoate) used in commercially available albumin preparations [20]. However, there are no definitive conclusions, and these issues should be addressed in further studies.

Regarding clinical outcomes, mostly retrospective studies were published in the first years following the debut of MARS. Most of them showed usefulness in the treatment of HE, and some even demonstrated improvement in terms of hemodynamic parameters. The few RCT evaluating survival showed conflicting results [21, 22]. These trials included studied a few patients diagnosed with acute-on-chronic liver failure. In a recent study of 27 patients who received MARS therapy for severe ALF, survival rate was 60% (n = 3/5) for patients with severe liver trauma, 78% (n = 7/9) for patients who used MARS as a bridge to transplantation, and 67% (n = 6/9) when MARS was used as definitive therapy for toxic ingestion or idiopathic liver failure [23].

Lastly, MARS has led us to discover its benefit in drug-induced liver injury (DILI) cases [24]. Statistically speaking, about 50% of cases of ALF are likely due to DILI in the United States [25, 26]. The standard of medical therapy (SMT) is the withdrawal of offending drugs and supportive therapy [27]. A review of the literature indicates several cases of reports of DILI involving several drugs. The most common offending drugs are acetaminophen, nonsteroidal anti-inflammatory drugs, isoniazid, and amoxicillin/clavulanate [28]. However, there are several potential hepatotoxic agents of DILI leading to ALF [29–31].

1.2.2 Fractionated plasma separation and adsorption—FPSA (Prometheus)

Falkenhagen et al. described the first method of FPSA for the use of ALF [32]. The device is shown in **Figure 4**. Prometheus uses endogenous albumin to pass through the circuit using the AlbuFow filter (molecular cut-off of 250 kDa) (**Figure 5**). Albumin is reactivated and returned to circulation using a neutral resin adsorber (Prometh 01) and an anion-exchange column (Prometh 02). Subsequently, the patient's blood then passes through a second circuit, where it is treated by conventional high-flux hemodialysis, eventually returning blood to the patient.

During the first decade of its use in the market, Prometheus showed better efficacy than MARS for both in vitro and in vivo trials in removing ammonia, bilirubin, or bile acids [33]. In 2009, Grodzicki et al. also showed a significant decline in serum ammonia, bilirubin, aspartate aminotransferase, alanine aminotransferase, urea, and creatinine with the use of Prometheus in patients with ALF [34]. Furthermore, Rifai et al. showed a decline in almost all 26 of the amino

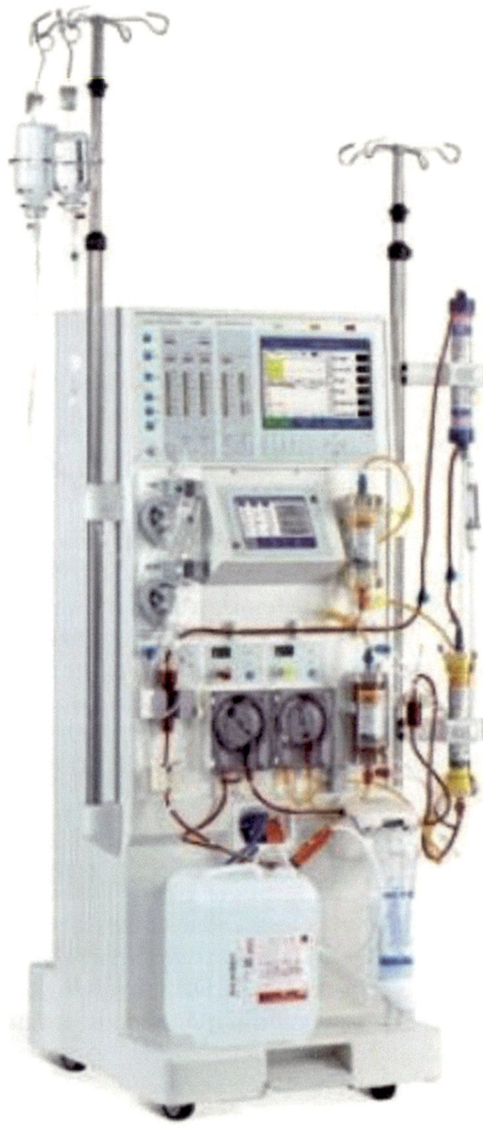

Figure 4.
Fractionated plasma separation and adsorption—FPSA (Prometheus). Adapted from http://dialize.lv. Slokas iela 84-1A, Rīga, LV-1007.

acids measured in nine patients with liver failure with a single treatment session. Prometheus is also hypothesized to improve the complications of HE due to the removal of amino acids such as glutamine, phenylamine, tyrosine, and tryptophan, which all have been noted to be contributing factors to HE, and thus, may help to improve outcomes in patients with liver failure [35]. In an experimental study of ALF by Ryska et al., Prometheus showed a significant decrease in intracranial pressure (ICP) in pigs to that of the control group (24 mmHg versus 29.8 mmHg, respectively, $p < 0.05$) suggesting that its use in the removal of amino acids in that contribute to the development of HE [36].

Rosen et al. also showed a significant reduction in most cytokines and tumor necrosis factor with Prometheus, potentially highlighting its possible role in the treatment of liver failure [37, 38]. Despite showing this drastic decrease, no other

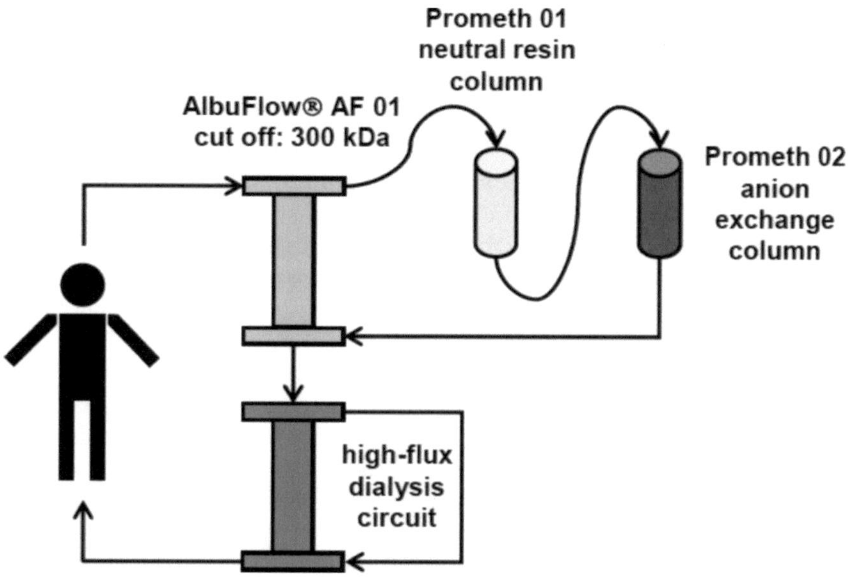

Figure 5.
Schema of Prometheus. Adapted from Karla et al. Extracorporeal Liver support devices for listed patients. Liver Transplantation 22839–8482016 AASLD.

improvement was seen aside from improvement of HE clinically. There was also note of a significant surge in hepatocyte growth factor (HGF) concentration, which stimulates liver regeneration. Similar to MARS, there was no significant impact shown in the cytokine profile, and further research needs to be done in this area of study.

In terms of survival and clinical outcomes, Laleman et al. published an article comparing SMT with MARS and Prometheus in a patient with acute-on-chronic liver failure and it showed MARS to have better outcomes in terms of hemodynamic parameters (mean arterial pressure, stroke volume, systemic resistance) [38]. Dethloff et al. also revealed similar findings in the improvement of mean arterial pressure in patients with decompensated liver cirrhosis with the MARS session as opposed to Prometheus and conventional hemodialysis [39]. Both of the modalities (MARS and Prometheus) decrease cytokines and inflammatory markers; however, there is no exact explanation for these hemodynamic changes.

Kribben et al. in 2012 conducted a multicentric RCT (HELIOS study) comparing Prometheus versus SMT in 145 patients with acute-on-chronic liver failure; the primary endpoints are survival at 28 days and 90 days [19]. The overall survival of the Prometheus group compared to the SMT group was 47% versus 38% but did not show any statistical significance.

In the subgroup analysis of patients with advanced liver disease (MELD >30), there was a significantly higher 90-day survival probability (48% versus 9%, $p < 0.05$) for the Prometheus group compared to SMT. This highlights a possible benefit of Prometheus for treating advance liver disease patients, although the small sample size of the group limits its generalizability to the population.

Over time, other studies derived differing conclusions in regard to its clinical benefit. Sentürk el al. compared the biochemical and clinical parameters for FPSA in patients with ALF and acute-on-chronic liver failure, and showed a significant improvement in the biochemical parameters in HE, although survival rates were not addressed in this study [40]. Similarly, Komardina et al. also showed hemodynamic and biochemical improvements with Prometheus in patients with ALF, but without any difference in survival outcomes [41].

1.2.3 Single-pass albumin dialysis (SPAD)

Single-pass albumin dialysis (SPAD) is a simple technique of blood purification without the sophisticated blood purification line and can be implemented in any intensive care unit applying a standard CRRT. The blood is passed across and dialyzed through a high-flux hollow-fiber hemodiafilter containing albumin-impregnated dialysate, as shown in **Figure 6**. Dialysate is discarded once it passes through the dialyzer, which uses high amounts of exogenous albumin, effectively making it significantly more expensive than MARS, which recycles endogenous albumin [17].

Sauer et al. studied SPAD and MARS, and both were shown to be better than continuous venovenous hemodiafiltration (CVVHD) in removing water-soluble and protein-bound compounds (bilirubin and bile acids) using 4.4% albumin dialysate solution [42]. Kortgen et al. also confirmed these results by comparing the detoxification capacity in patients with liver failure [43]. Both had a significant reduction in serum bilirubin levels, although MARS had a better result in lowering the urea and creatinine level. The limitation of the study was its retrospective and non-randomized nature, and fewer patients were in the SPAD group than there were in the MARS group.

Several studies were conducted to assess the efficacy of dialysate solution concentration for optimal results while carrying out SPAD. Churchwell et al. demonstrated that the highest effectiveness was achieved with 5% albumin dialysate and a larger polysulfone dialyzer (surface area 1.5 m^2). Subsequently, Schmuck et al. and Benyoub et al. demonstrated an optimal detoxification efficacy for albumin-bound substances such as bilirubin and bile acids with a 3–3.2% albumin concentration and a dialysate flow rate of 1000 mL/h using SPAD with a conventional CVVHD and a high-flux polysulfone hemodiafilter [44].

There were only a few case reports published for SPAD immediately after its introduction, and currently, there are no published studies that emphasize on demonstrating the clinical benefits of SPAD versus SMT in ALF. Two uncontrolled retrospective studies in pediatric and adult patients with ALF treated with SPAD as rescue therapy were previously done but neither had conclusive evidence showing their clinical effectiveness, although both noted its ease of use and absence of complications [45].

The most recent RCT done by Sponholz et al. comparing SPAD versus MARS demonstrated a similar decline in the total plasma bilirubin levels, without significant differences between these two LAD modalities [46]. However, the reduction in the total bile acids and γ-glutamyl transferase levels in the patient treated with

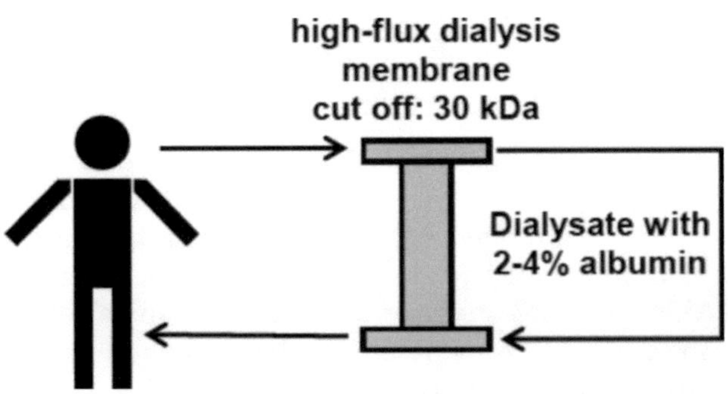

Figure 6.
Schema of SPAD. Adapted from Karla et al. Extracorporeal liver support devices for Listed patients. Liver Transplantation 22839–8482016.

SPAD was non-significant. Furthermore, the creatinine and urea levels were not significantly reduced with SPAD compared to those of MARS. The aforementioned results were differing in other studies, where there was a note of metabolic abnormalities with SPAD, such as a rise in lactate levels or a decline in calcium levels. This could be attributed possibly to the preferential use of citrate anticoagulation with a low dialysis flow rate. In these studies, The MARS and SPAD demonstrated a slight improvement in the HE and hemodynamic status.

Regardless of the ease of administration of SPAD as compared to MARS, the standard albumin dialysate concentration, dialysate flow rate, and standard of care are not yet fully established.

1.3 Other devices

New systems are currently being developed, building on previous knowledge of LADs.

Marangoni et al. described a high-efficiency MARS by incorporating a double adsorption system (double columns containing charcoal and another pair with ion-exchange resin) into the albumin circuit [47]. The detoxification potential of modified MARS was compared with that of the "classical" MARS in four patients with liver failure and demonstrated that "improved" MARS was potentially more efficient in reducing bilirubin and bile acids.

Another system currently being studied conducted by Akcan Arikan et al. presented the usefulness of high-flux CRRT for hyperammonemia, therapeutic plasma exchange for coagulopathy, and MARS for HE. This retrospective observational study showed that 15 pediatric patients with ALF or acute-on-chronic liver failure showed improvement in hepatic encephalopathy with these modalities [48].

More recently, Al-Chalabi et al. and Huber et al. published an animal model of ALF, and patients with liver failure respectively. A modified device called advanced organ support (ADVOS) was first presented in 2013, which included a dialysate circuit containing standard dialysate with a 2–4% albumin concentration, an extracorporeal blood circuit, and a third and last circuit where the albumin dialysate was separated into two parts. Each part would undergo a PH and temperature change before reaching the cation and anion filters, resulting in dialysates that have albumin that is free of toxins [49, 50]. This is accomplished by adding and removing acid or base. The dialysates containing toxin-free albumin then join with each other to reach the expected pH before entering the hemodialyzer again. Huber et al. also showed the same result with ADVOS in reducing bilirubin levels. However, no other studies were further published recently.

Some other modification techniques such as plasma diafiltration, plasma exchange, or therapeutic apheresis using a bilirubin adsorbent column were also published in literature anecdotally [51–53].

1.4 Bioartificial liver support devices

In the last 10 years, significant developments were made with bioartificial liver support devices. These systems are designed to be able to mimic the synthetic and regulatory functions of the liver, in conjunction with the use of LADs to detoxify the patient's plasma. Tumor cell lines, developing expandable progenitor cell populations, or primary human cells can be used, although the most widely used are xenogeneic derivations of primary porcine cells, due to their availability, although there is a risk of infection (i.e., porcine retrovirus infection) and metabolic incompatibility (i.e., graft-versus-host disease, drug-induced thrombocytopenia, complement clotting cascade activation).

1.4.1 Extracorporeal liver assist device (ELAD)

Extracorporeal liver assist device (ELAD) consists of hepatoblastoma C3A cell line, derived from human hepatoblastoma cell line HepG2. Cells are localized in the extra capillary space of a modified dialysis cartridge with a membrane cut-off of 70 kDa to prevent immunoglobulins, blood cells, and C3A tumorigenic cells from crossing [54].

This modality was first developed by Sussman et al. and was assessed in King's College Hospital in London in a pilot-controlled study done by Ellis et al. for patients with ALF who were judged to have >50% survival still and in those who were already indicated for LTx. Twenty-four patients were randomly divided into two groups of ELAD hemoperfusion or control. Overall survival in the ELAD hemoperfusion group was 7 of 9 (78%), and survival for the controls was unexpectedly high, 6 of 8 (75%). Due to the small sample size, the study failed to prove an improvement in the survival rate of patients with ALF [55].

Working off of the initial ELAD, Millis et al. studied a modified version of ELAD to determine the safety profile of the device for patients with fulminant hepatic failure [56]. All patients successfully had an LTx, with four out of the five patients surviving the 30-day survival endpoint of the study, with no noted biomechanical problems or hemodynamic instability. The authors concluded that ELAD is safe and can be conducted on a larger scale in multi-center RCTs.

1.4.2 Bioartificial liver—HepatAssist

Bioartificial liver (BAL) works on the concept of combining hepatocyte bioreactor with a column filled with cultured hepatocytes to mimic liver function. Arbios first described BAL devices, which the Food and Drug Administration approved for Phase I, II, and III clinical trials. In HepatAssist, the patient's blood is initially separated into plasma and cellular components. The plasma is then passed through a high-flow plasma circulation loop and then successively through a charcoal filter, oxygenator, heater, and a hollow fiber bioreactor containing 7 billion cryopreserved hepatocytes. The resulting processed plasma then combines again with the cellular components and sent back to the patient's blood [3].

In the study of Watanabe et al., 31 patients were enrolled in a Phase I study, with the goal of developing a BAL for patients with severe liver failure until they can be transplanted or recover spontaneously [57]. Sixteen out of 18 (89%) patients in group 1 were successfully bridged to LTx. The same goes for group 2 patients (n = 3); all were bridged successfully to transplantation, while group 3 (n = 10) had two who were supported to recovery and LTx. The remaining eight patients in group 3 expired since they were not candidates for LTx.

Other Phase II and III clinical trials from multiple centers across US and European centers involving 171 patients (86 controls and 85 treated) were conducted to study the efficacy of this device in patients with ALF. Inclusion criteria were patients with Stage III or IV HE or with primary non-function of the transplanted liver. The groups were randomized, receiving standard of care and daily treatment with HepatAssist for 7 hours. Results for this trial were inconclusive and failed to show an improvement in 30-day survival rates, although a good safety profile was noted.

Subgroup analysis indicated that the HepatAssist session might provide an improvement in survival rate in patients, especially with drug and chemical toxicity-induced liver failure [58]. Recently, according to Arbios Systems, Inc., there is a study underway to assess a version of HepatAssist with 15–20 billion porcine hepatocytes to be studied in Phase III clinical trials [3].

1.4.3 Modular extracorporeal liver support (MELS)

Modular extracorporeal liver support (MELS) was developed in Germany and is based on tailoring the extracorporeal therapy units to the clinical need of the patient. In a Phase I study using porcine hepatocytes-based BALs, eight patients with ALF showed that it might be beneficial as a bridge to a liver transplant. The limitations are its high cost and complicated design, which may become an obstacle for its wide availability [3].

1.4.4 Academic Medical Center (Amsterdam)-BAL

In contrary to other BAL support devices, this modality is incorporated with capillaries for oxygenation and viability [54]. Preliminary studies are promising; however, more extensive trials are needed to validate its efficacy.

When comparing MELS to AMC-BAL, both have shown comparable efficiency. Although in one study, it was demonstrated that ammonia and lidocaine removal was significantly higher in AMC-BAL as compared to MELS. However, LDH was observed to be considerably lower in MELS.

Several other liver support devices have been developed across the world such as the Hybrid-BAL (Nanjing, China), TECA-Hybrid Artificial Liver Support System (Beijing, China), the Bioartificial Hepatic Support (Udine, Italy), and the Radial Flow Bioreactor (Ferrara, Italy), although further research is required to assess their efficacy and safety [59].

2. Conclusion

ALF, despite being treated medically, is linked with high mortality. Due to longer wait time for liver donors in patients who require LTx, many patients with ALF will, unfortunately, die while waiting for a transplant. Therefore, a liver support system is necessary as a "bridge" to final treatment or until the liver regenerates upon removal of the inciting cause. Over the last 20 years, many artificial liver support systems with the potential to emerge as an ideal device with advances have been introduced. At present, whether BALs can reduce mortality in the ALF population remains controversial.

BALs incorporating human primary hepatocytes are the most suitable cells but are limited by low availability due to a shortage of donor organs. The development of an implantable liver system where hepatocytes can be cultured on substrates to mimic the lobular structure of the liver is promising. However, mimicking the vascular and biliary connections of the liver and recreating all of the necessary metabolic and biochemical functions of the liver will be challenging. As technology is continually evolving, only time will tell the future of these innovative liver assist devices and their possible impact on human culture and health and well-being of affected individuals.

Conflict of interest

None.

Abbreviations

ALD	artificial liver assist device
BLD	bioartificial liver assist device

MARS	molecular adsorbent recirculating system
ALF	acute liver failure
RCT	randomized clinical trial
SIRS	systemic inflammatory response syndrome
FPSA	fractionated plasma separation and adsorption
MELD	model for end-stage liver disease
CVVHD	continuous venovenous hemodiafiltration
SPAD	single-pass albumin dialysis
ELAD	extracorporeal liver assist device
MELS	modular extracorporeal liver support

Author details

Amrendra Kumar Mandal, Pavani Garlapati, Benjamin Tiongson and Vijay Gayam*
Department of Medicine, Interfaith Medical Center, Brooklyn, NY, USA

*Address all correspondence to: vgayam@interfaithmedical.com

References

[1] Naghavi M, Abajobir AA, Abbafati C, Abbas KM, Abd-Allah F, Abera SF, et al. Global, regional, and national age-sex specific mortality for 264 causes of death, 1980-2016: A systematic analysis for the Global Burden of Disease Study 2016. 2017;**390**(10100):1151-1210

[2] Bernal W, Wendon J. Acute liver failure. The New England Journal of Medicine. 2014;**370**(12):1170

[3] JJX R. Liver support technology–an update. Xenotransplantation. 2006;**13**(5):380-389

[4] Moreau R, Arroyo VJCG. Acute-on-chronic liver failure: a new clinical entity. Hepatology. 2015;**13**(5):836-841

[5] Koivusalo A-M, Teikari T, Höckerstedt K, Isoniemi HJ. Albumin dialysis has a favorable effect on amino acid profile in hepatic encephalopathy. Metabolic Brain Disease. 2008;**23**(4):387-398

[6] Guo LM, Liu JY, Xu DZ, Li BS, Han H, Wang LH, et al. Application of Molecular Adsorbents Recirculating System to remove NO and cytokines in severe liver failure patients with multiple organ dysfunction syndrome. Liver International. 2003;**23**:16-20

[7] Pless G, Sauer IM. Bioartificial liver: Current status. Transplantation Proceedings. 2005;**37**(9):3893-3895

[8] Qin G, Shao JG, Wang B, Shen Y, Zheng J, Liu XJ, et al. Artificial liver support system improves short- and long-term outcomes of patients with HBV-associated acute-on-chronic liver failure: A single-center experience. Medicine. 2014;**93**(28):e338

[9] Carpentier B, Gautier A, C L. Artificial and bioartificial liver devices: Present and future. Gut. 2009;**58**(12):1690-1702

[10] Patzer J. Principles of bound solute dialysis. Therapeutic Apheresis and Dialysis. 2006;**10**(2):118-124

[11] Stange J, Ramlow W, Mitzner S, Schmidt R, Klinkmann H. Dialysis against a recycled albumin solution enables the removal of albumin-bound toxins. Artificial Organs. 1993;**17**(9):809-813

[12] Liu Q. Role of cytokines in the pathophysiology of acute-on-chronic liver failure. Blood Purification. 2009;**28**(4):331-341

[13] Guo LM, Liu JY, Xu DZ, Li BS, Han H, Wang LH, et al. Application of molecular adsorbents recirculating system to remove NO and cytokines in severe liver failure patients with multiple organ dysfunction syndrome. Liver International. 2003;**23**(Suppl 3):16-20

[14] Stadlbauer V, Krisper P, Aigner R, Haditsch B, Jung A, Lackner C, et al. Effect of extracorporeal liver support by MARS and Prometheus on serum cytokines in acute-on-chronic liver failure. Critical Care (London, England). 2006;**10**(6):R169

[15] Donati G, La Manna G, Cianciolo G, Grandinetti V, Carretta E, Cappuccilli M, et al. Extracorporeal detoxification for hepatic failure using molecular adsorbent recirculating system: Depurative efficiency and clinical results in a long-term follow-up. Artificial Organs. 2014;**38**(2):125-134

[16] Dominik A, Stange J, Pfensig C, Borufka L, Weiss-Reining H, M E, et al. Reduction of Elevated Cytokine Levels in A cute/A cute-on-Chronic Liver Failure Using Super-Large Pore Albumin Dialysis Treatment: An In Vitro Study. Therapeutic Apheresis and Dialysis. 2014;**18**(4):347-352

[17] Gay M, Pares A, Carrascal M, Bosch-i-Crespo P, Gorga M, Mas A, et al. Proteomic analysis of polypeptides captured from blood during extracorporeal albumin dialysis in patients with cholestasis and resistant pruritus. PLoS One. 2011;**6**(7):e21850

[18] Uchino S, Fealy N, Baldwin I, Morimatsu H, Bellomo R. Continuous venovenous hemofiltration without anticoagulation. ASAIO Journal (American Society for Artificial Internal Organs: 1992). 2004;**50**(1):76-80

[19] Kribben A, Gerken G, Haag S, Herget-Rosenthal S, Treichel U, Betz C, et al. Effects of fractionated plasma separation and adsorption on survival in patients with acute-on-chronic liver failure. Gastroenterology. 2012;**142**(4):782-789.e3

[20] De Bruyn T, Meijers B, Evenepoel P, Laub R, Willems L, Augustijns P, et al. Stability of therapeutic albumin solutions used for molecular adsorbent recirculating system-based liver dialysis. Artificial Organs. 2012;**36**(1):29-41

[21] Heemann U, Treichel U, Loock J, Philipp T, Gerken G, Malago M, et al. Albumin dialysis in cirrhosis with superimposed acute liver injury: A prospective, controlled study. Hepatology (Baltimore, Md). 2002;**36** (4 Pt 1):949-958

[22] Sen S, Davies NA, Mookerjee RP, Cheshire LM, Hodges SJ, Williams R, et al. Pathophysiological effects of albumin dialysis in acute-on-chronic liver failure: A randomized controlled study. Liver Transplantation. 2004;**10**(9):1109-1119

[23] Hanish SI, Stein DM, Scalea JR, Essien EO, Thurman P, Hutson WR, et al. Molecular adsorbent recirculating system effectively replaces hepatic function in severe acute liver failure. Annals of Surgery. 2017;**266**(4):677-684

[24] Eapen J, Ayoola R, Subramanian RM. The efficacy of extracorporeal liver support with molecular adsorbent recirculating system in severe drug-induced liver injury. Oxford Medical Case Reports. 2018;**2018**(1):omx077

[25] Ostapowicz G, Fontana RJ, Schiodt FV, Larson A, Davern TJ, Han SH, et al. Results of a prospective study of acute liver failure at 17 tertiary care centers in the United States. Annals of Internal Medicine. 2002;**137**(12):947-954

[26] Reuben A, Koch DG, Lee WM. Drug-induced acute liver failure: results of a U.S. multicenter, prospective study. Hepatology (Baltimore, Md). 2010;**52**(6):2065-2076

[27] Diaz FC, Saez-Gonzalez E, Benlloch S, Alvarez-Sotomayor D, Conde I, Polo B, et al. Albumin dialysis with MARS for the treatment of anabolic steroid-induced cholestasis. Annals of Hepatology. 2016;**15**(6):939-943

[28] Larson AM, Polson J, Fontana RJ, Davern TJ, Lalani E, Hynan LS, et al. Acetaminophen-induced acute liver failure: Results of a United States multicenter, prospective study. Hepatology. 2005;**42**(6):1364-1372

[29] Gayam V, Khalid M, Dahal S, Garlapati P, Gill A. Hyperacute liver injury following intravenous fluconazole: A rare case of dose-independent hepatotoxicity. Journal of Family Medicine and Primary Care. 2018;7(2):451-454

[30] Gayam V, Khalid M, Dahal S, Garlapati P, Gill A, Alex R, et al. Fatal acute liver failure with intravenous Amiodarone: A case report and literature review. Gastroenterology Research. 2018;**11**(1):62-63

[31] Gayam V, Mandal AK, Khalid M, Shrestha B, Garlapati P, Khalid M.

Valproic acid induced acute liver injury resulting in hepatic encephalopathy- a case report and literature review. Journal of Community Hospital Internal Medicine Perspectives. 2018;**8**(5):311-314

[32] Falkenhagen D, Strobl W, Vogt G, Schrefl A, Linsberger I, Gerner FJ, et al. Fractionated plasma separation and adsorption system: A novel system for blood purification to remove albumin bound substances. Artificial Organs. 1999;**23**(1):81-86

[33] Evenepoel P, Laleman W, Wilmer A, Claes K, Kuypers D, Bammens B, et al. Prometheus versus molecular adsorbents recirculating system: Comparison of efficiency in two different liver detoxification devices. Artificial Organs. 2006;**30**(4):276-284

[34] Grodzicki M, Kotulski M, Leonowicz D, Zieniewicz K, Krawczyk M, editors. Results of treatment of acute liver failure patients with use of the prometheus FPSA system. Transplantation Proceedings; 2009

[35] Rifai K, Das A, Rosenau J, Ernst T, Kretschmer U, Haller H, et al. Changes in plasma amino acids during extracorporeal liver support by fractionated plasma separation and adsorption. Artificial Organs. 2010;**34**(2):166-170

[36] Ryska M, Laszikova E, Pantoflicek T, Ryska O, Prazak J, Koblihova E. Fractionated plasma separation and adsorption significantly decreases intracranial pressure in acute liver failure: Experimental study. European surgical research Europaische Chirurgische Forschung Recherches Chirurgicales Europeennes. 2009;**42**(4):230-235

[37] Rocen M, Kieslichova E, Merta D, Uchytilova E, Pavlova Y, Cap J, et al., editors. The effect of Prometheus device on laboratory markers of inflammation and tissue regeneration in acute liver failure management. Transplantation Proceedings; 2010

[38] Laleman W, Wilmer A, Evenepoel P, Elst IV, Zeegers M, Zaman Z, et al. Effect of the molecular adsorbent recirculating system and Prometheus devices on systemic haemodynamics and vasoactive agents in patients with acute-on-chronic alcoholic liver failure. Critical Care (London, England). 2006;**10**(4):R108

[39] Dethloff T, Tofteng F, Frederiksen HJ, Hojskov M, Hansen BA, Larsen FS. Effect of Prometheus liver assist system on systemic hemodynamics in patients with cirrhosis: A randomized controlled study. World Journal of Gastroenterology. 2008;**14**(13):2065-2071

[40] Senturk E, Esen F, Ozcan PE, Rifai K, Pinarbasi B, Cakar N, et al. The treatment of acute liver failure with fractionated plasma separation and adsorption system: Experience in 85 applications. Journal of Clinical Apheresis. 2010;**25**(4):195-201

[41] Komardina E, Yaroustovsky M, Abramyan M, Plyushch M. Prometheus therapy for the treatment of acute liver failure in patients after cardiac surgery. Kardiochirurgia i torakochirurgia polska = Polish Journal of Cardio-thoracic Surgery. 2017;**14**(4):230-235

[42] Sauer IM, Goetz M, Steffen I, Walter G, Kehr DC, Schwartlander R, et al. In vitro comparison of the molecular adsorbent recirculation system (MARS) and single-pass albumin dialysis (SPAD). Hepatology (Baltimore, Md). 2004;**39**(5):1408-1414

[43] Kortgen A, Rauchfuss F, Götz M, Settmacher U, Bauer M, Sponholz C, et al. Albumin dialysis in liver failure:

Comparison of molecular adsorbent recirculating system and single pass albumin dialysis—a retrospective analysis. Therapeutic Apheresis and Dialysis. 2009;**13**(5):419-425

[44] Benyoub K, Muller M, Bonnet A, Simon R, Gazon M, Duperret S, et al. Amounts of Bile Acids and Bilirubin Removed During Single-Pass Albumin Dialysis in Patients With Liver Failure. Therapeutic Apheresis and Dialysis. 2011;**15**(5):504-506

[45] Piechota M, Piechota A. An evaluation of the usefulness of extracorporeal liver support techniques in patients hospitalized in the ICU for severe liver dysfunction secondary to alcoholic liver disease. Hepatitis Monthly. 2016;**16**(7):e34127

[46] Sponholz C, Matthes K, Rupp D, Backaus W, Klammt S, Karailieva D, et al. Molecular adsorbent recirculating system and single-pass albumin dialysis in liver failure–a prospective, randomised crossover study. Critical Care (London, England). 2016;**20**:2

[47] Marangoni R, Bellati G, Castelli A, Romagnoli E. Development of high-efficiency molecular adsorbent recirculating system: Preliminary report. Artificial Organs. 2014;**38**(10):879-883

[48] Akcan Arikan A, Srivaths P, Himes RW, Tufan Pekkucuksen N, Lam F, Nguyen T, et al. Hybrid extracorporeal therapies as a bridge to pediatric liver transplantation. Pediatric Critical Care Medicine. 2018;**19**(7):e342-e3e9

[49] Al-Chalabi A, Matevossian E, von Thaden A, Schreiber C, Radermacher P, Huber W, et al. Evaluation of an ADVanced organ support (ADVOS) system in a two-hit porcine model of liver failure plus endotoxemia. Intensive Care Medicine Experimental. 2017;**5**(1):31

[50] Al-Chalabi A, Matevossian E, Thaden A-K v, Luppa P, Neiss A, Schuster T, et al. Evaluation of the Hepa wash(R) treatment in pigs with acute liver failure. BMC Gastroenterology. 2013;**13**:83

[51] Shen Y, Wang X-L, Wang B, Shao J-G, Liu Y-M, Qin Y, et al. Survival benefits with artificial liver support system for acute-on-chronic liver failure: a time series-based meta-analysis. Medicine (Baltimore). 2016;**95**(3):e2506

[52] Viggiano D, de Pascale E, Marinelli G, Pluvio C. A comparison among three different apheretic techniques for treatment of hyperbilirubinemia. Journal of Artificial Organs. 2018;**21**(1):110-116

[53] Nakae H, Eguchi Y, Saotome T, Yoshioka T, Yoshimura N, Kishi Y, et al. Multicenter study of plasma diafiltration in patients with acute liver failure. Therapeutic Apheresis and Dialysis. 2010;**14**(5):444-450

[54] Pless GJO. Artificial and bioartificial liver support. Organogenesis. 2007;**3**(1):20-24

[55] Ellis AJ, Hughes RD, Wendon JA, Dunne J, Langley PG, Kelly JH, et al. Pilot-controlledtrialoftheextracorporeal liver assist device in acute liver failure. Hepatology. 1996;**24**(6):1446-1451

[56] Millis JM, Cronin DC, Johnson R, Conjeevaram H, Conlin C, Trevino S, et al. Initial experience with the modified extracorporeal liver-assist device for patients with fulminant hepatic failure: System modifications and clinical impact. Transplantation. 2002;**74**(12):1735-1746

[57] Watanabe FD, Mullon C, Hewitt WR, Arkadopoulos N, Kahaku E, Eguchi S, et al. Clinical experience with a bioartificial liver in the

treatment of severe liver failure. A phase I clinical trial. Annals of Surgery. 1997;**225**(5):484

[58] Demetriou AA, Brown RS Jr, Busuttil RW, Fair J, McGuire BM, Rosenthal P, et al. Prospective, randomized, multicenter, controlled trial of a bioartificial liver in treating acute liver failure. Annals of Surgery. 2004;**239**(5):660

[59] Phua J, Lee KH. Liver support devices. Current Opinion in Critical care. 2008;**14**(2):208-215